NURSING SPECIALTY CROSSWORDS:

A FUN AND EFFECTIVE WAY TO STUDY FOR YOUR

LICENSURE EXAMS

By: Helene V. Molnar, LNHA, MHA

ALSO BY AUTHOR:

Healthcare Administration Specialty Crosswords: A Fun and Effective Approach to Studying for Licensure Exams.

DEDICATION:

This book is dedicated to my father, a retired LNHA and Professor at the University of Illinois, and my mother, a retired R.N. and state surveyor. Both provided the highest quality of care throughout their careers (and continue to do so through volunteerism) and inspired me to do the same. And to my children, Victoria Angelique and Justyn Aleksandr, my greatest source of joy and pride. And finally, to all healthcare professionals who have dedicated their lives to helping others.

#1

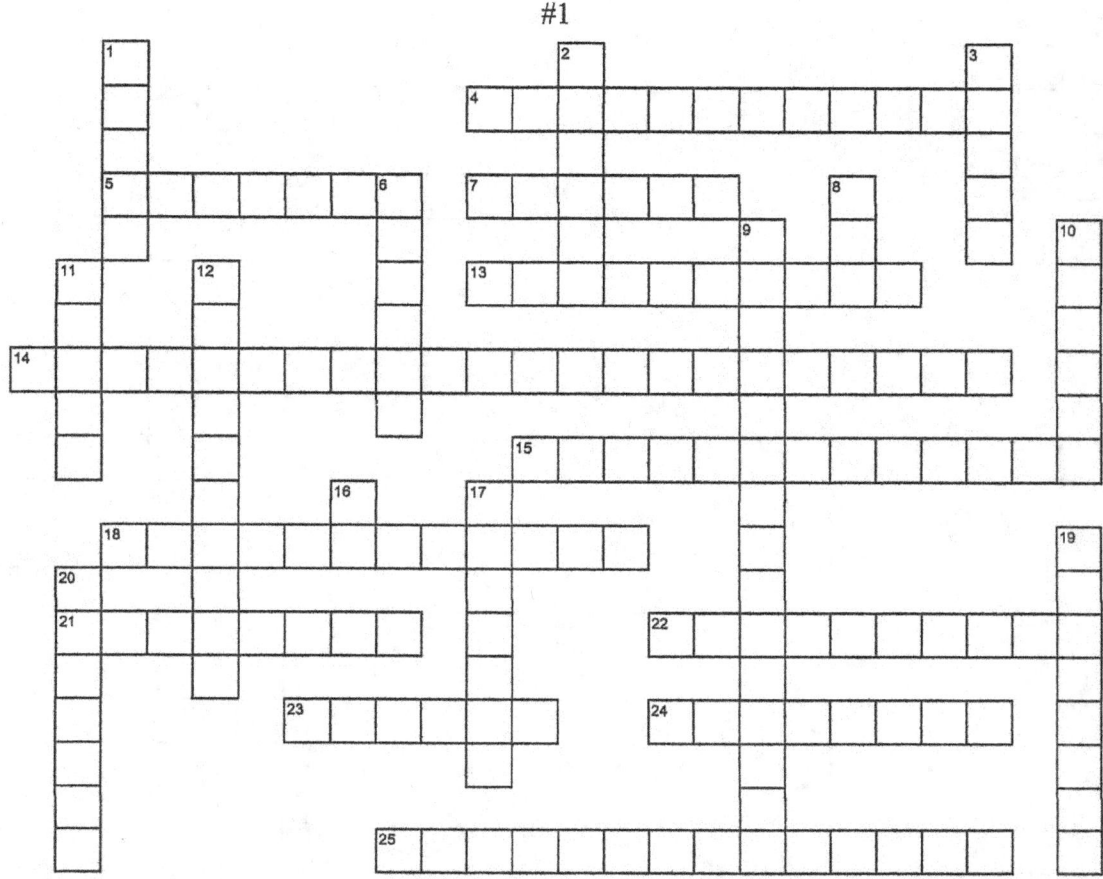

ACROSS

4 A major class of drugs used to relieve anxiety and tension.
5 Free from infectious material
7 A narcotic drug that is used for the treatment of pain
13 The muscle that flexes the forearm
14 A disease caused by bacteria or viruses due to immunosuppression (2 wds)
15 The vascular structure that attaches the fetus to the placenta in utero (2 wds)
18 The nonmylenated segment of the neuron (2 wds)
21 The accumulation of fluid
22 Composition of all layers of the skin, including the epidermis, dermis and corium.
23 The presence of a high blood cell count in the urine; frequently attributed to a bladder or urethra infection.
24 A disorder that affects the central nervous system, characterized by recurrent seizures
25 Small increase of the number of platelets in circulation

DOWN

1 Swelling in specific skin areas
2 The liquid that is secreted by the salivary glands and contains amylase.
3 Prefix that means "slow or decreased rate"
6 Sufffix meaning "points or projections"
8 Prefix meaning "one, singular"
9 The fragmentation of stones through ultrasound short waves, so that smaller pieces can be passed naturally (2 wds)
10 A thick and sticky substance, such as mucus
11 The dark center of the iris; it allows light rays to enter the eye.
12 Type of gland that secretes cerumen or earwax
16 Prefix that means "back" or "again"
17 The inability to perceive the sensation of touch
19 A skin disease characterized by patches without pigmentation
20 A bony process that extends out the back of the body of vertebrae.

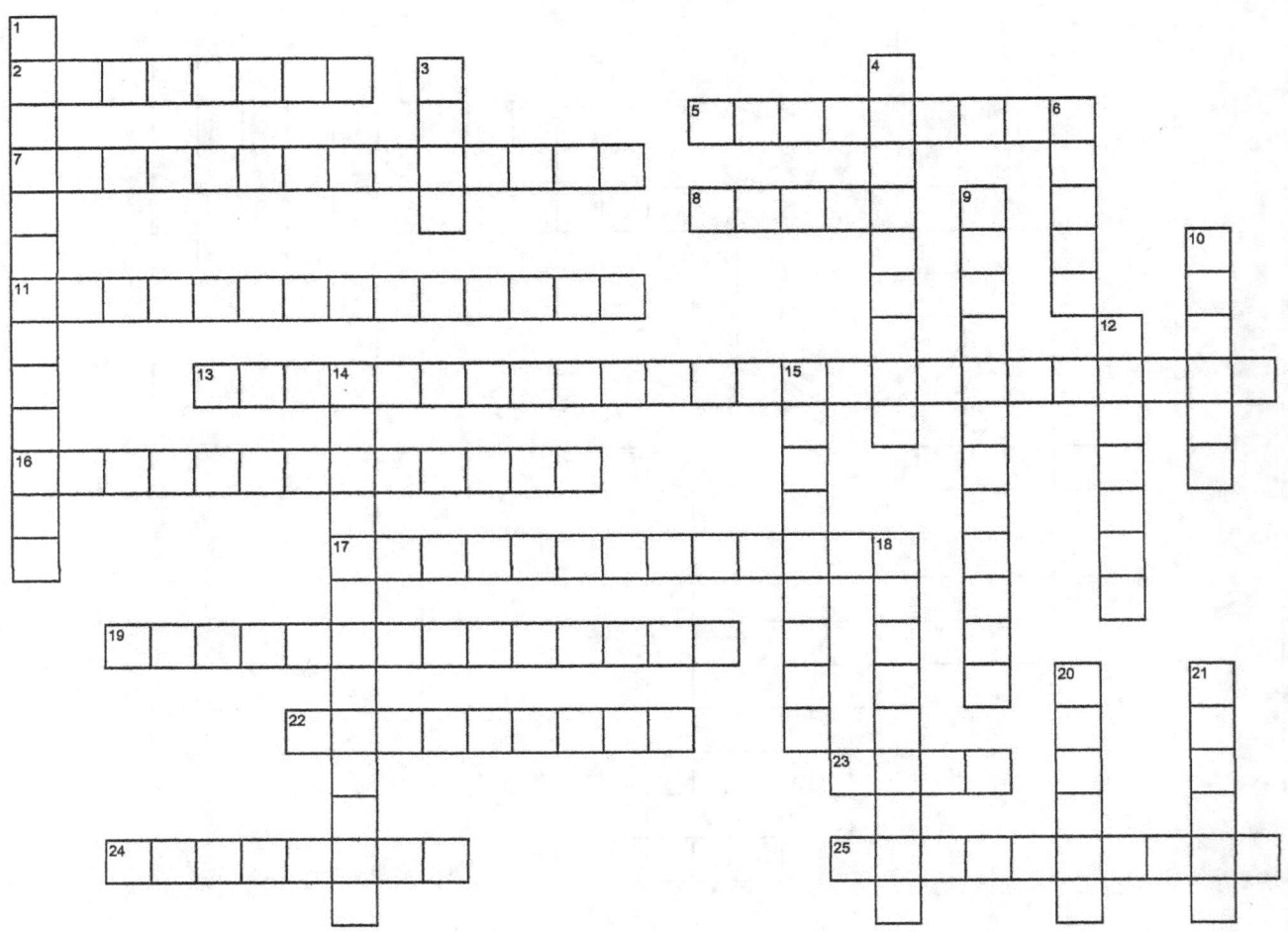

ACROSS

2 Lack of a heartbeat. Cardiac standstill.
5 A brace for this condition must be worn at all times, except for bathing, and is often worn continually for several months to a year.
7 Outpouching of the bowel wall.
8 Swelling of a body part
11 A radiological study of the gallbladder and bile ducts
13 Treatment for refractive errors of the eye; The cornea is heated to shrink collagen fibers, reshape the eye, and change the angle of the cornea in relation to the focal point (3 wds)
16 Term used to describe when the umbilical cord precedes the fetal presenting part. (2 wds)
17 The accumulation of serous fluid in a joint.
19 A life threatening complication of heart failure, which can develop in minutes. (2 wds)
22 To cut a hole in a cast or other material, in order to relieve pressure on either the skin or a bony prominence
23 Suffix that means "split"
24 Suffix that means "meal"
25 The muscle that extends and medially rotates the shoulder. (2 wds)

DOWN

1 The amount of blood that the heart expels per minute. (2 wds)
3 The fluid produced by the liver, stored in the gallbladder, and released into the duodenum to digest fats in foods.
4 A plasma measurement of viral RNA, usually done in serial fashion with human immunodeficiency disorder (2 wds)
6 An artificially created opening on the surface of the body. (an example is a tracheostomy).
9 The use of chemical agents to treat a disease (such as cancer).
10 The chin
12 The renal pelvis of the kidney collects urine from the ____.
14 Massive swelling of the lower extremities or genitalia. Also known as pachydermas.
15 This procedure allows direct visualization of a tumor in gastric cancer.
18 A tubular elastic mesh device that holds dressings in place on the trunk, head and extremities.
20 Respiratory disease characterized by increased airway irritability, narrowing and constriction of air passages.
21 Involuntary shaking of a body part, due to pathological states or side effects of medications.

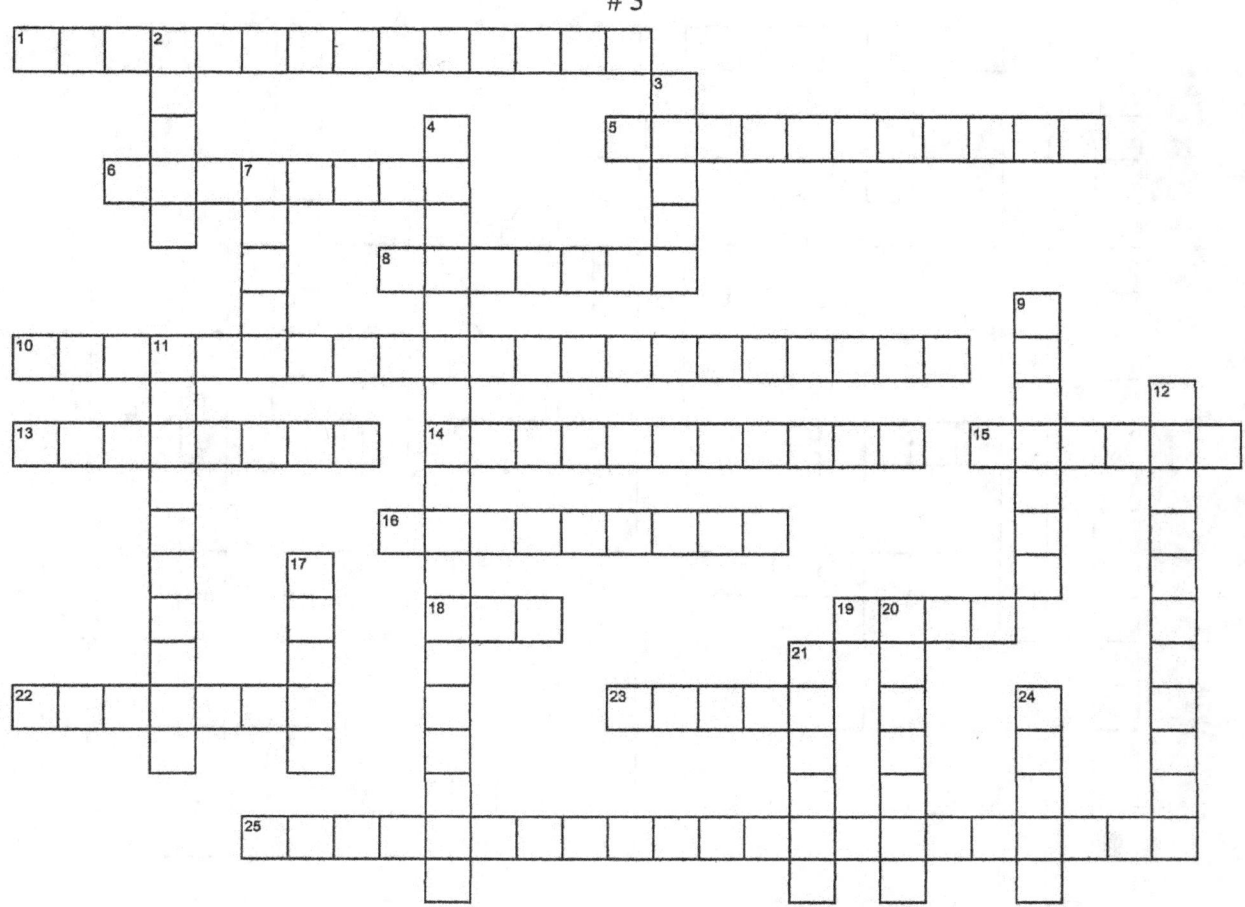

ACROSS

1 Narrowing or obstruction of the aortic outflow tract; causes significant reduction of blood flow from the left ventricle, resulting in decreased cardiac output. (2 wds)

5 Central venous access devices may be used for _____ therapy.

6 A boil.

8 A disaccharide found in milk of all mammals, made up of the monosaccharides glucose and galactose.

10 This test measures the fetal response to uterine contractions. (3 wds)

13 Yellow appearance of skin and sclera due to excess bilirubin.

14 A third-degree prolapse of the uterus and cervix, extending through the introitus.

15 Dark, tarry stools that contain digested blood due to bleeding from the esophagus or stomach.

16 The termination of menses and the ability to conceive.

18 Suffix that means "similar to".

19 Prefix that means "eight"

22 Tympanic membrane; the eardrum.

23 A non-elevated skin lesion larger than one centimeter in diameter.

25 A treatment for intractable seizure disorder, when electrical impulses are delivered for thirty seconds, every five minutes, by a device implanted in the anterior wall. (3 wds)

DOWN

2 The first tarsal bone and the largest of the bones of the ankle.

3 Facing downward

4 The enlargement of both the liver and the spleen.

7 The fleshy hanging part of the soft palate that activates the gag reflex when stimulated.

9 The condition of having a wide, open lumen.

11 Releasing a tendon from adhesions

12 Discomfort of the gastrointestinal tract, including heartburn, acid regurgitation, pain, nausea and vomiting.

17 Those with diabetes are prone to _____ insufficiency and ____ failure. (1 wd)

20 Renal calculi (kidney stones) are commonly composed of ____.

21 Suffix that means "pertaining to extreme fear".

24 Normal neonatal respirations are thirty to ____ beats per minute.

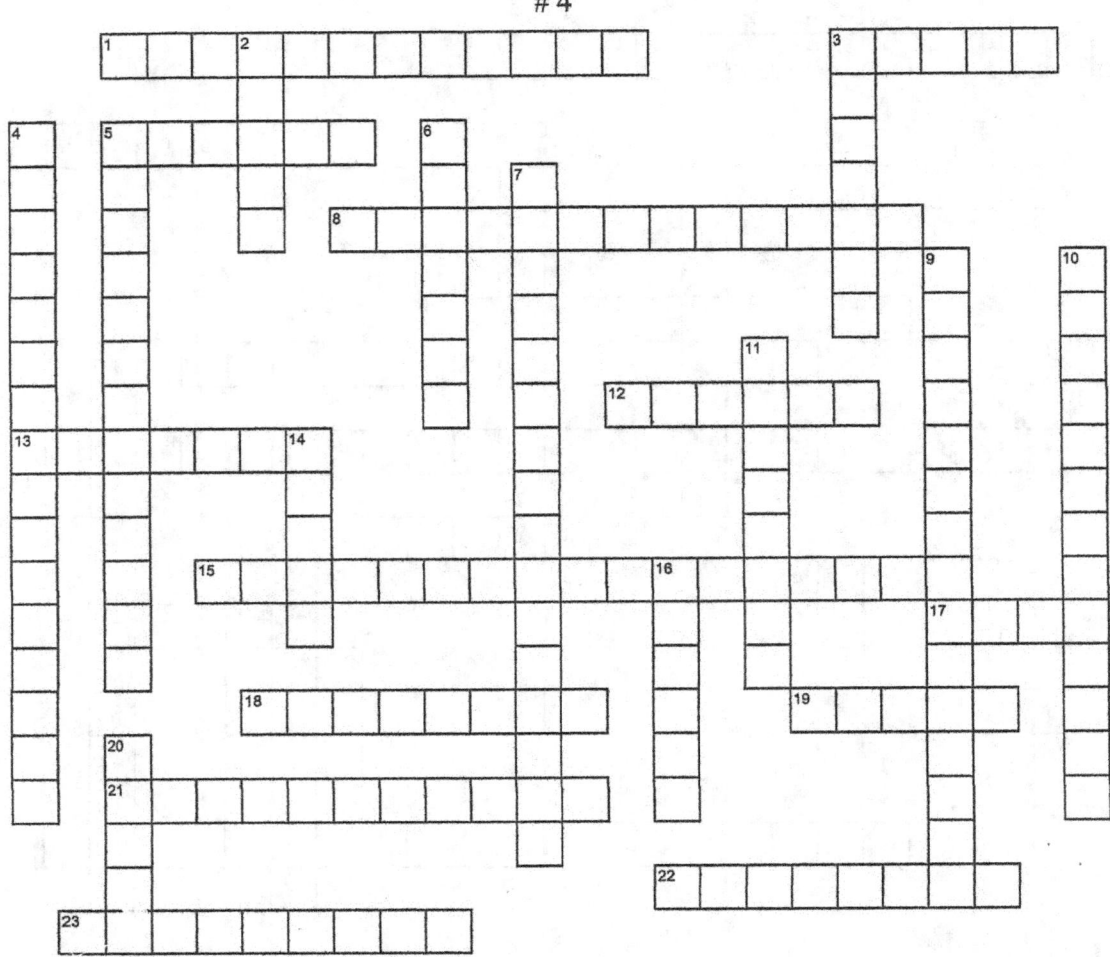

ACROSS

1 Failure to have regular, soft bowel movements.

3 Small bone of the anterior surface of the lower leg.

5 When administering blood or blood components, avoid using an existing line if the needle or catheter lumen is smaller than _____G.

8 An enlargement of the lymph nodes.

12 A fertilized ovum.

13 The recurrence of a disease after a period of remission or recovery.

15 A disturbance in thought process evidenced by inclusion of excessive, tangential and irrelevant information when asked a question. May be associated with schizophrenia and obsessive disorders.

17 Prefix meaning "down"

18 A nurse must report illegal, incompetent, or ___ practices.

19 Suffix meaning "sudden, involuntary contraction".

21 Damage to the muscles or nerves of the wrist that cause the wrist to be unable to extend.

22 Finding meaning through helping others.

23 Chamber of the inner ear.

DOWN

2 A cavityor space within a structure.

3 Lymphatic tissue located at the back of the thr

4 The tip of the catheter must be placed in the _____ for the catheter to be considered a central venous access device. (3 wds).

5 Conflicts involving three family members.

6 The long bone in the upper arm that articulates with the scapula at the shoulder joint and the head of the radius and ulna to form the elbow joint.

7 A deficiency of thrombocytes due to action or chemicals or drugs that damage stem cells in the bone marrow. This may also occur when leukemia cells take over and crowd the stem cells that produce thrombocytes.

9 Bactericidal antibiotics.

10 A nurse is responsible for assessing, monitoring and _____ the status of a client who is under his or her care.

11 Embryonic membranous tissue that produces the first red blood cell of the embryo. (2 wds)

14 _____ state allows an emancipated minor to consent to his or her own medical care and treatment.

16 A differential skin test using Giemsa stain with microscopic examination.

20 Type of therapy used in critically ill clients who require intensive therapy.

5

ACROSS

1 Primary sleep disorders may be categorized as dyssomnias or _____.
4 Found in the mouth, these are similar to facial milia. (2 wds).
7 A result of a gene mutation. (2 wds).
8 Contraction of the heart muscle.
12 ____ asthma is characterized by less than six attacks per year.
13 The most common adverse reactions to _____ include dermatitis, pruritus and stomatitis. (2 wds).
17 A surgical procedure used to re-attach a detached retina using cryotherapy to freeze the tissue and fix all three layers (sclera, choroid, and retina) together.
18 Between age ____ to nine months, an infant can self-feed him or herself crackers and a bottle.
21 These are used to treat noncompensatory tachycardia when the heart rate requires specific intervention.
22 Pityriasis rosea starts with a ____ and then erupts in a Christmas tree pattern on the trunk. (2 wds).
23 Opioid _____ block the effects of opioids.
24 Itching.

DOWN

1 The loss of eyelashes due to disease or chemotherapy.
2 A small, discolored spot or patch on the skin.
3 The functional unit of the nervous system responsible for conducting impulses.
5 Powders come in single-strength or _____-strength formulas.
6 The stages of grief include denial, anger, bargaining, depression and _____.
9 Prefix meaning "five"
10 Palate or roof of the mouth.
11 Communicating region between neurons.
14 The branch of medicine that focuses on the treatment of cancers.
15 An intramuscular injection for a child should contain no more than ____ ml. of solution.
16 This acts directly on skeletal muscle to decrease excitation and reduce muscle strength by interfering with intracellular calcium movement.
19 An end product of protein metabolism that is present in measurable quantities and ultimately excreted in urine. (2 wds).
20 An inflammation of the nasal mucous membrane.

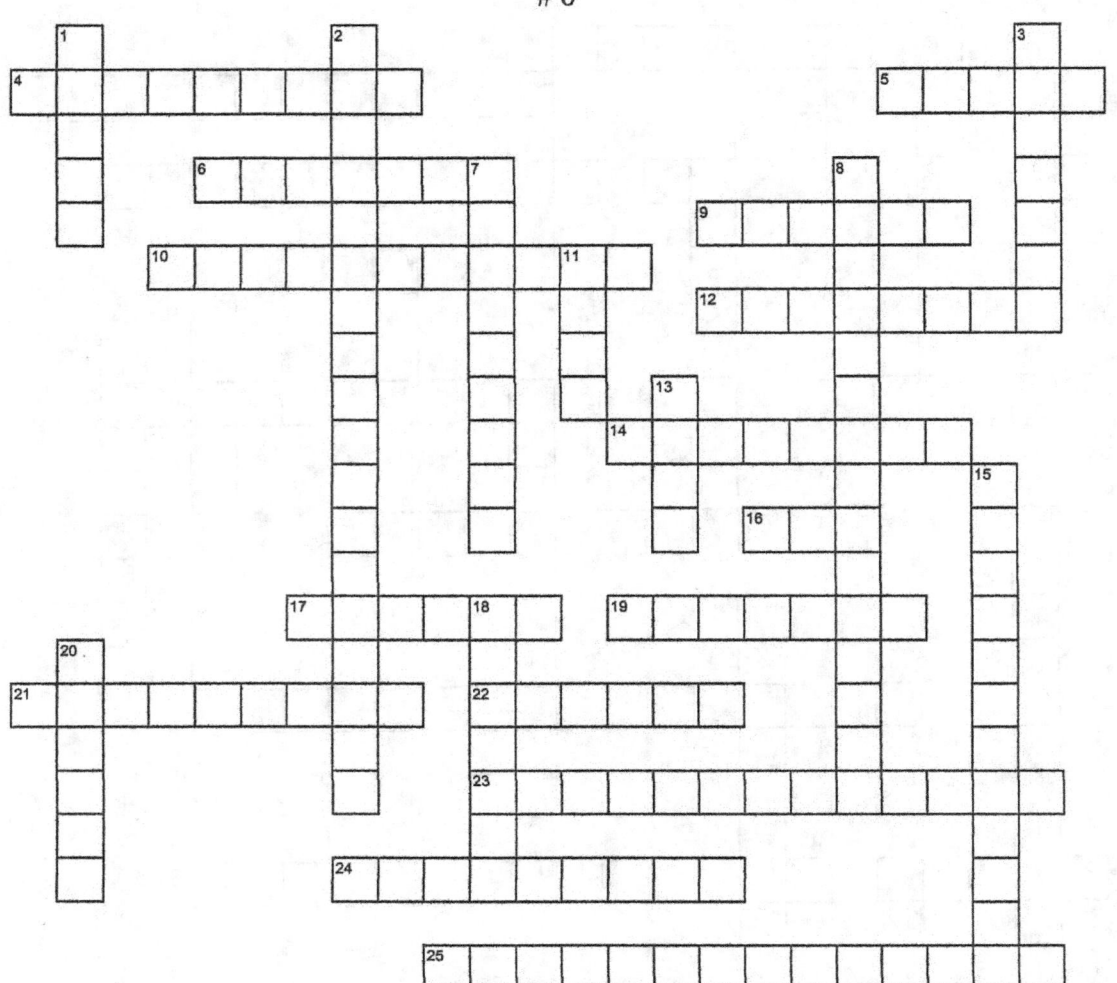

ACROSS

4 Promoting _____ is the priority during an acute exacerbation of Crohn's disease. (2 wds).

5 Suffix meaning "labor" or "to give birth".

6 This type of vest provides significant immobilization, including lateral flexion.

9 A raised lesion detectable by touch that is usually one centimeter or more in diameter.

10 A nonmalignant tumor of skeletal muscle tissue.

12 Trypsin breaks down _____.

14 Twisting of a loop of intestine around itself or around another segment of bowel, causing obstruction.

16 Suffix meaning "condition"

17 Going toward the middle.

19 Extending from the bladder to the urinary meatus, this transports urine from the bladder to the exterior of the body.

21 Testing the _____ helps assess cranial nerve X function. (2 wds).

22 After a hip replacement, the hip should not be flexed more than ____ degrees.

23 This is responsible for the majority of force for cardiac output. (2 wds).

24 _____ may be delivered by tube when dysphagia exists.

25 If the tongue or relaxed throat muscles are obstructing the airway, a _____ or oropharyngeal airway can be inserted.

DOWN

1 The point of central vision.

2 After a spinal cord injury, _____ may cause a higher level of injury. (3 wds).

3 Regulation of fluid volume by the _____ affects blood pressure.

7 A lack of appropriate and orderly development of an embryo.

8 Smooth-muscle cells found near the afferent and efferent arterioles adjacent to the glomerulus.

11 Prefix meaning "breast".

13 Stage of pressure ulcer that involves full-thickness skin loss, with the base of the ulcer covered by slough and yellow, tan, gray, green or brown eschar.

15 This is indicated by a rapid and bounding pulse and edema.

18 Type of rash that is ring-shaped.

20 Wrist.

7

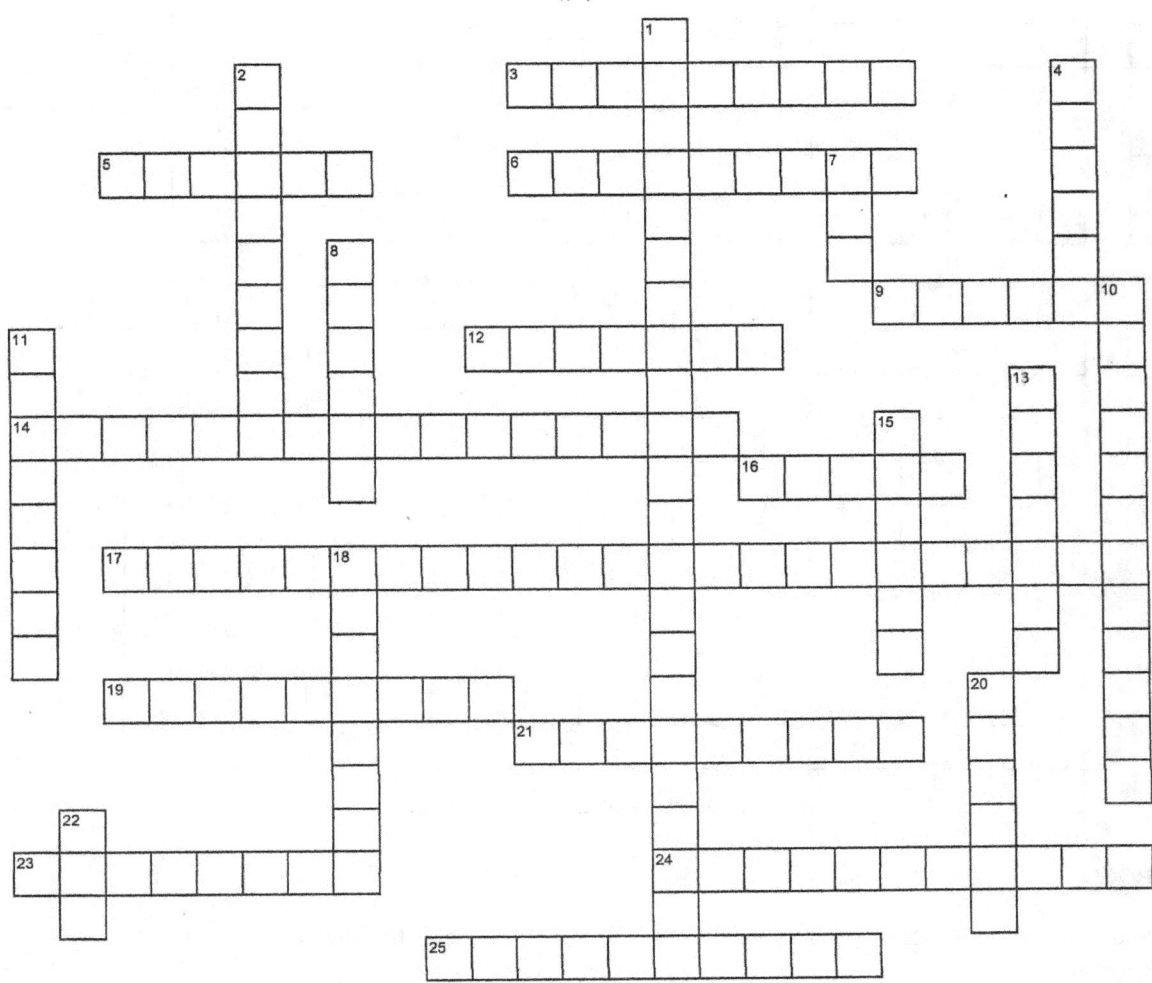

ACROSS

3 Abnormal or excessive hair growth on a female's face or body.

5 Peak incidence of iron deficiency anemia occurrence is between _____ and eighteen months of age.

6 Turning a body part inward.

9 White, semilunar area of nail near the root.

12 An eight-foot-long section of the small intestine.

14 Hemophilia B is also called factor IX deficiency, or _____. (2 wds).

16 How often should you induce vomiting if a victim has ingested a toxic chemical?

17 A fat and protein complex that removes excess cholesterol from arterial walls and transports it to the liver. (3 wds).

19 A defense mechanism commonly seen in clients with personality disorders in which the world is perceived as all good or all bad.

21 Dilation of the pupil.

23 Pus-filled lesions, such as acne.

24 Substances that can cause cancer.

25 The five bones that make up the hand.

DOWN

1 Brittle-bone disease characterized by sustaining multiple fractures throughout life from minimal trauma. (2 wds).

2 Cancer, carcinoma, endangering health or life.

4 Pertaining to the seven individual bones that make up the ankle.

7 Prefix meaning "pertaining to the ear or auditory function"

8 Linear depressions of the skin.

10 These are associated with rectal bleeding and pain with bowel movements. (2 wds).

11 An enzyme that breaks down nucleic acid.

13 Weight twenty percent above the recommended weight for sex and height.

15 Elevated, firm hyperplasia with ill-defined borders. A scar site.

18 These allow normal fluid to drain from the middle ear, improve ventilation, and permit pressure to equalize in the middle ear. (2 wds).

20 Mucus secreted by the walls of the respiratory tract.

22 Suffix meaning "tissue" or "structure"

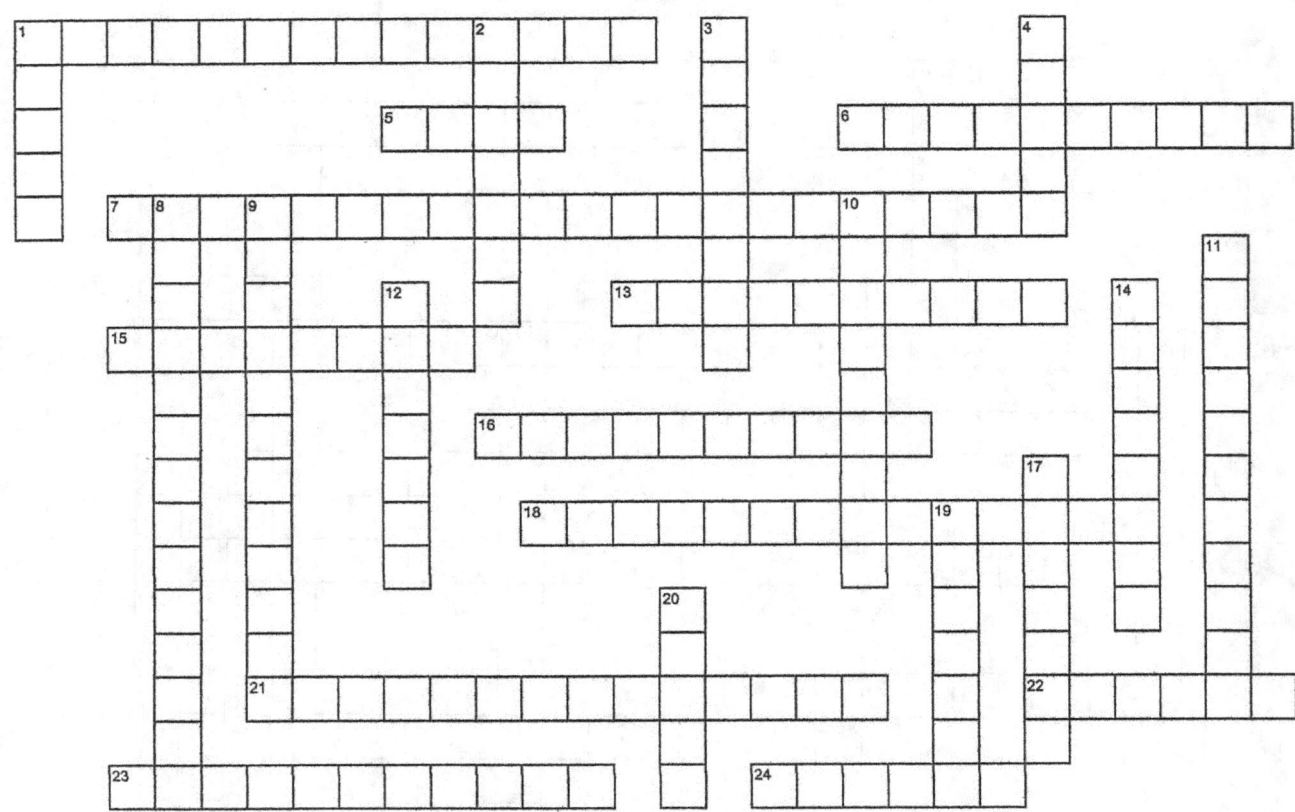

ACROSS

1 Blood vessel that brings oxygenated blood to the brain. (2 wds).
5 Suffix meaning "movement"
6 A volvulus is a type of _____ obstruction.
7 An autoimmune disease causing an inflamed thyroid gland. (2 wds).
13 Removal of a tube, especially an endotracheal tube.
15 Cystitis symptoms include dysurai, frequency, urgency, and _____.
16 There are three main types of T cells: killer, helper and _____ T cells.
18 This terms refers to visual acuity of 20/150 or less. (2 wds).
21 The method of increasing force and effectiveness of chest muscles by placing the palm of the hand on the abdominal musculature below the ribs during expiration and then removing the hand during inspiration. (2 wds).
22 Pertaining to the lips of the vagina or face.
23 This type of care refers to care of a pregnant woman during labor.
24 About _____% of blood cells are T cells.

DOWN

1 A standardized measurement of the concentration of a substance in a solution, often used to measure the presence of immune response to vaccinations.
2 Fibrous bands or cords that attach muscle to bone or muscle to other body parts.
3 _____ asthma is characterized by several attacks per month.
4 Suffix meaning "hearing".
8 The redistribution of blood flow to areas of greatest need. Also, self-management of emotions and behavior during periods of stress.
9 This is caused by weakness of the diaphragmatic muscle and increased intra-abdominal (not intrathoracic) pressure. (2 wds).
10 The identification of a pathological state of disorder.
11 Chronic, mild bipolar disorder in which the patient has mild mood swings, with periods of symptom-free intervals for months at a time.
12 Pertaining to bile, gall.
14 This is the most consistent clinical sign of tricuspid atresia.
17 Having an elevated temperature.
19 The movement of the fetal presenting part through the pelvis.
20 Prefix meaning "large" or "elongated"

#9

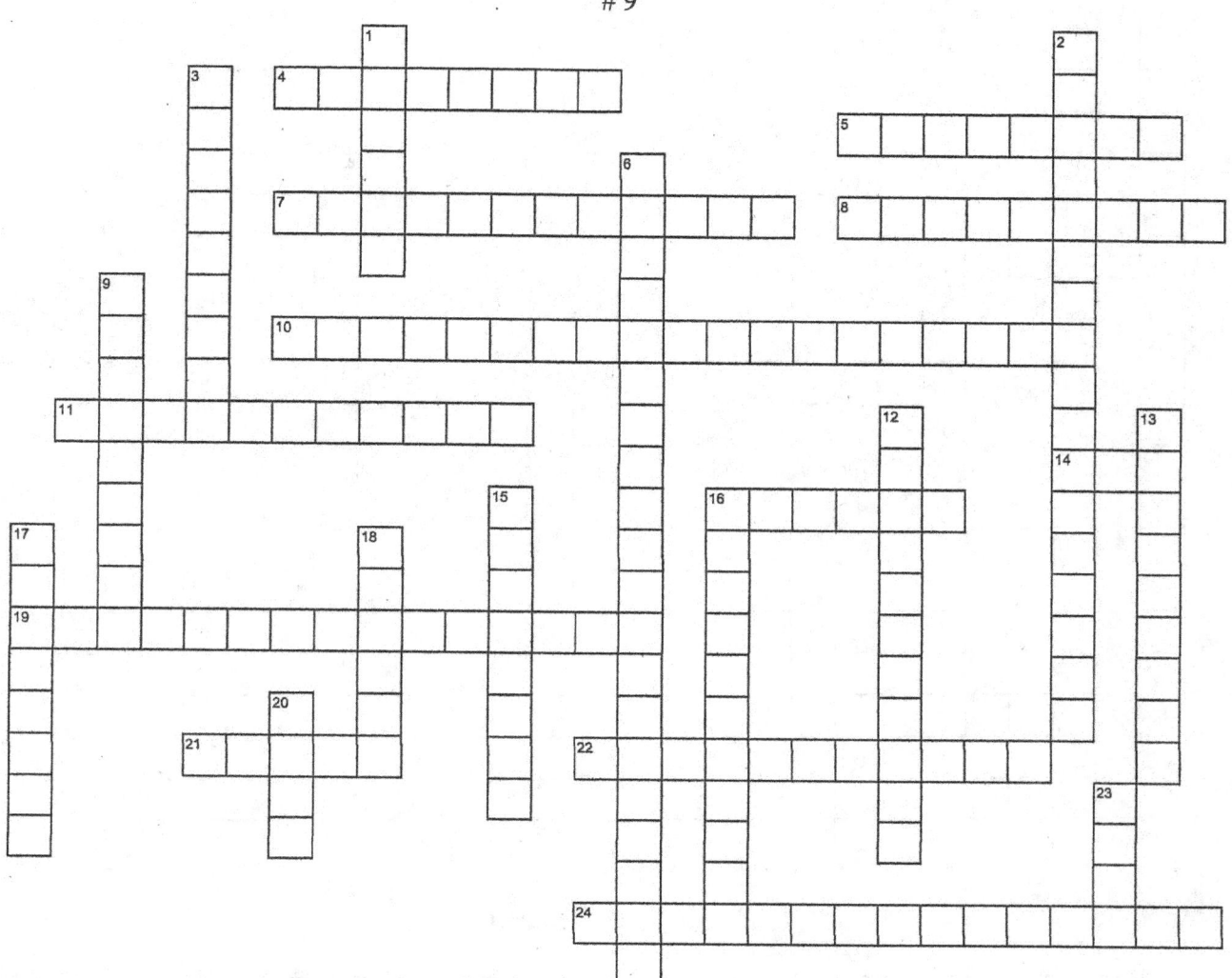

ACROSS

4 The surgical resection of a tendon.

5 The spread of disease from animals to humans.

7 The right eye. (2 wds).

8 An autoimmune skin disease characterized by white, scaly plaques.

10 A surgical procedure of cutting into tissue to drain fluid. (3 wds).

11 Chronic indigestion of lead produces effects on the central nervous, renal, and _____ systems.

14 Being prepared for emergencies is the responsibility of _____ health care workers.

16 Prefix meaning "opposing" or "against"

19 Analysis of _____ is characteristic of Freudian psychoanalysis. (2 wds).

21 For an _____ year old (or a child who is 4'9" tall), seat belts fit properly when the lap belt lays across the upper thighs and the shoulder belt fits across the chest.

22 A _____ host is one that is at risk for getting an infection.

24 The organism responsible for an infection. (2 wds).

DOWN

1 Section of the stomach that terminates at the pylorus.

2 Substances that may react with pressure or temperature changes. (2 wds).

3 In asthma, this results from areas of the lung not being well-perfused.

6 Sometimes, these are needed in order to rid blood of lead quickly. (2 wds).

9 Muscular dystrophy is hereditary and acquired through a _____ sex-linked trait.

12 These are characterized by abnormal, unpleasant motor or verbal arousals and behaviors that occur during sleep.

13 This is a fast-acting bronchodilator for the treatment of asthma.

15 Fat-filled cells in subcutaneous tissue.

16 A hamstring release is done only when there is a knee flexion _____.

17 An antigen found on the surface of red blood cells called Rh-positive. An absence of this antigen is indicated by the term Rh-negative. (2 wds).

18 A hollow joint or acetabulum.

20 Suffix meaning "sudden, severe pain".

23 Suffix meaning "body".

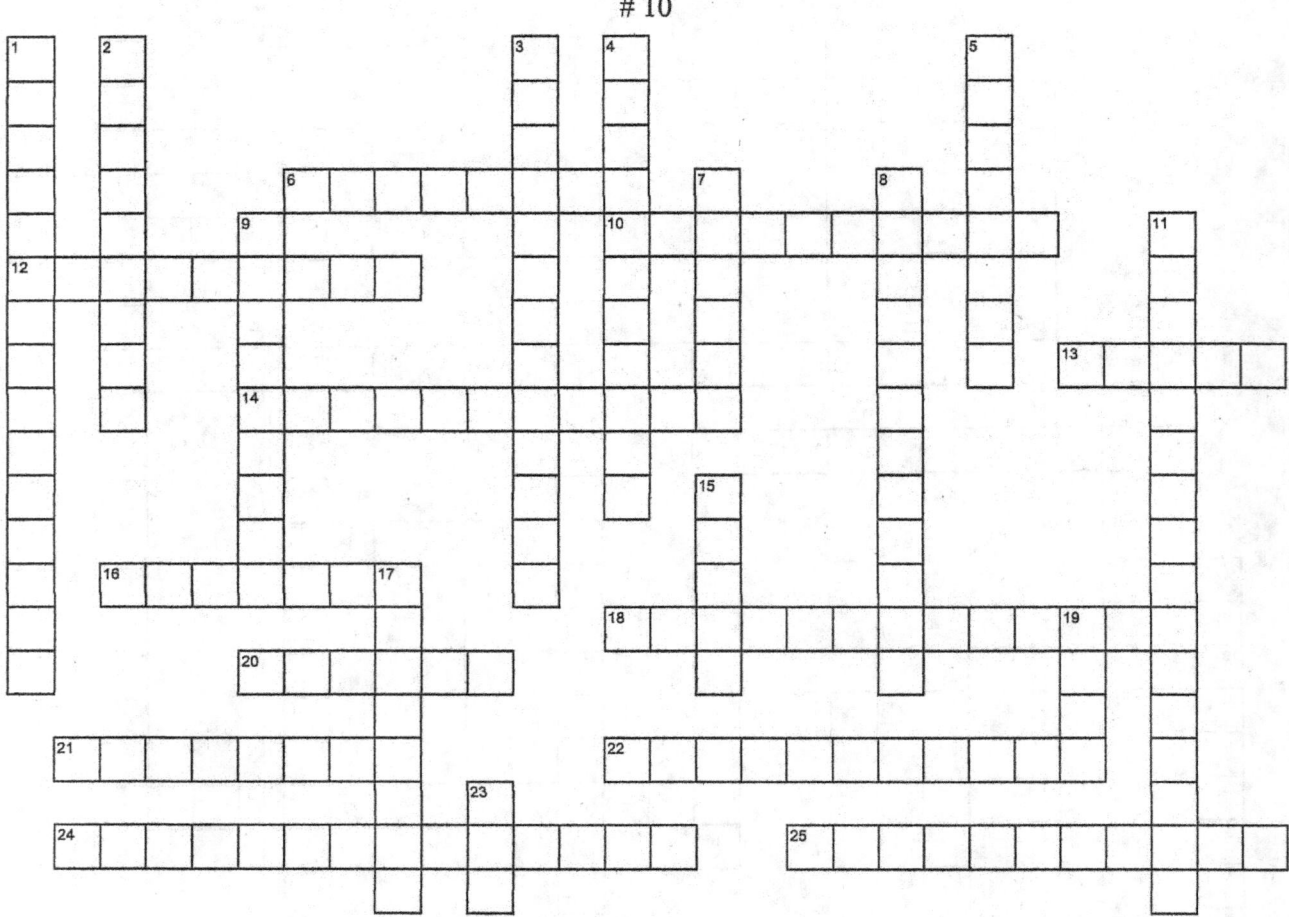

ACROSS

6 Joints are characterized into three types: suture, vertebral, and _____.
10 Lacking natural teeth.
12 Serum antibody formed in response to a biological toxin that works to counteract a specific poisonous substance.
13 Prefix meaning "pertaining to tears".
14 To divide into two branches.
16 Resembling a socket of a joint. The depressed or indented articular surface.
18 Sexual maturity in males and females is classified according to _____, named after the original researcher on sexual maturity. (2 wds).
20 A digestive enzyme produced by the pancreas to emulsify fat globules in the duodenum.
21 One of four parts.
22 Fear of germs.
24 Muscles of the upper chest and shoulders. (2 wds).
25 Part of the abdominal aorta from which arteries arise to take blood to the stomach, small intestine, liver, gallbladder, and pancreas. (2 wds).

DOWN

1 Immune response maintained by antibodies. Antigens stimulate the production of an antibody. (2 wds).
2 Sense of smell, or the act of smelling.
3 This, as well as a gastroscopy are used to view upper GI structures. (2 wds).
4 Bluish discoloration of the periumbilical area from subcutaneous intraperitoneal hemorrhagic pancreatitis. (2 wds).
5 Skin elevations that contain pus.
7 Not malignant. A condition of mild intensity.
8 The main cause of acute pancreatitis in males. (2 wds).
9 The anterior portion of the brain including the telencephalon and diencephalon.
11 Spongy or lattice-like bone formation located in the epiphyses of developing bone. (2 wds).
15 An area where two bones come together.
17 Relaxation of the heart, allowing it to refill with blood for the next contraction.
19 Suffix meaning "substance that holds matter together".
23 Visual coordination is usually resolved by age ____ months.

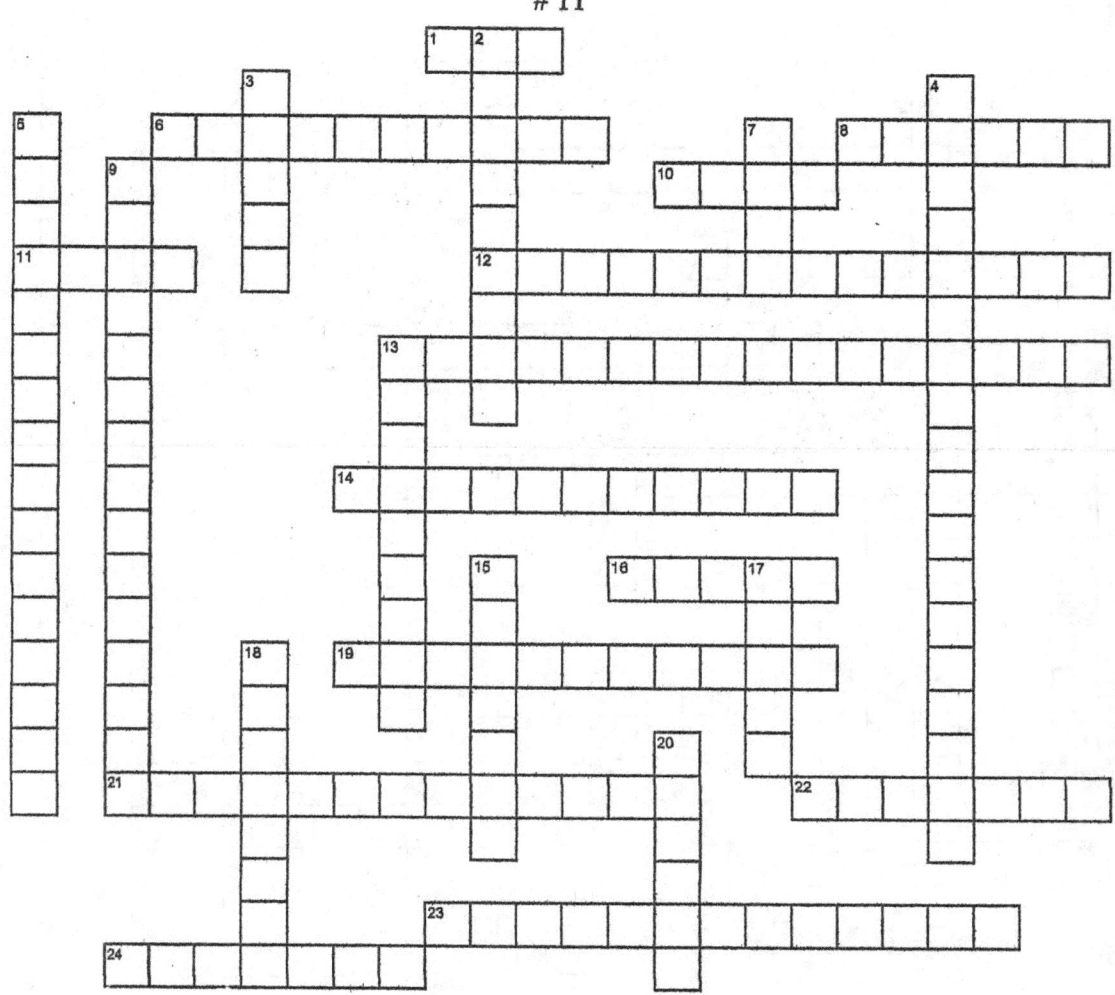

ACROSS

1 Prefix meaning "blood".
6 A harmful, destructive, or fatal condition.
8 Suffix meaning "excessive discharge or flow".
10 Suffix meaning "having the manner or structure of".
11 The _____ reflex disappears around age four months.
12 A shortened _____ may cause a child to walk on his or her toes. (2 wds).
13 With _____, the tympanic membrane may present as bright red or yellow, bulging or retracted. (3 wds).
14 Urination.
16 A narrow or tubular channel.
19 Branch of spinal nerves that passes on the back surface to innervate skin, muscle, and bones of the vertebral column. (2 wds).
21 This is the definitive test for tuberculosis. (2 wds).
22 Pertaining to the side.
23 A crescent-shaped bone of the wrist. (2 wds).
24 A child's _____ attain the adult number of nephrons (approximately one million in each) shortly after birth.

DOWN

2 A flexible, muscular tube leading from the pharynx to the stomach.
3 A barking cough and inspiratory stridor are noted with _____.
4 Necrotic, painful rashes are associated with the bite of a _____. (3 wds).
5 Narrowing at the entrance of the pulmonary artery represents _____. (2 wds).
7 True or false: Various special nipples are used for infants with cleft lip or palate, because normal nursery nipples are not effective.
9 Small vesicles on the genital area with itching indicate _____. (2 wds).
13 A state of complete physical and psychological dependence on a substance.
15 An erythematous rash after a fever is characteristic of _____.
17 Intense, sharp, severe symptoms followed by a short course of illness.
18 This may cause maternal tachycardia.
20 Abnormal backward flow of fluid.

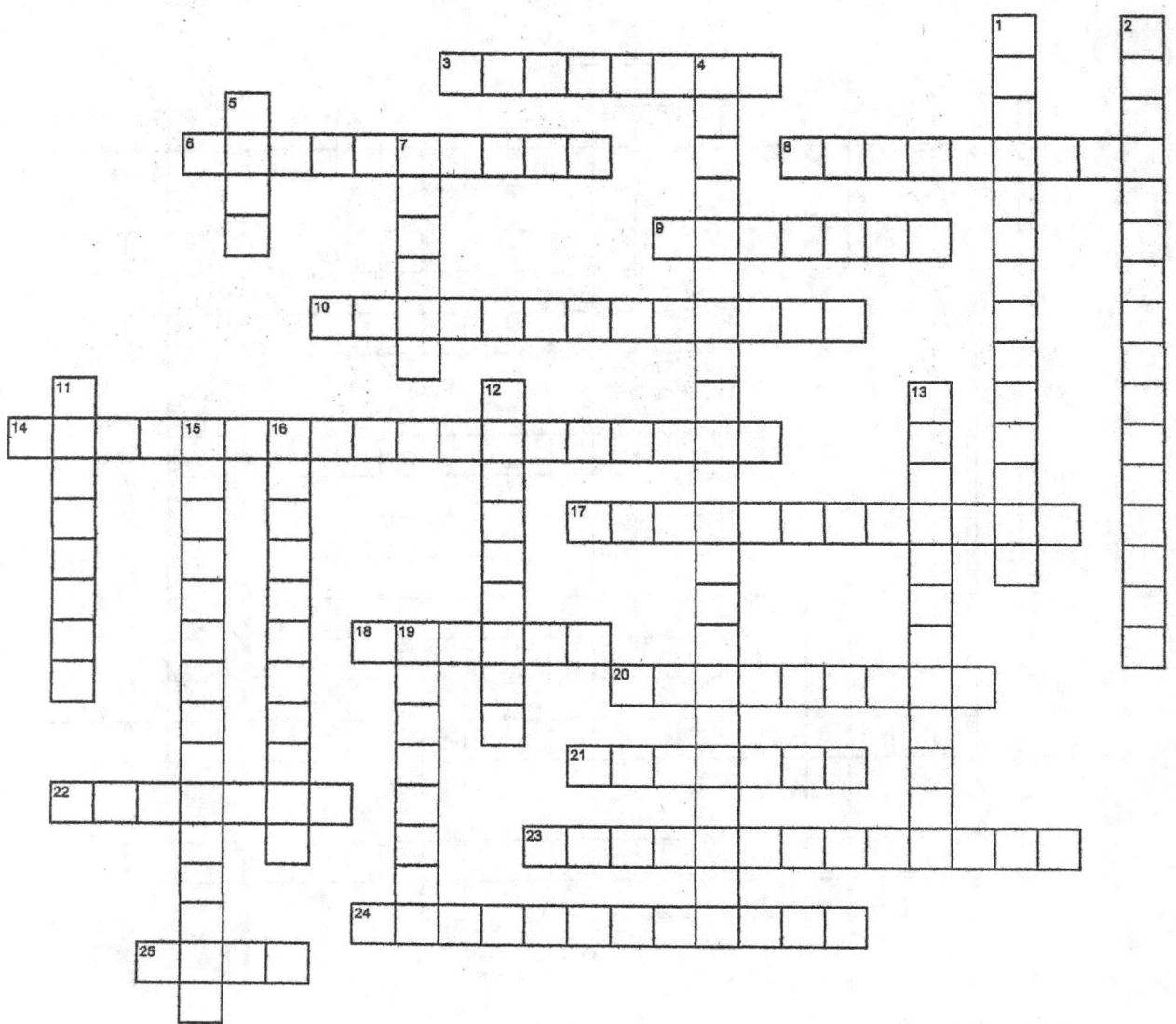

ACROSS

3 Pain that follows the pathway of the sciatic nerve, caused by compression or trauma of the nerve or its roots.

6 Injection of anesthetic into peripheral nerves or nerve trunks to interrupt sensation. (2 wds).

8 An open expression of previously suppressed feelings.

9 A cleavage in the surface of skin.

10 Suturing of the fascia that covers the surface of a muscle.

14 A measurement of the volume of air after forced expiration. (3 wds).

17 Paralysis of all four limbs caused by a spinal cord lesion.

18 A hollow space in a body organ or structure. Regarding dentition, this term identifies erosion of dental structure.

20 The use of an object to become sexually aroused.

21 Yellow coloration of the conjunctivae which makes the sclerae also appear yellow.

22 Loss of the ability to comprehend sensory input despite normal sensory function.

23 Malabsorption disorder caused by gluten sensitivity. (2 wds).

24 A machine that acts as an artificial kidney during dialysis.

25 Suffix meaning "stone".

DOWN

1 Infection of the lacrimal sac of the eye.

2 A clinical observation scale used to document level of consciousness. (3 wds).

4 This is based on drug interaction. One drug may be given to complement the effects of another. (3 wds).

5 Prefix meaning "one half".

7 Bleeding into tissue.

11 The _____, which form urine, continue to mature throughout early childhood.

12 A linear, papular, vesicular rash indicates exposure to _____. (2 wds).

13 Damage from Alzheimer's-type dementia is _____.

15 Movement of particles within an electric field toward a cathode or anode.

16 Parasomnias are _____ or behavioral reactions during sleep.

19 Distention of a bodily cavity with gas.

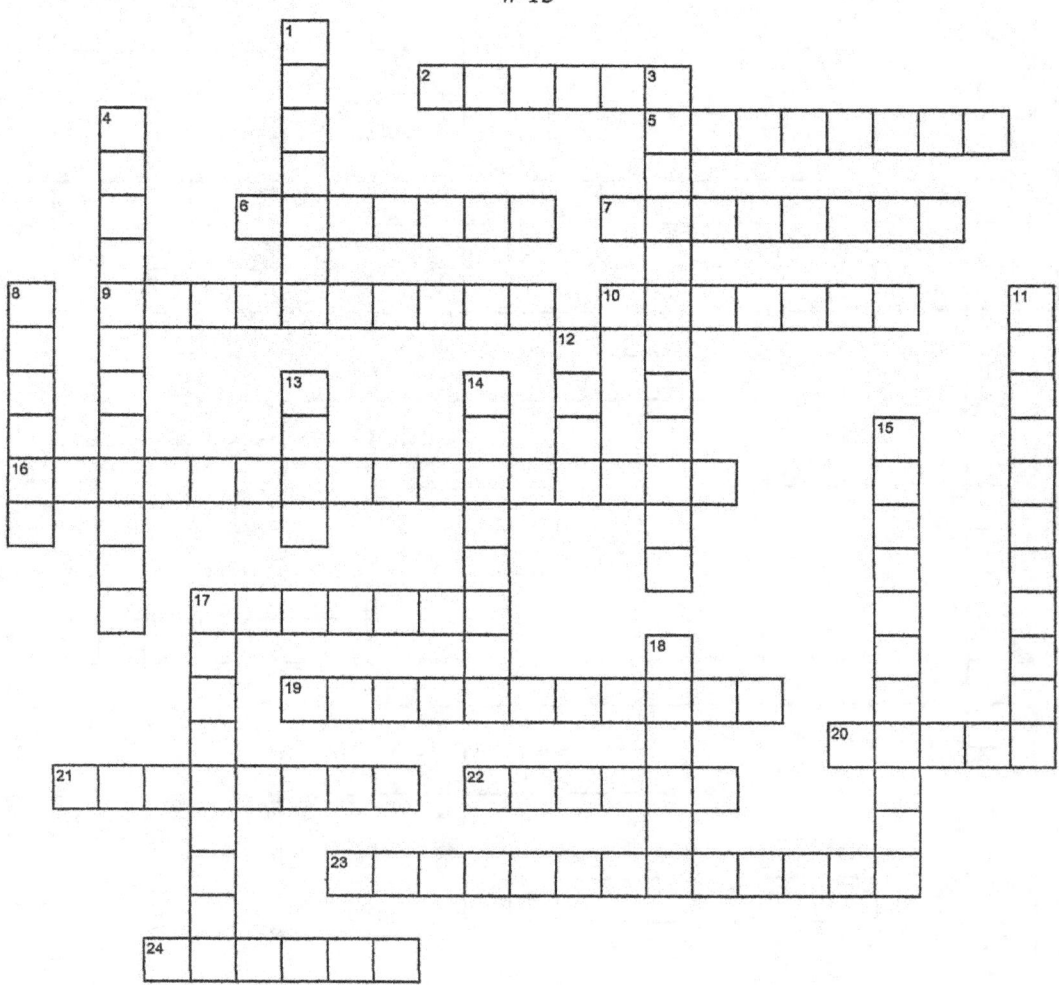

ACROSS

2 The anterior bone of the lower leg that extends from the knee and terminates at the lateral aspect of the ankle.
5 Near the center or point of origin.
6 A childhood disease caused by inadequate vitamin D intake.
7 First stool produced by newborn babies.
9 A device used to determine the specific gravity of liquid by comparison to water.
10 Denoting the flow of sweat.
16 Stiff and awkward muscle control caused by a central nervous system disorder. (2 wds).
17 Expelled food or chyme.
19 Mental confusion associated with gross sedation and brain disorders.
20 Suffix meaning "system composed of".
21 Pertaining to the chest.
22 A hollow muscular organ of the female reproductive tract where a fertilized ovum implants and develops into a fetus.
23 A group of motor disorders caused by damage to motor centers of the cerebral cortex, cerebellum, or basal ganglia during fetal development, childbirth, or early infancy. (2 wds)
24 Suffix meaning "short"

DOWN

1 Dizziness while not moving, and ringing in the ears in quiet environments.
3 The process of clearly perceiving one's own personality.
4 Surgical reconstruction of the jaw.
8 Suffix meaning "to crush".
11 Ischemia and necrosis of tissue with bacterial infection causing cellulitis in adjacent tissues. (2 wds).
12 Suffix meaning "suspension or fixation by surgical intervention"
13 Suffix meaning "state of".
14 Artificial procedure used to replace normal kidney filtering by using an external filtration system.
15 Surgical insertion of a permanent feeding tube through the abdominal wall into the jejunum.
17 A device for changing liquid medications to a gaseous state for the purpose of inhalation.
18 A detailed, prescribed order of actions.

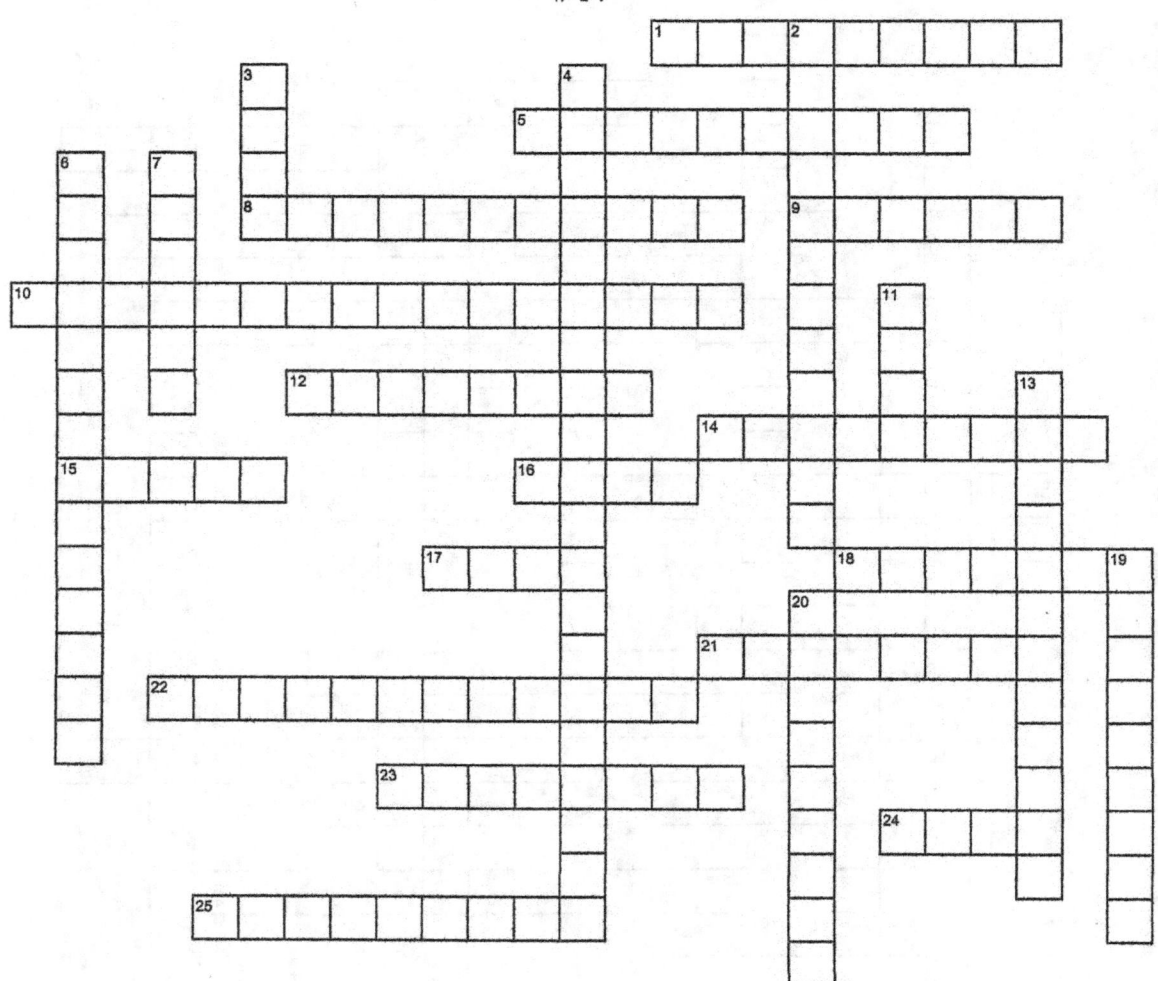

ACROSS

1 This may be indicated by a hard, painless, red defined lesion.
5 Skin inflammation from any source.
8 Series of contractions producing emission of two to five ml of semen from the male urethra.
9 The area furthest from the opening.
10 An inherited growth disorder of bone and cartilage that leads to skeletal malformation and dwarfism.
12 Audible whistling breath sound often associated with asthma or airway constriction.
14 Production of milk by the breasts following pregnancy.
15 Prefix meaning "false".
16 True or false: Sound discrimination is present at birth.
17 Suffix meaning "middle".
18 A resonant cough described as ____ is the most characteristic sign of croup.
21 A crescent-shaped, fibrocartilaginous structure of the knee, acromioclavicular, and temporomandibular, and sternoclavicular joints.
22 Muscular weakness in all four extremiities.
23 Having two points or parts.
24 A firm structural attachment, often the lowest part of the organ.
25 The kidneys are responsible for excreting ____.

DOWN

2 A saclike structure from which hair grows. (2 wds).
3 Most pediatric burns occur to children younger than age ____.
4 Lead intoxification produces damage to the _____ that is difficult to repair. (3 wds).
6 The small tip at the inferior end of the sternum. (2 wds).
7 One of two large, bean-shaped organs located in the flank region of the back that are responsible for filtering waste products out of the blood and for formation of urine.
11 Cleft or fissure.
13 These are consistent with measles. (2 wds).
19 A response from the throat that causes retching. (2 wds).
20 A term applied to cancerous cells that revert to a less developed state in arrangement and structure.

15

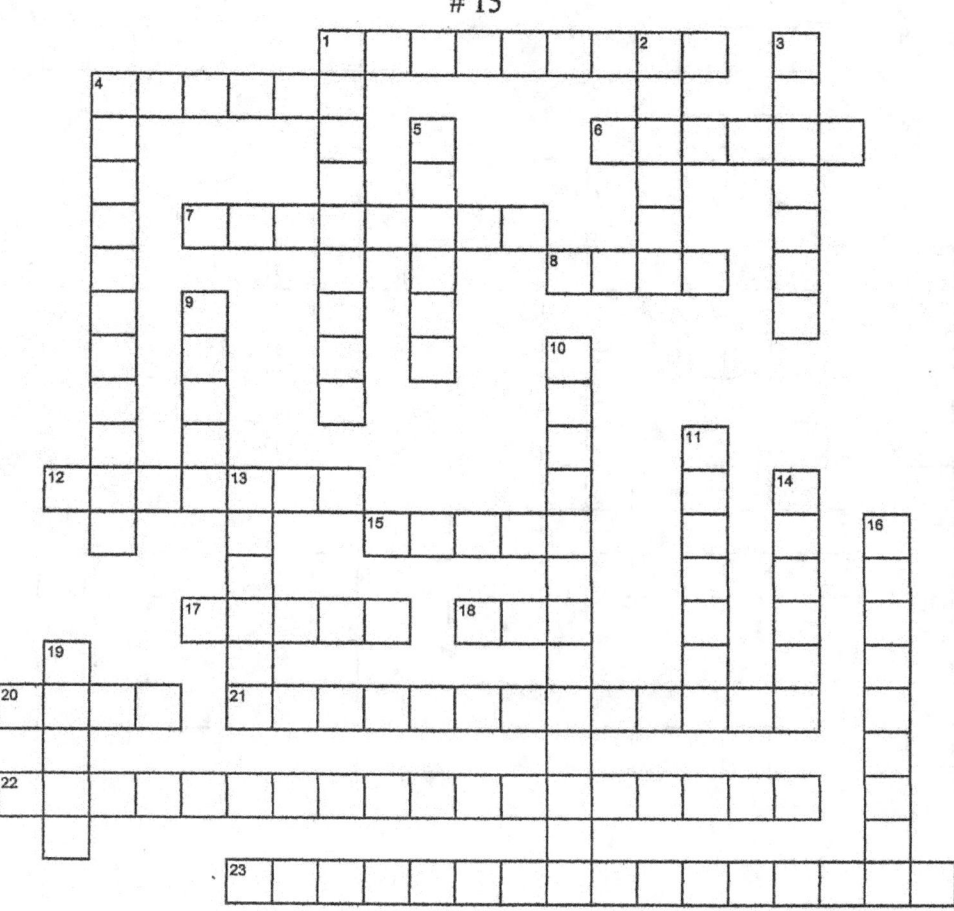

ACROSS

1 Skin disorder with groups of bulla.
4 The avoidance of death's inevitability, and the first step of the grieving process.
6 The three stages of Alzheimer's-type dementia are mild, moderate, and _____.
7 Paired occurrences, such as heart rhythms.
8 Suffix meaning "record of".
12 The study of structures of the human body.
15 Suffix meaning "something that produces movement.
17 The three leading causes of accidental death in children are motor vehicle accidents, drowning, and ____.
18 Prefix meaning "twice" or "double".
20 Suffix meaning "study of"
21 Removal of fluid from the thoracic cavity, usually due to cancer or pneumonia.
22 The four cavities within the cerebrum containing cerebrospinal fluid. (2 wds).
23 A solution that has an infective agent that has been killed or substantially weakened and does not produce disease. (2 wds).

DOWN

1 These are used to prevent bleeding caused by thrombocytopenia.
2 Excessive urea and nitrogenous wastes in the blood.
3 This type of pain lasts six months or longer, and is ongoing.
4 Removal of necrotic tissue to foster the regeneration of healthy tissue.
5 An enlargement of the thyroid gland.
9 Acne vulgaris primarily affects adolescents, but lesions may appear as early as age ____.
10 A peripheral nerve that conveys impulses from the central nervous system to the peripheral nerves. (2 wds).
11 These are responsible for regulating the acid-base balance.
13 Hidden. Not observable by the naked eye. Often used in reference to bleeding in the gastrointestinal tract.
14 Bone of the lateral forearm that is aligned with the thumb.
16 Any accumulation of fluid around the testicle.
19 A natural depression on a body surface such as a bone.

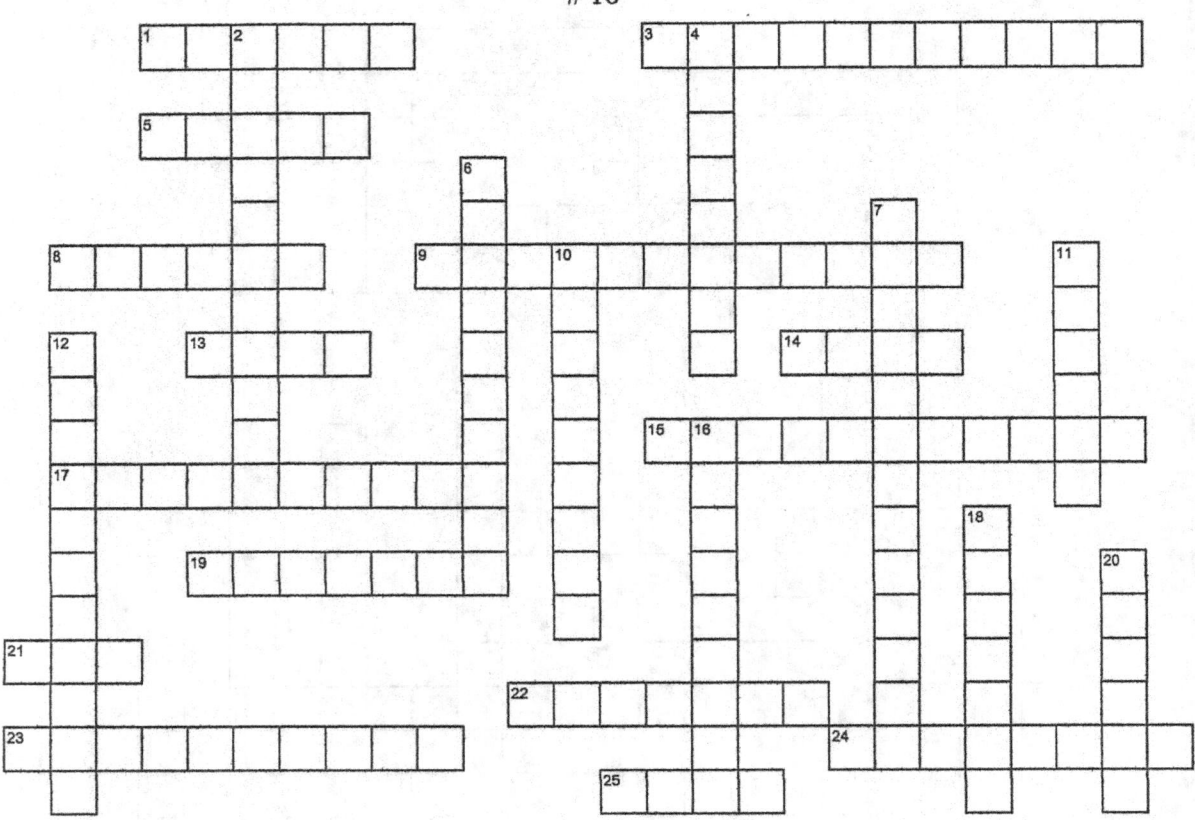

ACROSS

1 The _____ grasp reflex disappears around age three-four months.
3 Excessive uterine bleeding during menstruation.
5 A branching structure from a larger anatomical structure such as a nerve or blood vessel.
8 Suffix meaning "related to hearing"
9 Repetition of phrases and words in writing, indicative of brain or psychaitric pathology.
13 Suffix meaning "bulging" or "hernia".
14 True or false: Paralysis may occur in lead toxicity as toxic damage to the brain progresses.
15 Surgical repair of a tendon to restore functionality.
17 The branch of medicine focused on the care of women during pregnancy, delivery, and the postpartum period.
19 The small, rounded bone situated at the front of the knee. Also known as the kneecap.
21 Ribonucleic acid. (3 init's).
22 Pharmacological agent that combines with receptors to initiate drug actions.
23 An area of hardened tissue, caused by various pathological states.
24 Suffix meaning "puncture".
25 Prefix meaning "strange" or "odd".

DOWN

2 A bull's eye rash is a classic symptom of _____ and is located primarly at the site of the bite. (2 wds).
4 A negatively charged subatomic particle.
6 Pharmacological agents used to block nerve sensations.
7 Valve between the left atrium and the left ventricle. (e.g., mitral valve). (2 wds).
10 True labor contractions are felt initially in the _____ and radiate to the abdomen in a wavelike motion. (2 wds).
11 The incubation period of varicella is ten to _____ days
12 An inability to voluntarily control bowel movements or bladder function.
16 The weakening of connective tissue in the lower eyelid in older patients causing the eyelid to turn outward, exposing the conjunctiva and causing dryness and chronic conjunctivitis.
18 Use of a Z-shaped surgical incision to reduce tension on a scar produced by normal movement of a body part.
20 A tract of myelinated nerves among the arched floor of teh lateral ventricles, connecting the hippocampus in each temporal lobe to the thalamus and each amygdaloid body.

17

ACROSS

1 Pertaining to the abdomen.

5 A medical device used to encourage a patient to inhale and sustain inspiratory volume to exercise lungs and prevent pulmonary complications. (2 wds).

8 A congenital deformity of the bony thorax in which the sternum, particularly the xyphoid process, is bent inward, creating a hollow depression in the anterior chest. (2 wds).

9 Facial bones that form the lateral edges of the eye sockets and cheekbones. (2 wds).

13 Entrance of air into a blood vessel, most often a vein, during trauma or medical procedures. A large amount of air may result in death. (2 wds).

14 Pertaining to having two sides.

16 The clinical sign of _____ is perianal itching that increases at night.

17 Tissue graft from a distant species.

18 Koplik's spots, as well as a descending maculopapular rash, are diagnostic of _____.

21 Painful spasm of anal sphincter, ineffective straining at stool associated with inflammatory bowel disease, or IBS.

23 The most commonly implicated cause of acute pancreatitis in women. (2 wds).

24 Poisonous or destructive to the kidney.

25 Borrelia burgdorferi is responsible for _____. (2 wds).

DOWN

2 Individuals, families, adn other subgroupings of people who are associated because of singular social, personal, or health care needs. A group or population.

3 A section of bowel located at the first portion of the large intestine that terminates at the appendix.

4 Thi is the most common adverse reaction of those undergoing radiation therapy.

6 Fresh frozen _____ is used to treat coagulation factor deficiencies, warfarin reversal, and thrombotic thrombocytopenic purpura.

7 Normal menstruation.

10 Massive, generalized body edema associated with right-sided heart failure.

11 Anatomical landmark of the right lung. (2 wds).

12 Bruising in a linear pattern on the skin.

15 Intense, unreasonable fear of a specific object or situation.

19 Suffix meaning "small".

20 Pertaining to the urinary bladder.

22 Genetic inflammatory skin disorder.

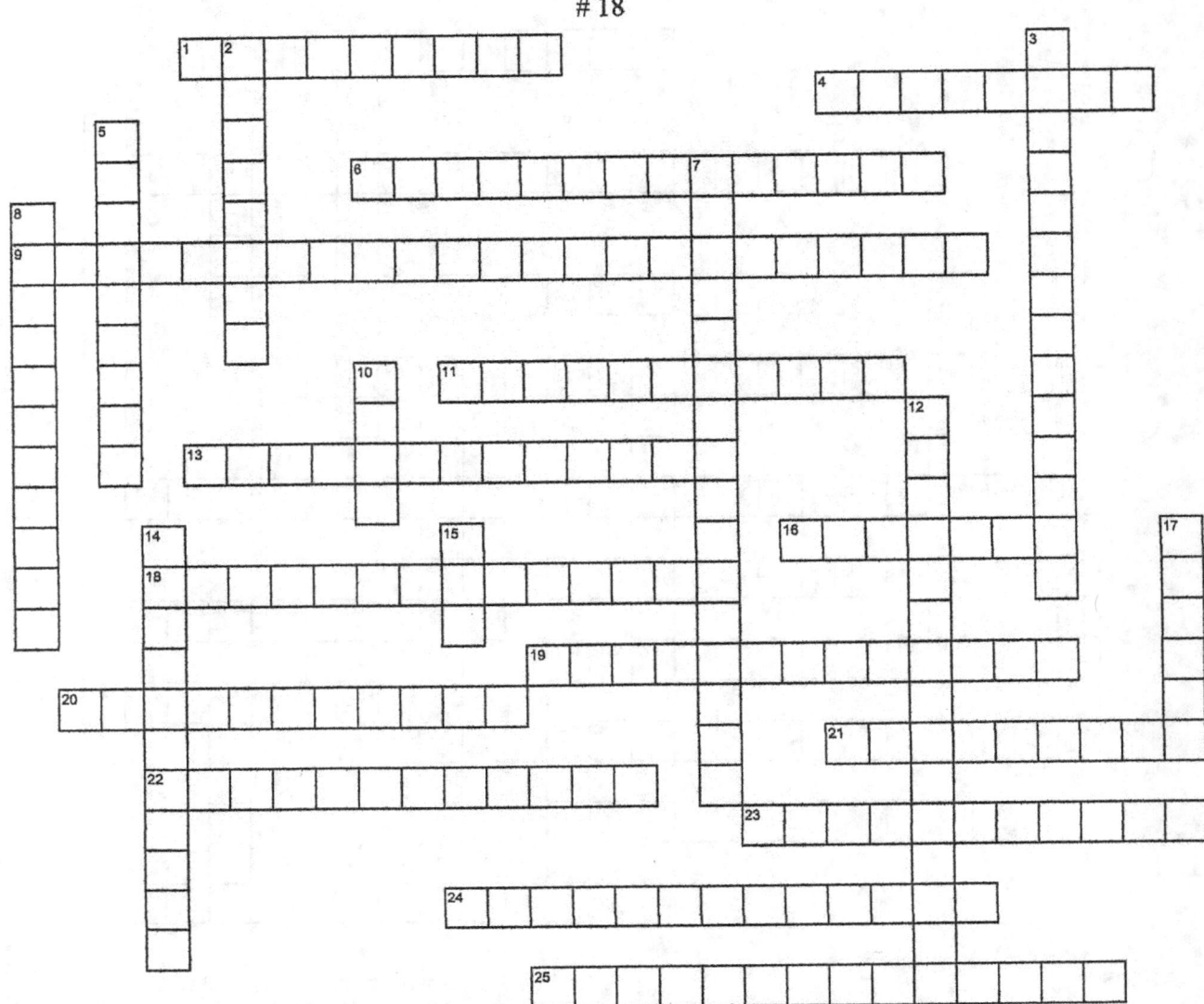

ACROSS

1 Movement away from the center.
4 Conduction or activity moving outward.
6 17-ketosteroids test is a 24-hour urine test to detect steroidal metabolites of androgenic and _____ hormones.
9 A rigid, plastic-tipped device used to aspirate secretions from the mouth and throat. (3 wds).
11 Protrusion of the meninges through bone, forming a filled cyst.
13 Surgical excision of the tonsils.
16 Fold of skin at the nail root. (eponychium).
18 Major blood vessel supplying blood to the abdominal organs. (2 wds).
19 Use of electromagnetic induction to artificially produce a fever in order to treat a primary pathology.
20 The tissue of the central nervous system consisting mainly of myelinated nerve fibers. (2 wds).
21 Extremely dry skin.
22 Surgical fixation of the cecum.
23 Skin infection caused by lice infestation.
24 Abnormal accumulation of cerebrospinal fluid in the ventricles of the brain as a result of developmental anomalies, infection, or tumor.
25 Lack of effective contractions during labor. (2 wds).

DOWN

2 The tubular structure that bile flows through.
3 Linked neurons that transmit electrical and chemical messages between the body and central nervous system. (3 wds).
5 Prolonged drowsiness, sedation, or sleepiness, often the result of disease or medications.
7 A malignant tumor of striated muscle.
8 The facial muscle that draws the corner of the mouth upward and outward.
10 Prefix meaning "inadequate number" or "few".
12 A slanting-angle break in bone. (2 wds).
14 Excision of the fascia that covers the surface of a muscle.
15 Suffix meaning "pertaining to".
17 The musculomembranous tube that connects the cervix uteri and the vulva.

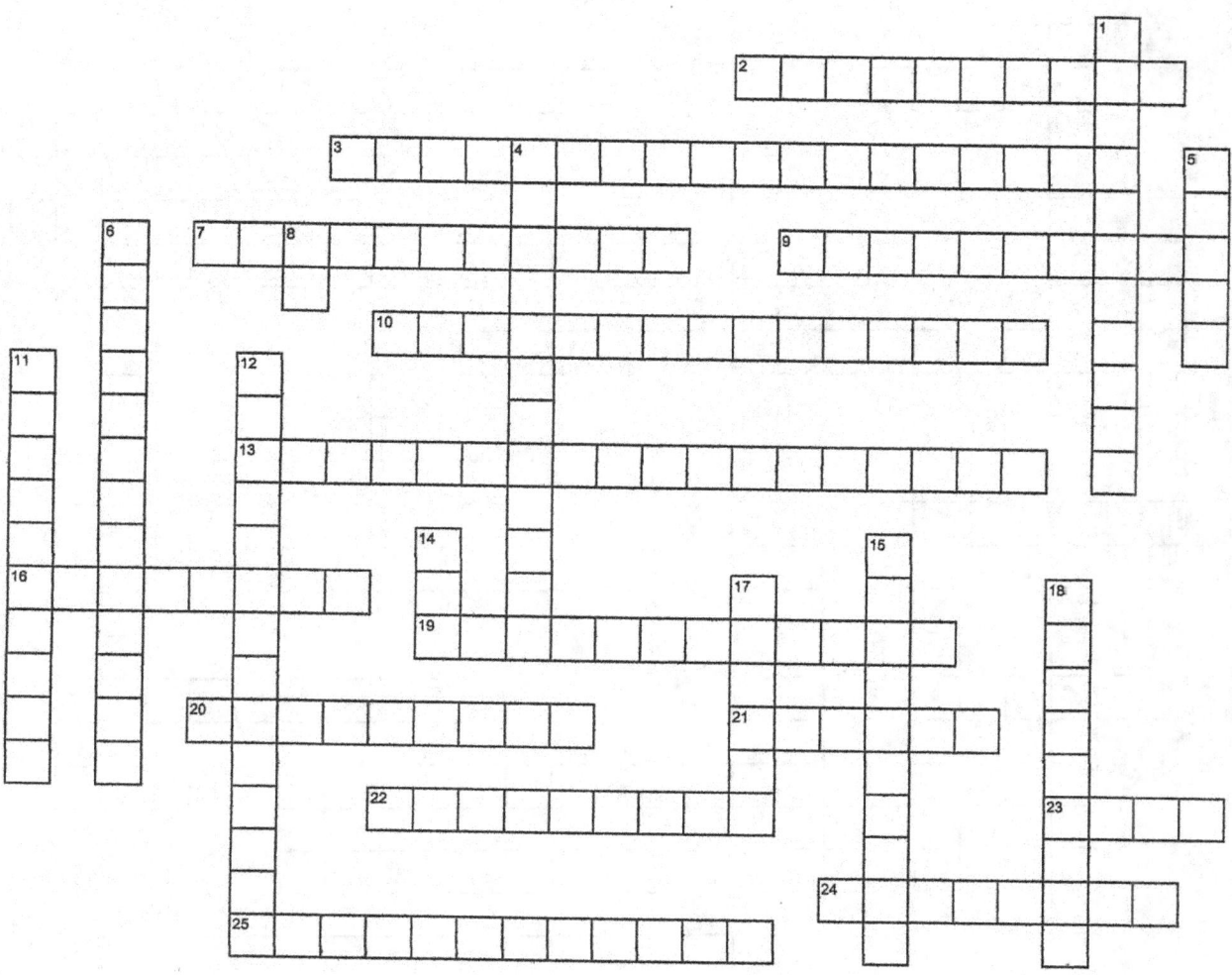

ACROSS

2 Inflammation of connective tissue, especially of the subcutaneous tissue.

3 A fleshy abnormal growth in the intestine or other tissues characterized by a thin stalk supporting a ball-shaped, irregular top. (2 wds).

7 Affecting the development of a fetus, as in transmitting or causing malformation.

9 Caused by a pathogen such as virus or bacteria.

10 Abnormal protrusion of an organ through the abdominal musculature. (2 wds).

13 Immune reaction due to formation of antibodies to a pathogenic organism. (2 wds).

16 An abnormal, goatlike sound observed during auscultation of the chest as the patient speaks in a normal fashion, associated with pleural effusion and pneumonia.

19 Loss of body function or part due to surgical intervention, disease, or degenerative condition.

20 Speech that includes a jumble of seemingly unrelated words. (May be associated with thought disorders). (2 wds).

21 Tumor of glial cells graded by degree of invasion.

22 The midsection or shaft of a long cylindrical bone.

23 Suffix meaning "state of".

24 Development of male secondary sex characteristics in a female.

25 A peptide responsible for the regulation and inhibition of hormones by various neuroendocrine cells in the brain and gastrointestinal tract.

DOWN

1 Profuse sweating.

4 Pertaining to the uterus and bladder.

5 A shallow depression in a bone or tissue.

6 The inability to comprehend or demonstrate insight into a highly emotional subject. (aka, emotional blind spot). (2 wds).

8 Abbreviation for "prescription".

11 A greenish bile pigment. Gall substance.

12 Acute and fulminating destruction of muscle tissue, possibly fatal.

14 Abbreviation for "nothing by mouth".

15 Congenital malformation where hands and/or feet are directly attached to the trunk.

17 Structural deformation of being bent or turned outward. (Usually describes extremities).

18 Pertaining to the prostate gland.

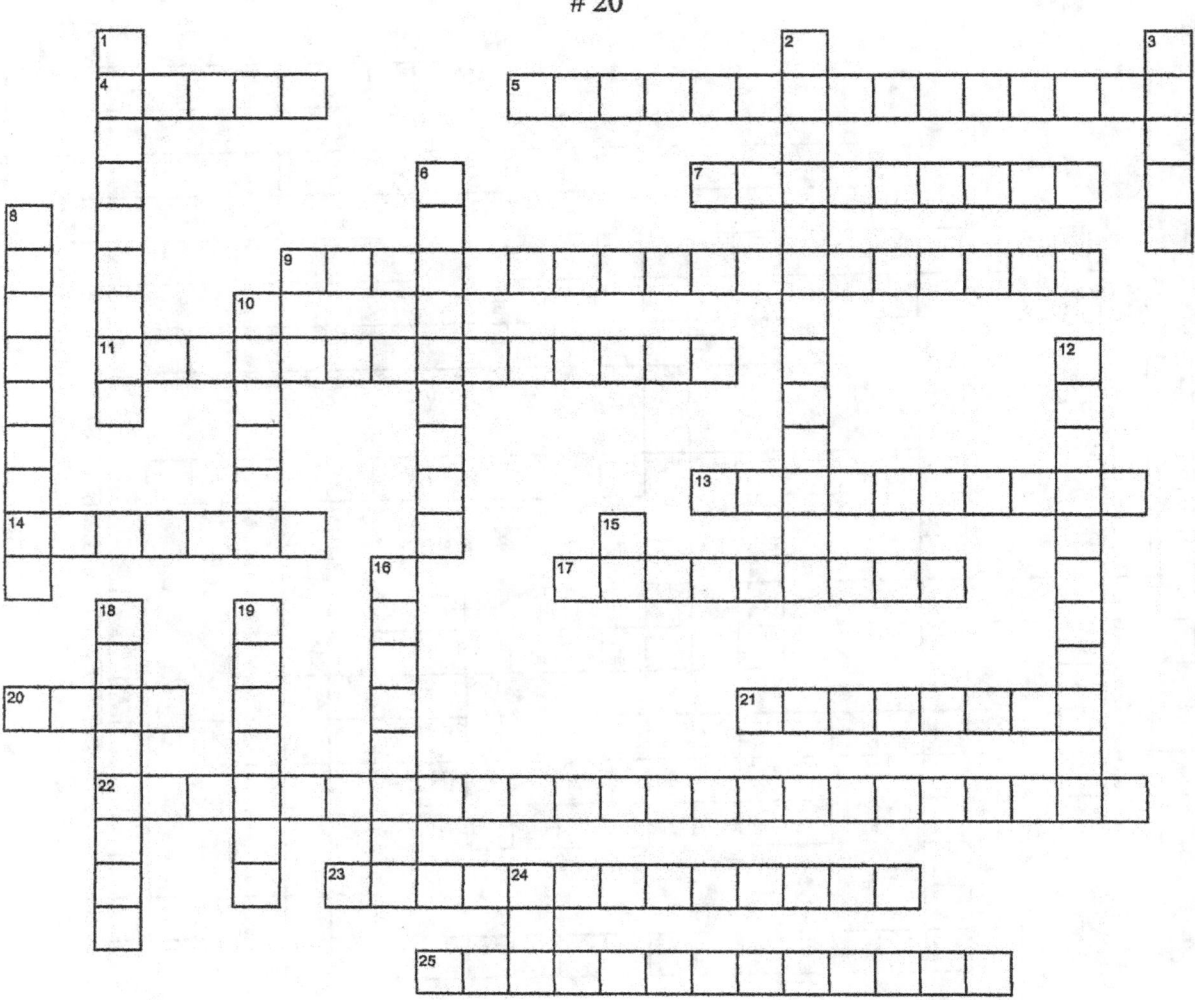

ACROSS

4 Prefix meaning "voice" or "sound".
5 Muscle that moves the scapula against the thorax. (2 wds).
7 Infrequent breathing that causes less oxygen to enter the lungs.
9 Body positioned erect, standing, facing forward, arms at sides, palms forward, and toes pointing forward. (2 wds).
11 Surgical removal of a small segment of the suspect lesion for microscopic examination. (2 wds).
13 Pertaining to the middle intestine attachment to the jejunum and iliac.
14 Relating to the tongue.
17 Constant, persistent, uncontrollable thoughts associated with anxiety and psychotic disorders.
20 Prefix meaning "change", "going beyond normal development".
21 Beneath or lower. (In reference to structures).
22 A structure that carries lymph toward the periphery. (3 wds).
23 Loss of all memories. (2 wds).
25 One of the posterior lateral muscles of the thigh included in the hamstring group that causes external rotation and flexion of the hip when contracted. (2 wds).

DOWN

1 Pertaining to spermatozoon.
2 Fungal infection of the vagina.
3 Use of electromagnetic radiation to penetrate body parts and produce images used for diagnosis and treatment of a variety of conditions.
6 Pertaining to or involving the skin.
8 A curved, muscular membrane that divides the thoracic and abdominal cavities.
10 Benign, fatty tumor.
12 Gluten enteropathy. A food allergy to the gluten in wheat that causes tissues of the small intestine to become damaged by the allergic response. (2 wds).
15 Prefix meaning "away from".
16 Pertaining to the end boundary, especially a disease from which a patient cannot recover or that is likely to cause death.
18 Suffix meaning "slipping".
19 Forceps that are used to remove small bone fragments.
24 Abbreviation for "airway, breathing, circulation".

21

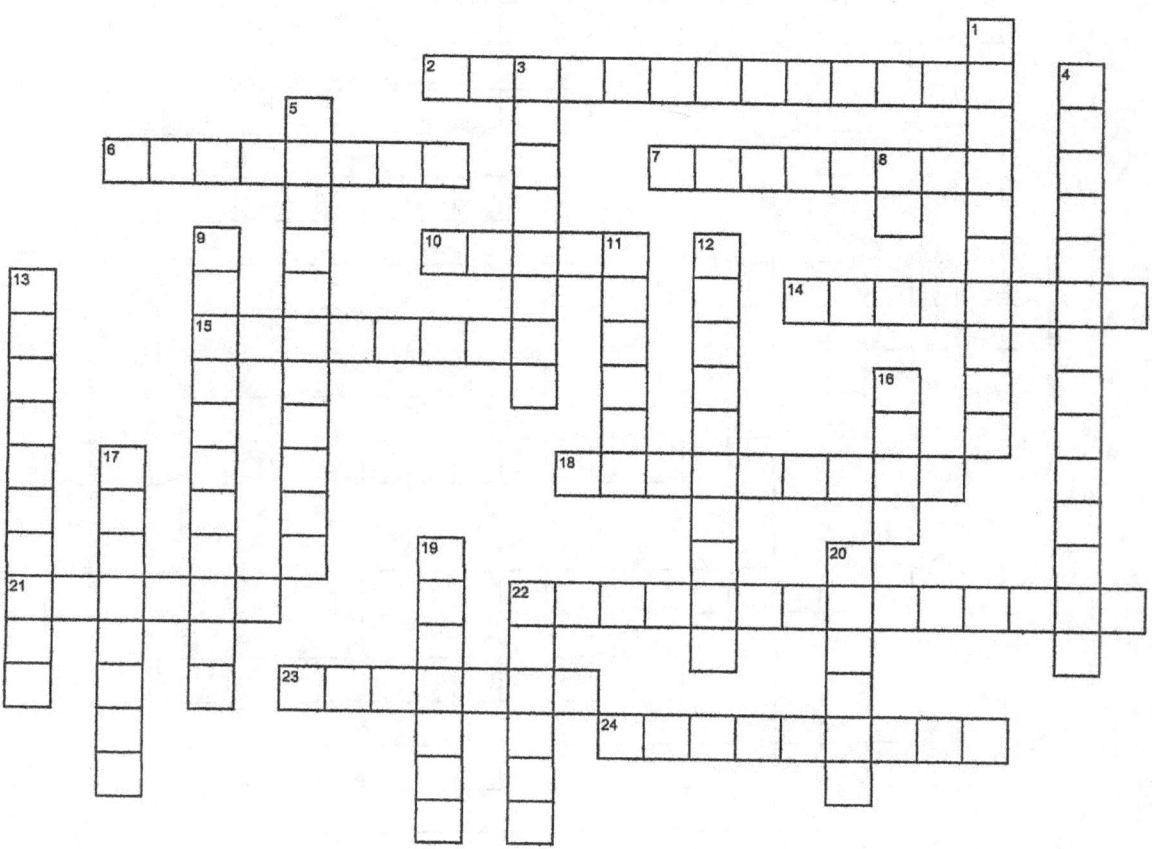

ACROSS

2 This is the most common cause of death for clients with systemic lupus erythematosus. (2 wds).
6 Eyelid.
7 Increased intraocular pressure because the aqueous humor cannot circulate freely.
10 The right lung has _____ lobes.
14 Highly toxic or intense disease-producing quality of a pathogen.
15 Male gonad which functions to produce sperm and testosterone.
18 Surgical destruction of the vagus (X) nerve interrupting the impulses transmitted to the stomach and intestines.
21 Reduction in the amount of hemoglobin in the blood, thus decreasing the oxygen-carrying capacity of the blood.
22 The facial muscle that circles the mouth. (2 wds).
23 Suffix meaning "condition of softening".
24 End product from the breakdown of old red blood cells.

DOWN

1 Entire transformation of energy and chemicals occurring within living cells, consisting of anabolism and catabolism.
3 Abnormally frequent and loose, watery stools with increased peristalsis caused by an infection (bacteria, viruses), irritable bowel syndrome, ulcerative colitis, lactose intolerance, or a drug side effect.
4 The dilation of the renal pelvis and calyces of one or both kidneys due to mechanical obstruction of the flow of urine by tumor, calculus, or inflammation or obstruction of the prostate or edema.
5 The space between the lungs.
8 Bone.
9 Slowed or incomplete development or function.
11 The unabsorbed food fragments that are passed through the digestive tract.
12 Type of transplant from the same individual.
13 A collective term for the ciliary body of the eye. (2 wds).
16 Suffix meaning "condition" or "increased".
17 Largest portion of the brain.
19 An opening in a bone through which nerves, blood vessels, and other structures pass.
20 Frontal portion of ear cartilage near the auditory canal.
22 Prefix meaning "backward".

22

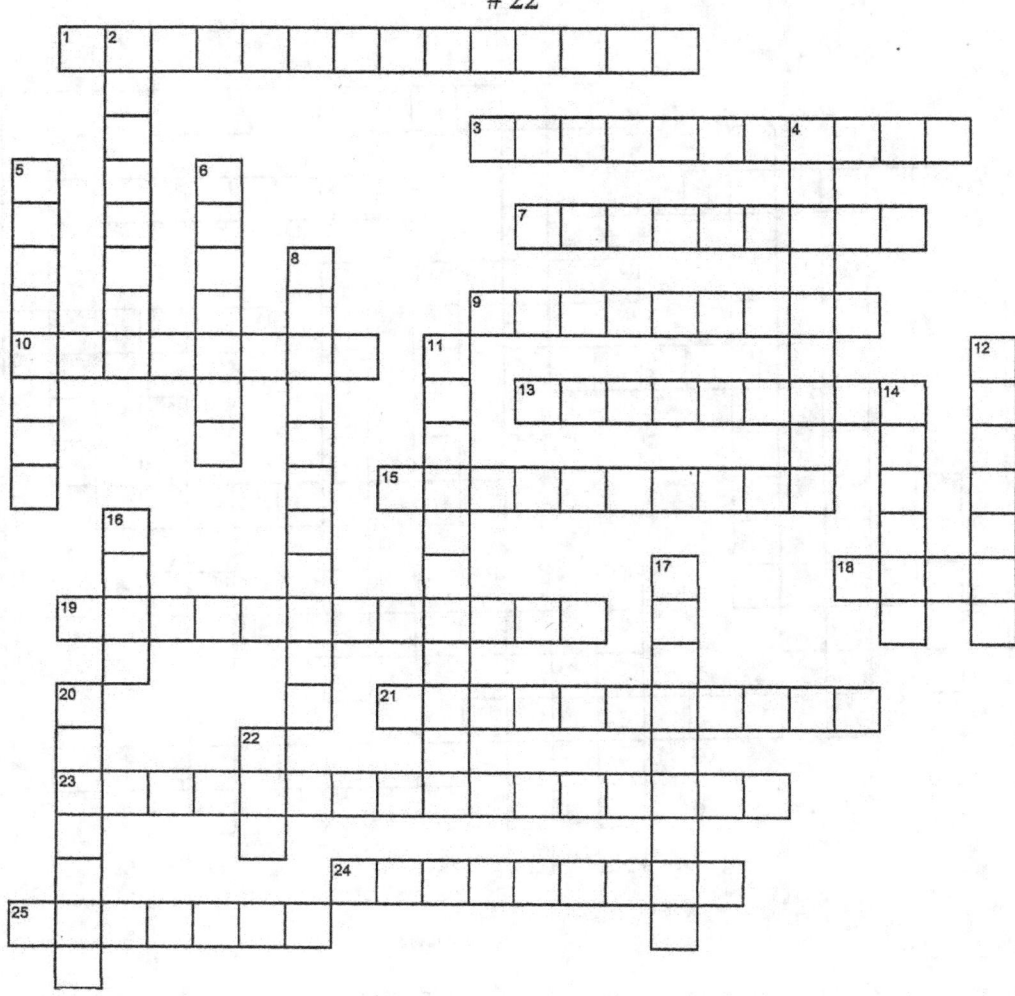

ACROSS

1 Semireclining in bed, with head of bed elevated. (2 wds).

3 This type of therapy is used on patients with chronic conditions that do not resolve.

7 The most common cause of ophthalmia neonatorum, and a major cause of pneumonia in infants during the first three months of life.

9 Movement of molecules in a solution or a gas from an area of high concentration to one of low concentration.

10 Type of fracture in which the bone is broken into separate pieces.

13 Substances that cause other substances to change and burn.

15 Substances that cause damage and burns when they contact the skin or eyes.

18 True or false: Respiratory infection may be fatal for patients with muscular dystrophy due to poor chest expansion and decreased ability to mobilize secretions.

19 In patients with _____, maintenance of airway and breathing take top priority.

21 Signs of sepsis include elevated temperature, increased heart rate, and increased _____ rate.

23 No weight on the extremity, and extremity must be elevated. (2 wds).

24 The primary complication of osteoporosis is ____.

25 Primary prevention of osteoporosis includes maintaining optimal _____ intake.

DOWN

2 An infection occurs when an _____ enters the body and the body's immune system is unable to fight it off, causing illness.

4 Hormone that promotes male secondary sex characteristics.

5 These may decrease digoxin absorption.

6 Innermost area of an organ or structure.

8 A drug _____ occurs when a drug is given with or shortly after another drug, and the effect of either or both drugs either increases or decreases.

11 A patient's next of kin can only sign a consent form if the patient is deemed _____.

12 Waxy substance produced by glands in the external auditory meatus which functions to protect it from infection by trapping microorganisms.

14 The fibrous tissue that forms the outer protective covering over the eyeball.

16 Circular, external opening of the rectum, controlled by the anal sphincter.

17 Limited to a specific region or body part.

20 _____ and dried fruit are high in potassium.

22 Suffix meaning "production" or "origin".

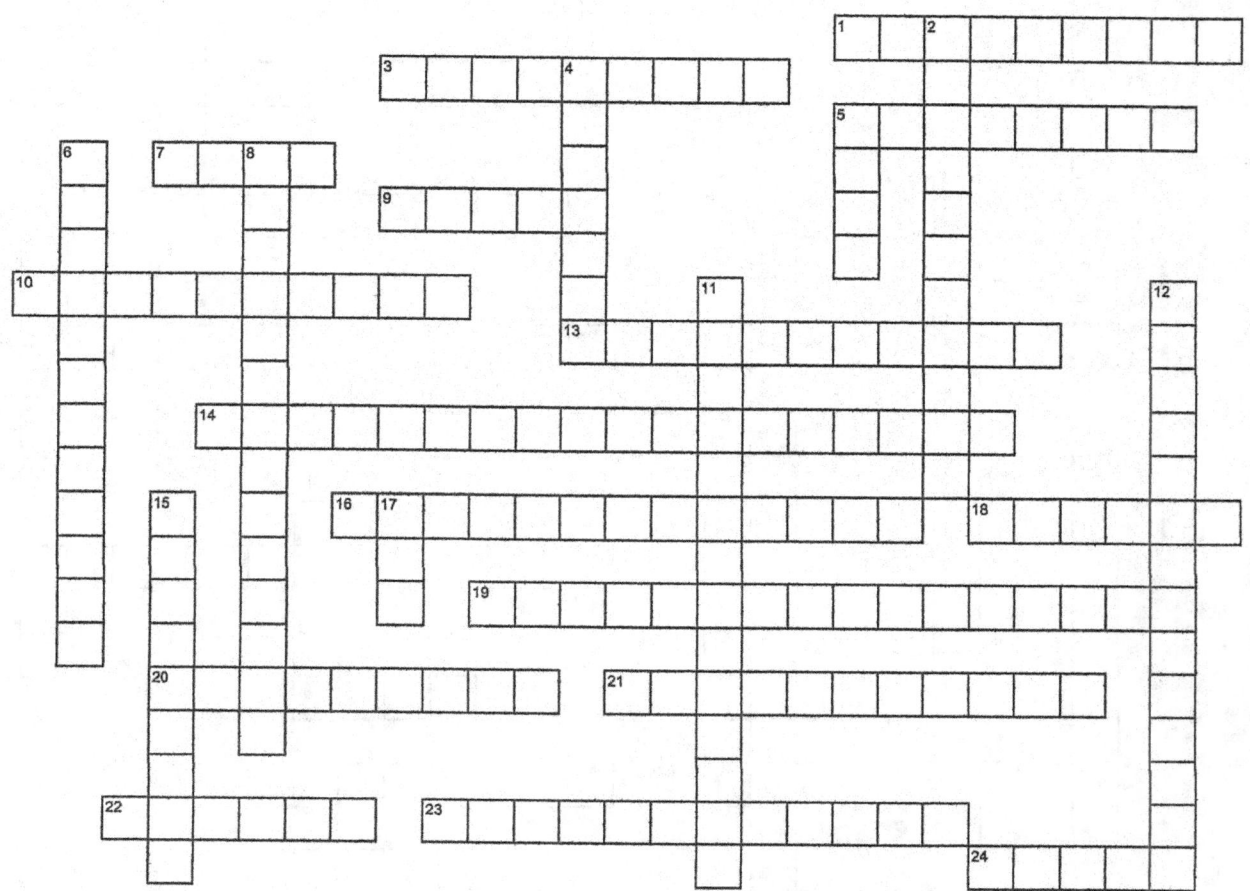

ACROSS

1 Therapeutic use of electromagnetic ultrasound waves to heat muscle tissue.

3 Cervical discharge with redness and edema indicates _____.

5 These can be either hypothermic or hyperthermic with meningitis.

7 Prefix meaning "circular".

9 Largest artery, that arises from the left ventricle.

10 This will decrease uric acid levels and decrease stress on joints. (2 wds).

13 Pertaining to the emission of semen from the male urethra.

14 Fibrosis of the renal glomeruli.

16 Concussion is associated with brief loss of _____.

18 Milk, ice cream and _____ are rich in calcium.

19 Protrusion of the bowel or abdominal structures occurring along the suture line of a prior surgical incision. (2 wds).

20 A surgical procedure in which tissue is scraped away using a curette.

21 Surgical repair of the nose to correct a defect or to change its appearance.

22 The _____ stage of labor is one to four hours after birth.

23 Formation of a stone in the body.

24 Prefix meaning "near" or "close proximity".

DOWN

2 Fear of crowds or public places which causes individuals to resist leaving home even for important or urgent medical care.

4 Feeling unwell, often the first sign of illness.

5 The purpose of the halo vest is to immobilize the ____, and to improve mobility.

6 A small depression in the center of the macula, directly opposite the pupil, where the greatest visual acuity lies. (2 wds).

8 A central landmark depression on the surface of the liver. (2 wds).

11 Left eye. (2 wds).

12 Congenital absence of major bile ducts. (also known as neonatal hepatitis). (2 wds).

15 Movement away from the center.

17 Suffix meaning "carbohydrate".

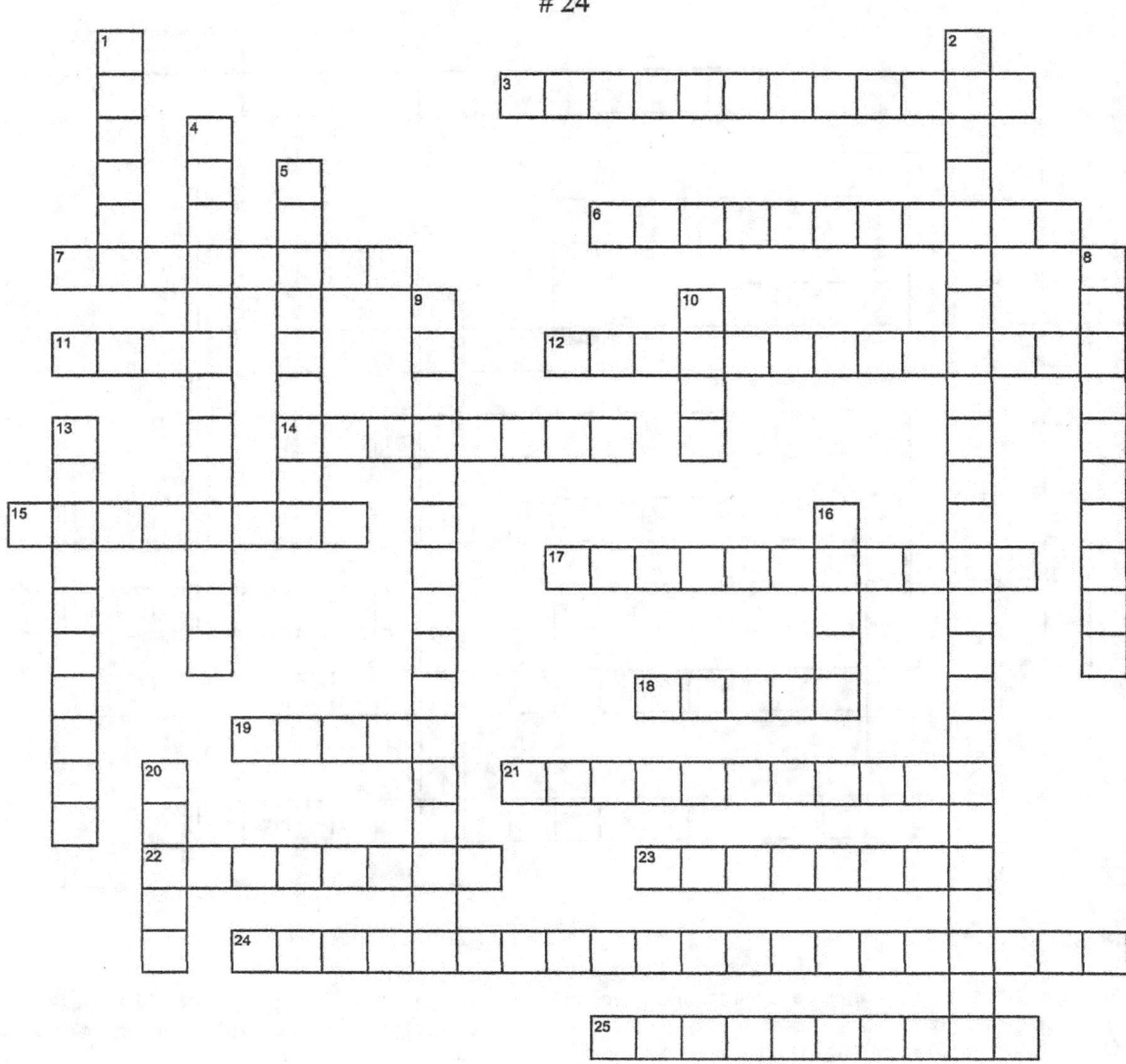

ACROSS

3 Brain structure containing the thalamus and hypothalamus.
6 Tactile hallucination or sensation that small insects are crawling under the skin. (may be associated with alcohol detoxification).
7 Sweat production and excretion.
11 Prefix meaning "blue in color", or "lacking oxygen".
12 Increased sensitivity to stimulation such as pressure or touch, resulting in pain.
14 Inflammation of the uterus.
15 Hereditary absence of melanin pigment in the body.
17 Difficult or painful eating or swallowing.
18 Prefix meaning "small".
19 Projections from the surface of the gastric mucosa.
21 Surgical revision or complete excision of the tongue.
22 Summary statement of research article that identifies the purpose, methodology, findings and conclusions.
23 Toward or in the direction of the head.
24 Abnormal skin-thickening caused by viral infection. (2 wds).
25 Discharge from the mucous membrane of the nose.

DOWN

1 paintful intermittent muscle spasms frequently associated with calcium imbalance.
2 Hypersection of gastric acid and formation of gastric ulcers, associated with nonbeta cell tumors of the pancreatic isles. (3 wds).
4 Endometrial tissue. (2 wds).
5 Involuntary rhythmic ocular movements, particularly when looking to the side. (each back-and-forth motion is known as a beat).
8 Demonstrating the ability to stretch.
9 An aqueous solution of hydrogen chloride. (2 wds).
10 Prefix meaning "pertaining to the cornea or to a horny substance of the skin".
13 A rapidly developing malignant neoplasm of the kidney of unknown etiology, seen in infants and children before age five. (2 wds).
16 Prefix meaning "light".
20 Suffix meaning "immature cell".

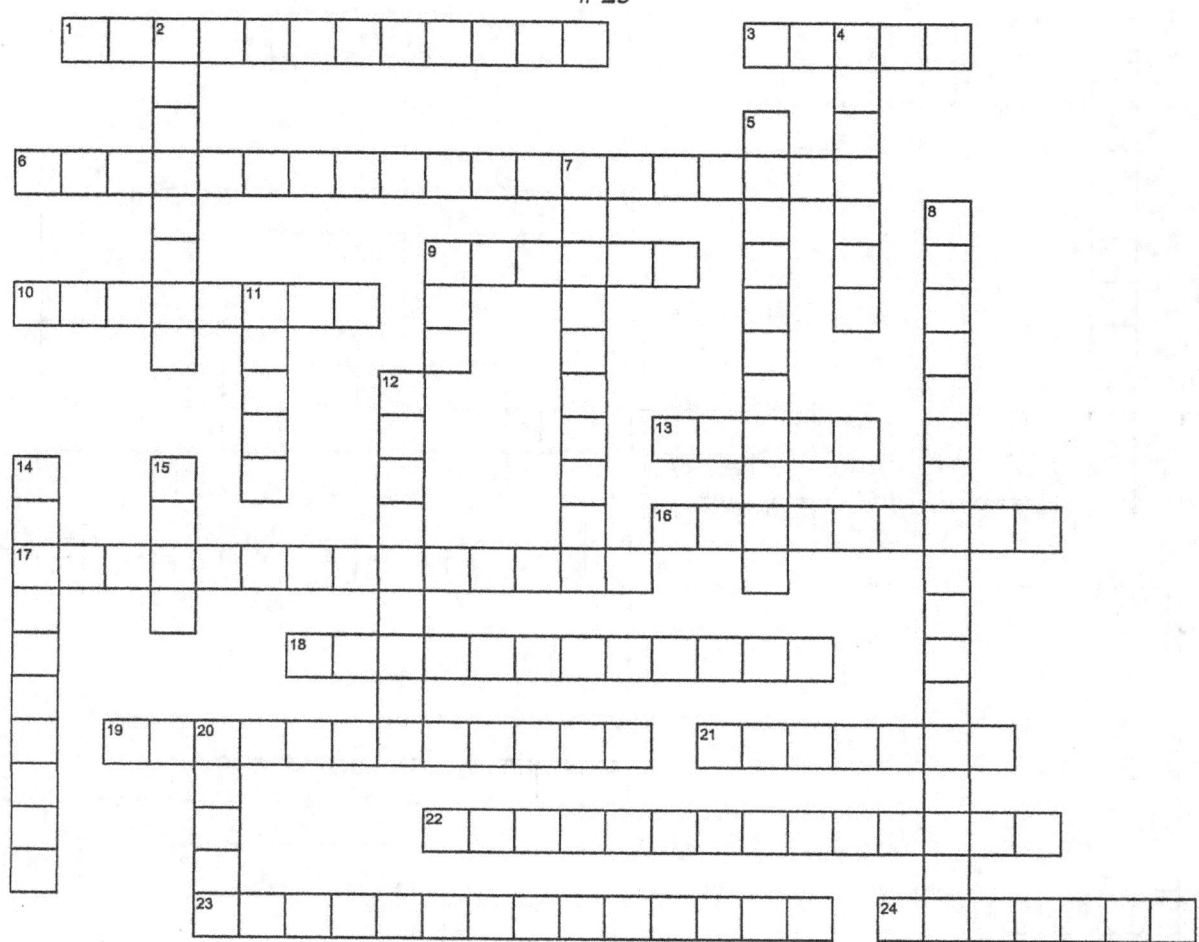

ACROSS

1 Decreased quantity of sperm in the ejaculate.
3 Prefix meaning "above" or "elevated"
6 Health alteration due to exposure or activities associated with work activity or job. (2 wds).
9 Suffix meaning "pertaining to digestion".
10 The inability to write due to cerebral pathology.
13 Prefix meaning "four".
16 Invented, fabricated words, whose meaning are only known to the speaker.
17 Physician who specializes in treating inflammatory and degenerative diseases of connective tissues and joints.
18 A woman who has never been pregnant.
19 A fibrous layer that encases the entire joint. (2 wds).
21 Respiratory and circulatory depression (including orthostatic hypotension) is the major hazard of _____.
22 Purplish-brown vascular malignancy first observed on the skin and mucous membranes, although it may become systemic. Often associated with AIDS. (2 wds).
23 Pertaining to the region of the body including the abdomen, pelvis, and hip bone.
24 Infection with the bacillus Clostridium tetani in deep puncture wounds, characterized by gross muscular rigidity, severe muscle spasms, respiratory failure and death.

DOWN

2 Pertaining to the groin.
4 Pertaining to the diaphragm.
5 Medical procedure that injects a vaccine into the body.
7 These involve excessive sleep or difficulty initiating and maintaining sleep.
8 Characteristics that increase the likelihood of development of heart disease, stroke, and diabetes whereby the individual processes three out of five known risk factors (hypertension, abdominal obesity, elevated triglycerides, low HDL, and elevated fasting glucose). (2 wds).
9 Prefix meaning "through" or "extremely".
11 Thin membranous folds of tissue that partially occlude the ostium of the vagina.
12 The repetition of words heard. (associated with schizophrenia).
14 A potassium-depleting diuretic that can cause hypokalemia.
15 True or false: Thoughtless or reckless spending is a common symptom of a manic episode.
20 Prefix meaning "under", "below" or "beneath"

26

ACROSS

2 A large, fluid-filled blister that is usually one centimeter or more in diameter.
4 Gastric _____ may be needed periodically to ensure patency of the nasogastric tube.
7 Headache.
8 A venous access device inserted into the subclavian vein, used to infuse medications, fluids, and other agents as well as to measure venous pressure. (2 wds).
14 This virus causes herpes zoster. (2 wds).
18 A burn injury causes a _____ state resulting in protein and lipid catabolism that affects wound healing.
19 Palpable vibration. Crackles from body cavities or joints.
20 A patient with _____ needs more steroids than the body produces. (2 wds).
21 These are associated with an allergic reaction. (3 wds).
22 A _____ rash usually has widely distributed scattered lesions.

DOWN

1 Inflammation of the liver due to a viral infection. (2 wds).
2 Surgical revision of the eyelid.
3 Killed or attenuated bacterial or viral cells or cell fragments used to trigger the production of antibodies and memory B lymphocytes specific to that pathogen. (Used to prevent diseases).
5 Gonorrhea always occurs with symptoms.
6 Uncomfortable physical symptoms that occur when use of a sedative, pain drug or illegal narcotic is stopped suddenly in a patient who is physically tolerant. (2 wds).
7 An inflammatory disorder that results from contact with an irritant. (2 wds).
9 A surgical procedure to obtain a tissue sample of a mass, tumor, or skin lesion for the purpose of cellular study.
10 A localized dilation of the wall of a blood vessel.
11 Insufficient production of tears because of eye irritation, associated with the aging process, or an ectropion of the eyelid.
12 Failure of the tricuspid valve to develop, leaving no communication between the right atrium and right ventricle. (2 wds).
13 Inflammation of the cerebellum.
14 A narrow wafer of bone that forms the inferior part of the nasal septum that continues posteriorly to the cranium, where it joins the sphenoid bone.
15 To connect two vessels, often blood vessels or bowel segments, to allow continuous flow.
16 All of the interal organs of the various body cavities.
17 Extremely severe vomiting.

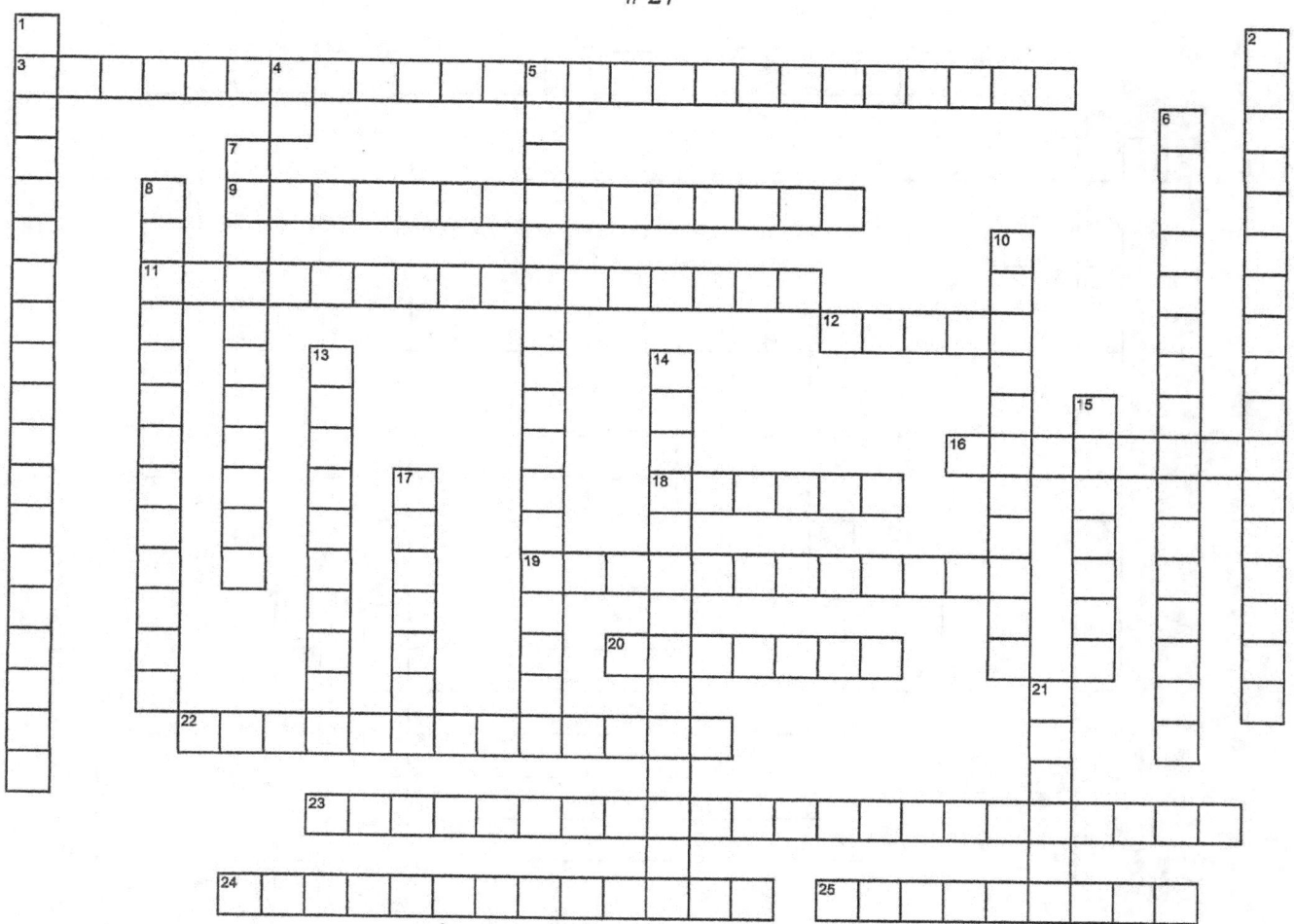

ACROSS

3 Plastic surgical procedure to remove excess soft palate, uvula, and other structures of the throat to resolve sleep apnea and intractable snoring.

9 The passage formed by the junction of the duct of the seminal vesicles and ductus deferens through which semen enters the urethra. (2 wds).

11 Assessment of intraocular pressure using a burst of air rebounding off the cornea without the instrument touching the patient's eye. (3 wds).

12 External structure of the ear.

16 Bluish skin and mucous membranes resulting from lack of oxygen in the blood.

18 Pertaining to the abdominal cavity.

19 Serous fluid in the fallopian tube.

20 A saclike structure that acts as a receptacle for secretions.

22 A large opening at the base of the cranium near the occipital bone that the spinal cord passes through as it connects with the medulla oblongata. (2 wds).

23 Force exerted by the circulating blood on the arterial walls during ventricular relaxation and filling. (3 wds).

24 Presence of increased intracranial and extracellular fluid in teh white matter of the brain. (2 wds).

25 The resistance of a substance to change in shape or flow due to molecular cohesion, such as liquids.

DOWN

1 Skin tags. (2 wds).

2 The 3-methoxy-4-hydroxymandelic acid test is a urine test used to determine possible _____. (2 wds).

4 Suffix meaning "pertaining or related to".

5 A hereditary disease of the central nervous system characterized by bizarre involuntary movements and progressive dementia. (2 wds).

6 Deficit in the ability to comprehend sounds or written words due to damage to the temporal lobe by trauma or stroke. (2 wds).

7 Loss of one-fourth of teh visual field.

8 Fear of death.

10 Extreme, immediate, hypersensitive reaction to an antigen, protein, or drug with systemic effects including bronchospasm, peripheral edema, and laryngeal edema. It can be life threatening.

13 Form of rosacea affecting the nose.

14 Smooth muscle of the internal organs. (2 wds).

15 Inflammation of the nail matrix or bed.

17 The bony structure of the thoracic skeleton that is formed by the twelve arched pairs of bone that insert on the sternum. (2 wds).

21 Suffix meaning "to grow".

28

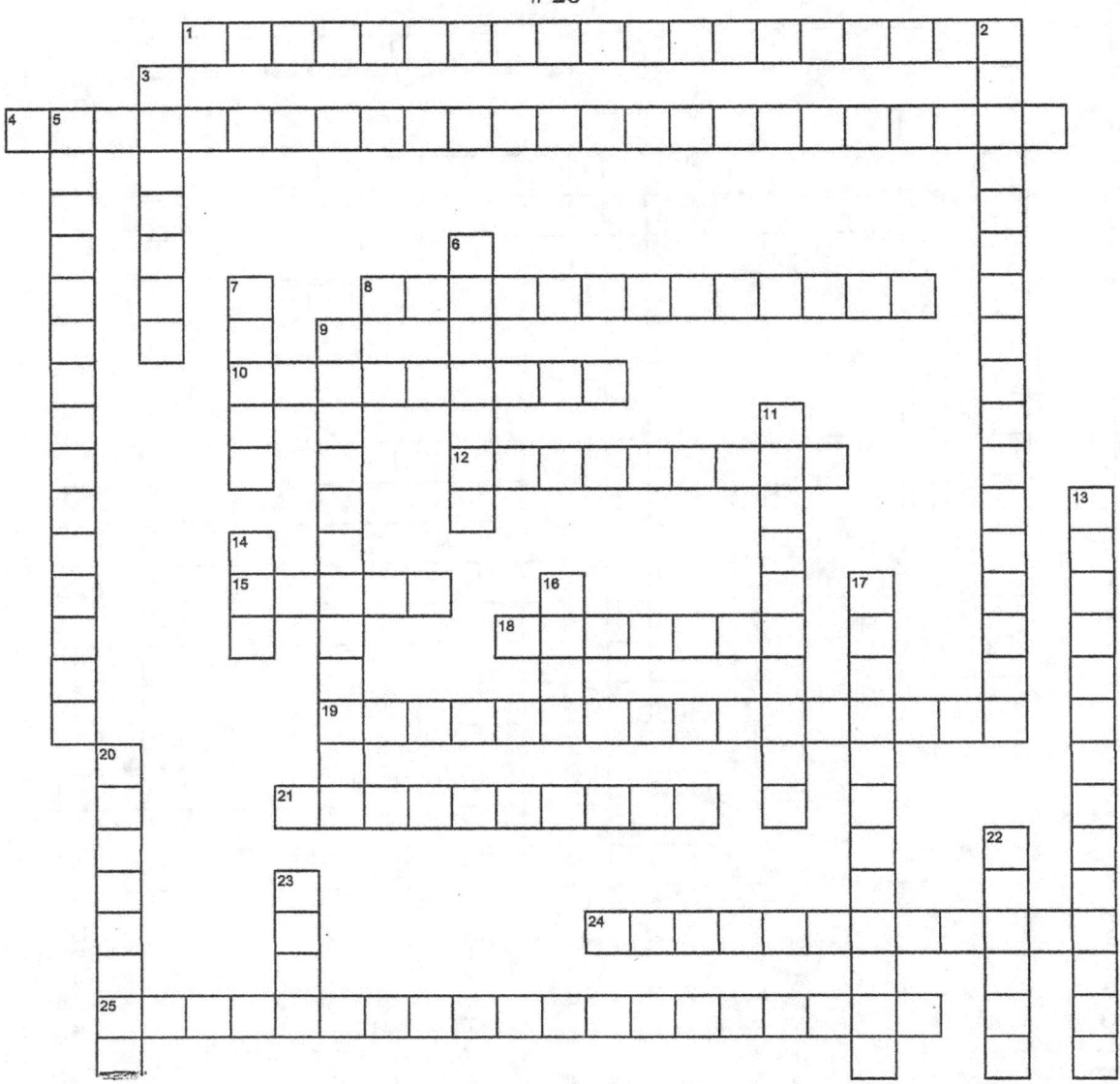

ACROSS

1 Assessment of bone conduction of sound by placing a vibrating tuning fork at the midpoint of the forehead to determine if sound is heard equally in both ears. (4 wds).

4 Major blood supply of the intestine. (3 wds).

8 The depression in the scapula into which the head of the humerus fits. (2 wds).

10 An acute infection of the lung parenchyma.

12 Congenital form of hypothyroidism, formally called cretinism.

15 Suffix meaning "instrument used for measurement".

18 State of movement.

19 The curved segment of the ulna, known as the elbow. (2 wds).

21 A precursor of pepsin that exists in granular form in the gastric glands.

24 Abnormally small liver.

25 Layer directly on the outside of the heart muscle. (2 wds).

DOWN

2 These are used to reduce dislocations, subluxations, pain and spasm in cervical spinal cord injuries. They are NOT used to reduce intracranial pressure, prevent deep vein thrombosis, or improve neurologic outcome. (3 wds).

3 Protein associated with hair and nails.

5 Opening in bone through which nerves or blood vessels pass. (2 wds).

6 Relating to the anterior portion of the cranium or forehead.

7 Prefix meaning "having a curvature or hump".

9 Sex hormone responsible for masculine characteristics.

11 Presence of glucose in the urine.

13 Anatomical portion of the cerebral cortex associated with the processing of impulses pertaining to smell.

14 Suffix meaning "tumor".

16 An eating disorder characterized by craving nonfood items such as clay or paste.

17 To go through the skin.

20 The largest vein, the _____, has no valves. (2 wds).

22 To dull or decrease perception of pain.

23 True or false: A dilated aorta causes a murmur.

29

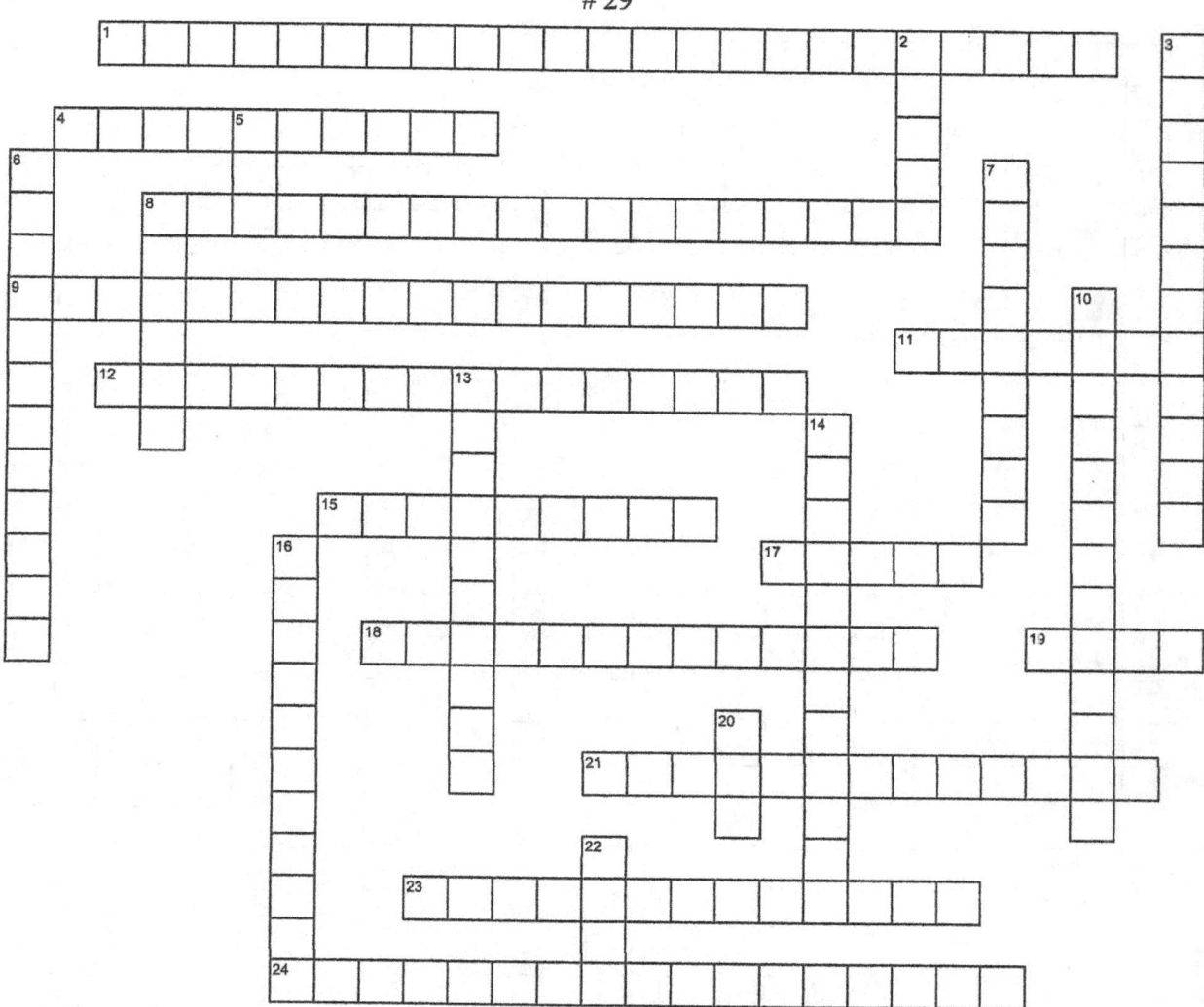

ACROSS

1 Brain damage with gross short-term memory disruption due to chronic alcoholism and thiamine deficiency. (2 wds).
4 A large group of viruses that cause upper respiratory infections.
8 Two leading causes of diabetes insipidus are hypothalamic or pituitary tumors, and _____. (3 wds).
9 Thyroid hormone.
11 A barium swallow looks at the _____ and the duodenum.
12 Periods of apnea alternating with breaths of the same depth. (2 wds).
15 In renal failure, the kidneys are no longer able to excrete _____, resulting in hyperkalemia.
17 Suffix meaning "process of measurement".
18 The maximum volume of air that can be exhaled following the deepest inhalation. (2 wds).
19 Prefix meaning "fingernails".
21 This occurs when endometrial cells are seeded throughout the pelvis and is not a sexually transmitted disease.
23 Excessive thyroid hormone levels indicate _____ (also known as hyperthyroidism). (2 wds).
24 Pain on deep palpation and release. (2 wds).

DOWN

2 Genetalia of the male, composed of erectile tissue.
3 Nail-biting.
5 Prefix meaning "shoulder or upper arm".
6 Hematemesis, malnourishment, and pain with eating are consistent with a _____. (2 wds).
7 Unit of measurement equaling one-millionth of a gram.
8 The portion of an organ resembling a neck.
10 This results from an obstruction of a duct of the Bartholin gland.
13 The process of drawing air into the lungs.
14 Nerve that stimulates the diaphragm to contract, thereby initiating respiration. (2 wds).
16 Malnutrition in children caused by inadequate intake of calories and protein.
20 A vasectomy can be reversed. Its success rate is _____.
22 Oxygenated blood returns to the _____ atrium.

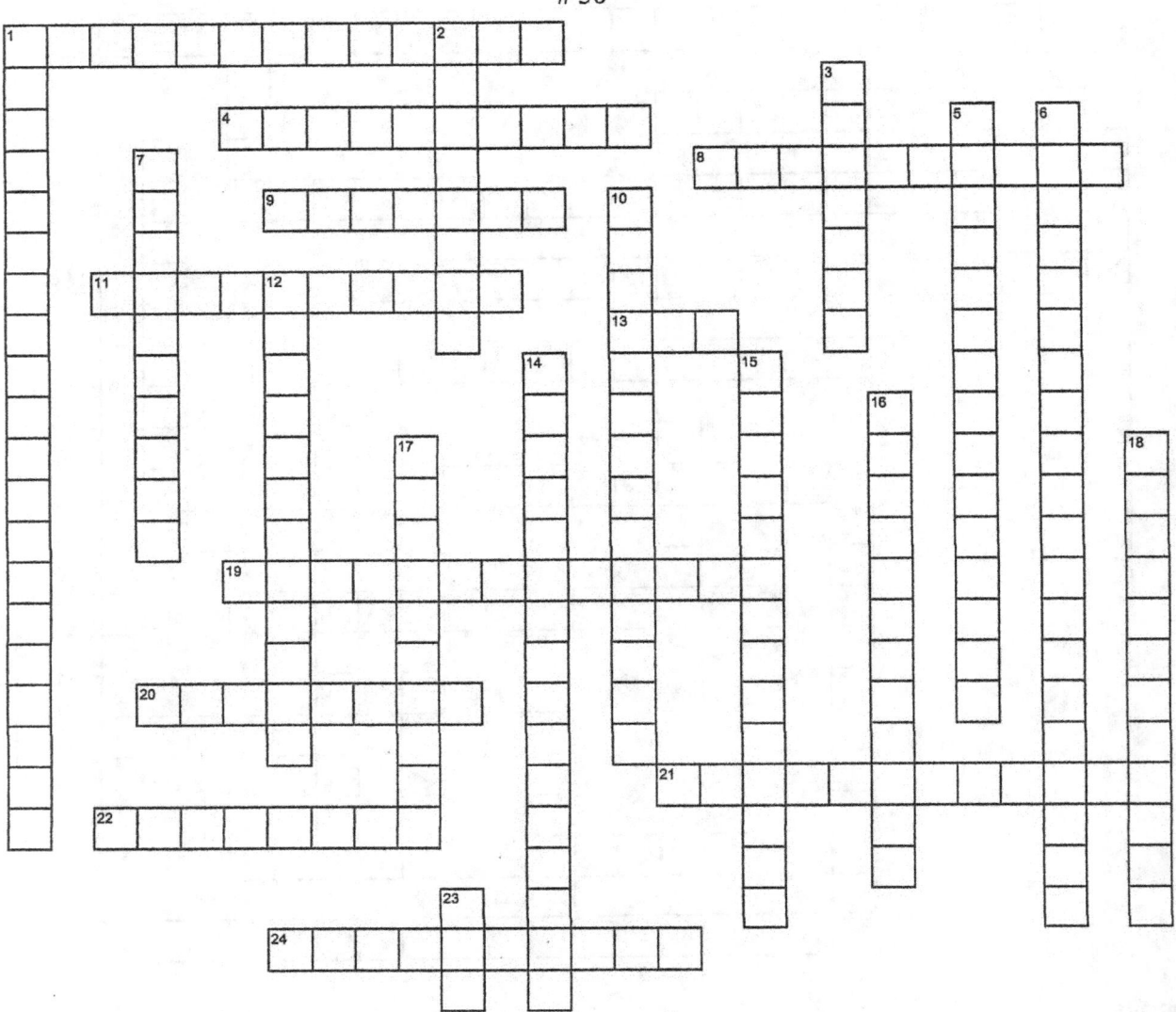

ACROSS

1 Lymph nodes located in the neck. (2 wds).
4 Sudden, painful, involuntary contraction of the muscles associated with the blood vessels.
8 Objective measures of key body parameters, such as temperature, pulse and blood pressure. (2 wds).
9 Referring to the buttocks.
11 Portion of a bone where growth occurs, situated between the diaphysis and epiphysis.
13 Prefix meaning "distress" or "choke".
19 Subjective sensation of smell experienced just prior to the onset of seizure activity. (2 wds).
20 Condition of having many ulcers with purulent drainage.
21 Surgical repair of the lip, usually because of a laceration.
22 Pancreatic hormone from alpha cells that elevates blood glucose.
24 Inflammation of the cervix.

DOWN

1 Movement or growth of cells from their usual location by means of unusual growth. (2 wds).
2 Paralysis involving both arms or both legs.
3 A skin ulcer associated with infection with syphillis.
5 Readiness of a drug to produce an effect in the circulation at the target site.
6 Muscle that turns the eye downward. (3 wds).
7 Muscle that rotates the arms laterally. (2 wds).
10 Formation of a hard crust on the skin, often with a horny shape.
12 Paralysis of the diaphram.
14 Liver disorder due to obstructed bile ducts. (2 wds).
15 Damage to heart valves as a result of rheumatic fever. (2 wds).
16 Surgical removal of one or both ovaries.
17 Tapping the finger of one hand, spread over a large body cavity to detect characteristics of underlying structures. Also, use of a cupped hand to strike the chest and various lung fields in order to break up mucus for expectoration or suctioning.
18 Destruction of tissue by electric current.
23 Prefix meaning "away from".

#31

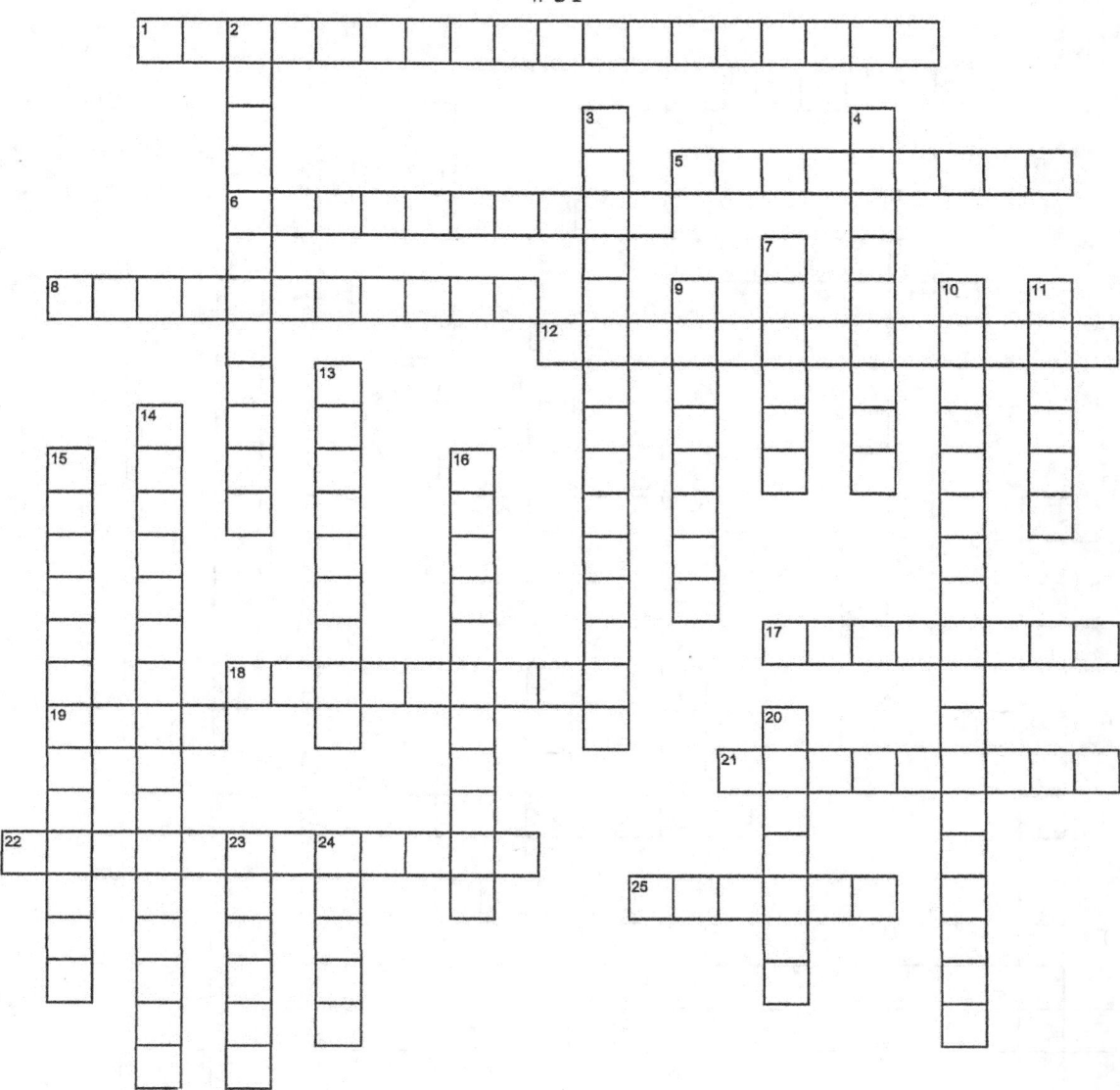

ACROSS

1 Passage of electrical impulses of the heart through abnormal pathways. (2 wds).

5 A small, firm, painless lump near the edge of the eyelid.

6 Brain waves seen on electroencephalography. Most often found in children, but may also be found in adults who are under emotional stress. (2 wds).

8 Hemorrhaging from the ovary.

12 Narrowed lumen of a blood vessel.

17 Gray matter on either side of the third ventricle of the brain that acts as a relay station for impulses from the sensory nerves and sends them to specific cortical areas of the brain.

18 Abnormal condition of the lips characterized by fissures and sores, frequently associated with vitamin B-complex deficiency.

19 Prefix meaning "pertaining to the urinary bladder or sac".

21 A pharmacological agent that increases the strength of heart muscle contraction.

22 Profuse bleeding from the nose.

25 A solid, raised lesion that is usually less than one centimeter in diameter.

DOWN

2 Soluble, inorganic ions, such as sodium and chloride, found in body fluids.

3 Protrusion or displacement of the uterus through the vaginal canal. (2 wds).

4 The rash with _____ is typically a maculopapular vesicular rash.

7 A cavity containing pus and surrounded by inflamed tissue.

9 A small, pea-sized bone located in the wrist.

10 Trochlear nerve. Innervates the sensory and motor function of the superior oblique muscle of the eye. (CN IV) (3 wds).

11 Suffix meaning "thirst".

13 Stings from _____ are associated with a stinger, pain, and erythema.

14 A metabolic disorder resulting from the chronic and excessive production of cortisol by the adrenal cortex. (2 wds).

15 Abnormally small size of the brain.

16 Excretion of fructose in the urine.

20 A painful, cracklike lesion of the skin that extends at least into the dermis.

23 The relative measurement of an impulse or activity in relation to time.

24 A flat, U-shaped bone that does not touch any other bones but functions as a bony bridge that anchors the muscles of the tongue.

32

ACROSS

4 A pharmacologic agent used to paralyze the ciliary muscle for examination or treatment.

7 The vocal apparatus of the larynx, including the vocal folds, vocal cords, vocal muscles and adjacent structures of the throat.

8 Sexual desire disorders include hypoactive sexual desire disorder and sexual ____ disorder.

10 An impaired ability to make decisions, perform voluntary actions, react emotionally or verbally. Commonly associated with bilateral frontal lobe disease.

14 Removing the vitreous humor and replacing it with a synthetic substitute.

15 Small, circular bone with two flat surfaces. Acts as a cushion to decrease impact during body movements.

16 Teardrop vesicles of varicella-zoster virus on an erythematous base generally begin on the ____, face, and scalp, with minimal involvement of the extremities.

17 Suffix meaning "to drive away".

18 Respiratory disease characterized by a collapsed alveoli due to the lack of surfactant, a subtance produced by the lungs to keep the alveoli inflated. (2 wds).

19 Inflammation of the urinary bladder and ureters resulting from bacterial infection, tumor or calculus.

20 Exposing one's genitals, and occasionally, masturbating in public.

21 A formula or set of rules for diagnosis and treatment of a disease.

22 Channel that drains lymph from the upper chest and neck. (2 wds).

23 Inability to see. Blindness.

DOWN

1 Lacking pigmentation of the skin, eyes, and hair.

2 Pruritic papules, vesicles, and linear burrows are diagnostic for _____.

3 A male has a persistent or recurrent inability to attain or maintain an adequate erection until completion of sexual activity. (3 wds).

4 Hand, foot, and mouth disease (often associated with yellow ulcers of the hands and feet) is caused by _____.

5 The liquid portion within the cell membrane.

6 Outer layer of the cerebrum. (2 wds).

7 An inflammatory disease of the kidney typically occurring one to two weeks after a streptococcal bacterial infection. (symptoms include hematuria and proteinuria).

9 Air hunger. Rapid and deep respirations without pause. (2 wds).

11 Blood test for unconjugated, conjugated, and total bilirubin levels. (2 wds).

12 The study of cells.

13 Dementia can easily be mistaken for _____, so cause must always be thoroughly investigated.

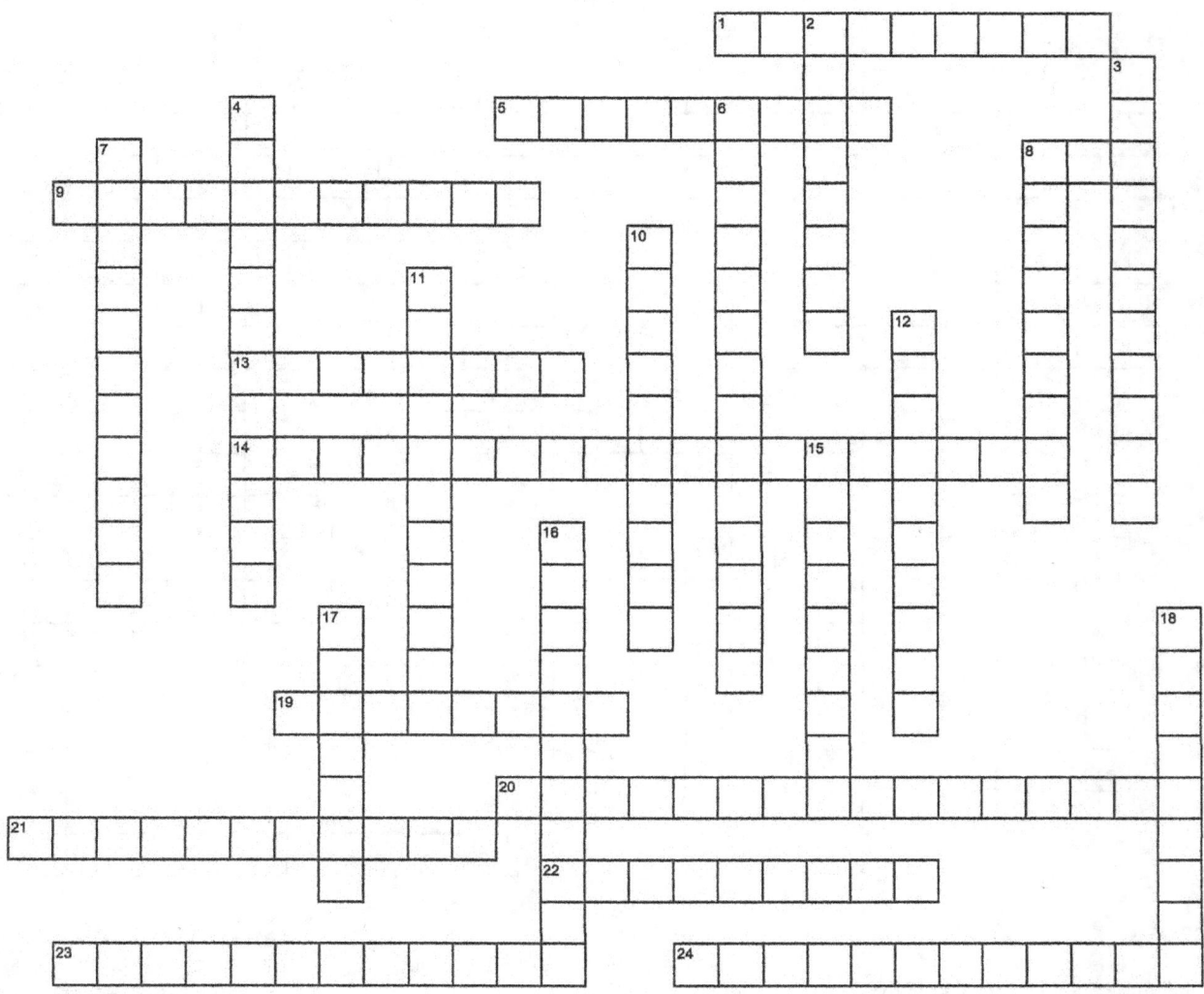

ACROSS

1 Inflammation of the tongue which may be caused by irritation from food, infection, or vitamin B deficiency.

5 Hives marked by redness and swelling wheals.

8 Light-sensitive cell. Sensitive to all levels of light, but not to color.

9 The duct through which bile from the gallbladder passes into the common bile duct. (2 wds).

13 Harsh, rattling, or whistling sound in lung fields.

14 Actions taken to stop transmission of infectious agents by exposure to airborne droplet spray, including air filtration systems and masks. (2 wds).

19 Destruction of tissue or function by surgery, electrocautery, or radio frequency.

20 Sound produced by the heart during late systole due to ventricular atrial systole and decreased ventricular compliances. (3 wds).

21 The study of the muscles and body movement.

22 A sexually transmitted infection with Haemophilus ducreyi that causes open, painful genital sores.

23 Ingrown fingernail or toenail.

24 Pain in the groin area due to trauma, tumors, or infection.

DOWN

2 Scant or inadequate urine production.

3 A mineralocorticoid steroid hormone that stimulates the renal tubule in the kidneys to retain water and sodium.

4 Uterine bleeding at times other than the regular menstrual period.

6 Chest pain that radiates to the left shoulder. (2 wds).

7 Abnormally high level of carbon dioxide in the arterial blood.

8 A method to assess hearing by air conduction by holding a vibrating tuning fork at the base of the mastoid process and the prongs near the ear. (2 wds).

10 A mercury compound used to preserve pharmacological agents and vaccines.

11 Loss of functionality of the ciliary muscle of the eye due to denervation or medication.

12 Sudden, well-defined, large area of edema often due to an allergy to foods or drugs.

15 Yellow pigment found in urine.

16 Spherical or oval-shaped bacterium, occurring in pairs.

17 Red measles.

18 An inability to experience pleasure from any activity.

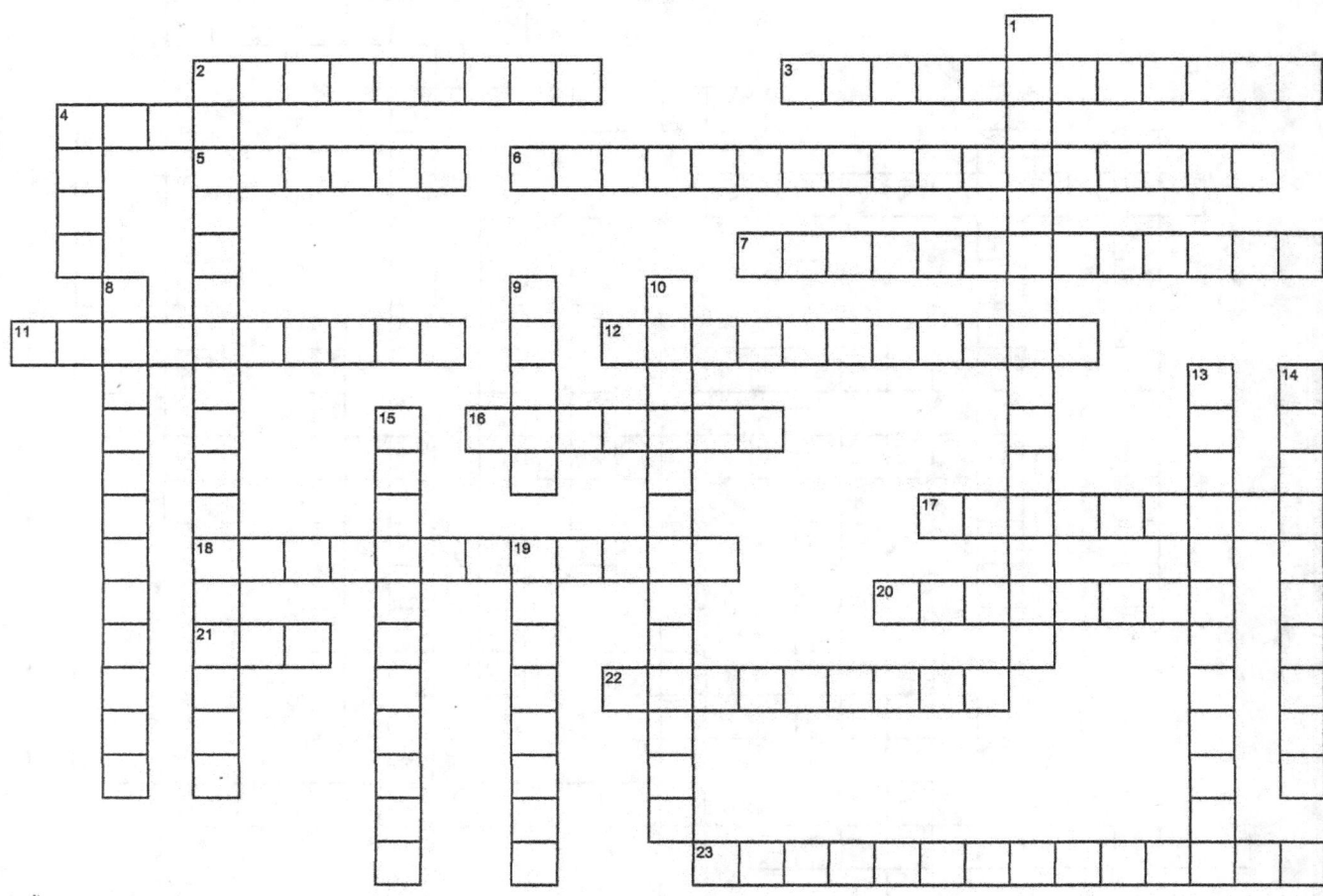

ACROSS

2 Inflammation and cracking of the lips and corners of the mouth due to nutritional deficiency, infection or allergies.

3 Collective term for structures involved in the delivery of bile from the liver to the duodenum. Includes the gallbladder, hepatic ducts, cystic ducts, and common bile ducts. (2 wds).

4 Suffix meaning "pertaining to a cell".

5 Suffix meaning "sudden outpouring of drainage".

6 Brain damage due to nutritional deficits associated with chronic alcoholism, characterized by severe impairment of short-term memory. (2 wds).

7 Abnormally high level of calcium in the blood.

11 Examination of urine.

12 Lack of skin elasticity as a result of death. (2 wds).

16 Chronic, noninfectious skin disorder marked by redness on the cheeks, nose, and chin.

17 Herniation or protrusion of the urinary bladder into the vagina.

18 Substance being infused or passing into tissue or organs.

20 Visual disturbance where single objects are perceived as two objects. Caused by increased intracranial pressure or by multiple sclerosis that affects nerve conduction.

21 Prefix meaning "white color" or "lacking of normal pigments".

22 Organisms such as bacteria that thrive in the urinary bladder or urine.

23 Surgical correction of a refractive error by reshaping the deep layer of the cornea.

DOWN

1 Muscle that covers the frontal bone. (2 wds).

2 Concept that one hemisphere of the brain exercises greater control or influence for functions such as speech, analytical thinking, mathematics, spatial perception and motor control. (2 wds).

4 Suffix meaning "head".

8 Areas in the right and left occipital lobes of the brain that merge images from both eyes to create a single image that is right side up and in its original horizontal direction. (2 wds).

9 Redness which is often associated with infection or inflammation.

10 An external device applied to the throat to amplify breath sounds in patients following surgical removal of the larynx.

13 Atoms or groups of atoms that can cause damage to cells. (2 wds).

14 Congenital defect of eyelid formation. Eyelid is either absent or reduced in size.

15 An autosomal recessive genetic disease that causes inadequate production of hemoglobin.

19 Wearing down of a surface, such as skin, by rubbing or scraping.

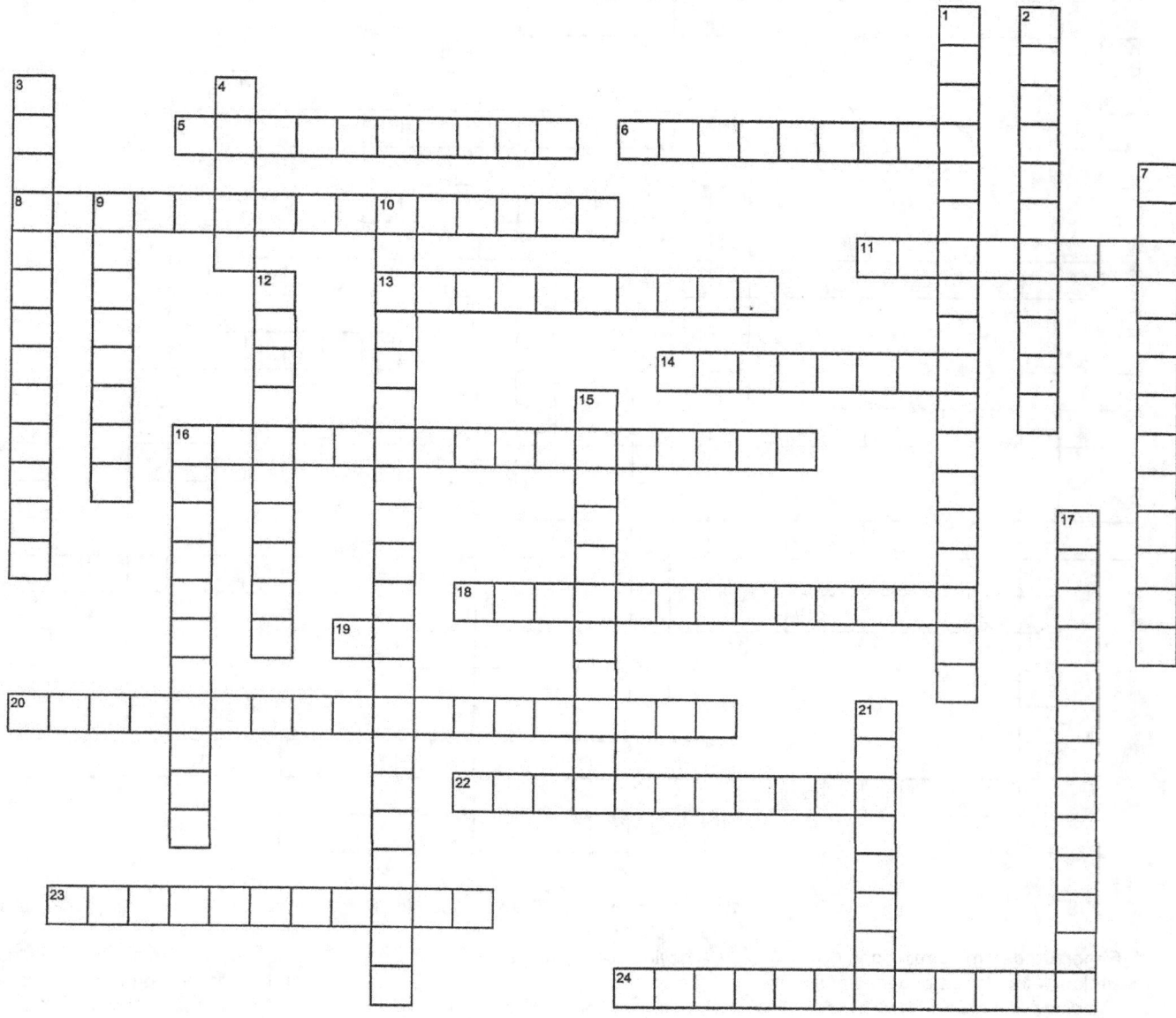

ACROSS

5 Energy-yielding conversion of glucose to lactic acid in the tissues.
6 To remove an arm or leg by surgical amputation.
8 The muscle that turns the eye downward and toward the midline of the visual field. (2 wds).
11 Suffix meaning "head".
13 Refraining from certain behaviors, activities, foods or beverages.
14 Painful urination , often associated with a urinary tract infection.
16 A canal in the midbrain that contains cerebrospinal fluid and connects the third and fourth ventricles. (2 wds).
18 Clear, gel-like substance that fills the posterior cavity of the eye. (2 wds).
19 Suffix meaning "structure" or "thing".
20 Use of an electrode to apply high-frequency, short electrical currents to destroy tissue by drying.
22 Deformation of the nail bed with thin, concave edges. Often associated with iron deficient anemia. (Also known as "spooning" of the nails).
23 Destruction of unwanted tissue by the use of electrical current in the form of sparks.
24 Formation of sugar from fats and proteins.

DOWN

1 A sheath located between the tendon of the infraspinatus muscle and the capsule of the shoulder joint. (2 wds).
2 Displacement of the end of a bone from its normal position within a joint.
3 A hollow, flexible tube inserted into a blood vessel to withdraw or instill fluids.
4 Suffix meaning "painful condition".
7 Response associated with increased intracranial pressure or compromised circulation in the brain stem. (Characterized by hypertension, increased systolic pressure with widened pulse pressure, bradycardia, and irregular respirations). (2 wds).
9 An elongated connective structure that attaches two parts.
10 Surgical fixation of the urethrovesical junction and the bladder neck to an elevated retropubic position to alleviate stress incontinence. (3 wds).
12 Process by which digested food nutrients move through villi of the small intestine into the blood.
15 Pertaining to the vulva and rectal area.
16 Surgical removal of osteophytes. The scraping away of bony irregularities.
17 Fungal infection of the cornea.
21 Breakage of bone due to injury or disease process.

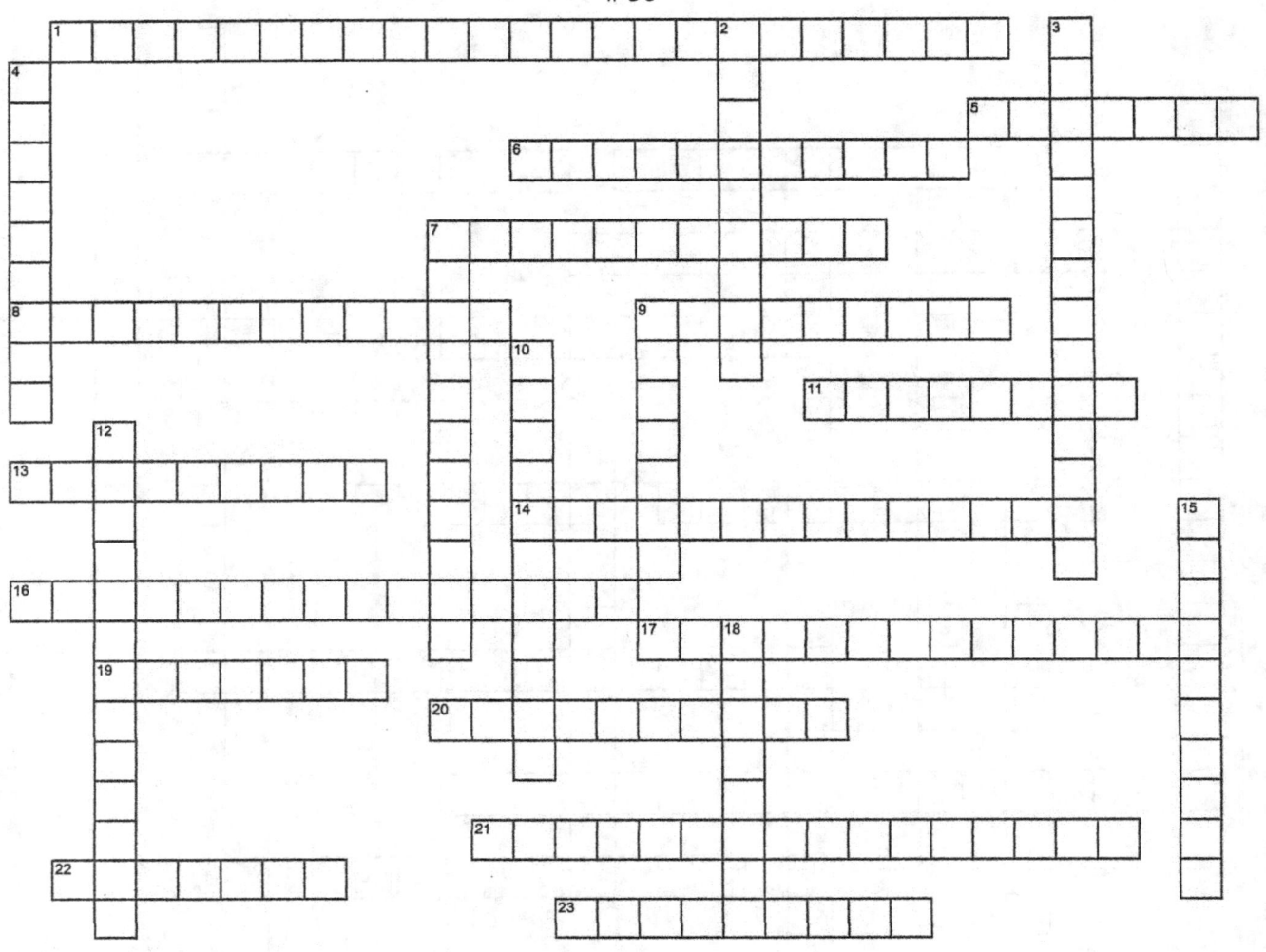

ACROSS

1 Generalized term pertaining to all strokes without regard to the underlying pathology or mechanism. (2 wds).
5 A rose- or red-colored rash.
6 Involuntary spasm or twitching of the diaphragm.
7 Loosening of a nail from the nail bed.
8 Formation of new blood vessels.
9 Incision in a spinal nerve root to relieve intractable pain.
11 Suffix meaning "protection" or "preventative measure".
13 Red pigment of the rods which is bleached by daylight.
14 Sensory sites that are stimulated by the rise in temperature.
16 Malignant neoplasm of the vulva, most often squamous cell type, with the greatest incidence in women ages sixty-five to seventy years. (2 wds).
17 Network of nerves in the cervical region. (2 wds).

19 Suffix meaning "sudden outpouring of drainage".
20 A device used to measure blood levels of glucose.
21 Sudden and premature separation of the placenta from the site of uterine attachment due to bleeding between the placenta and uterine wall. (2 wds).
22 Viral infection, also known as German measles.
23 Presence of excessive amounts of ketone bodies occurring as a result of uncontrolled metabolic conditions such as diabetes mellitus or starvation.

DOWN

2 Destruction of living cells.
3 Brain dysfunction involving a brief loss of consciousness without motor involvement. (2 wds).
4 Type of muscles that contract or relax in response to conscious thought.
7 Diminished thirst sensation.

9 A tear, break, or protrusion of an organ or body tissue.
10 Abnormal grating sounds detected during auscultation when pleura or pericardial tissues are inflamed. (2 wds).
12 Palpable vibration in the chest wall produced by voice sounds due to consolidates or congestion. (2 wds).
15 The study of the function of the body.
18 One of the basic movements of a joint.; having a quality of turning around an axis.

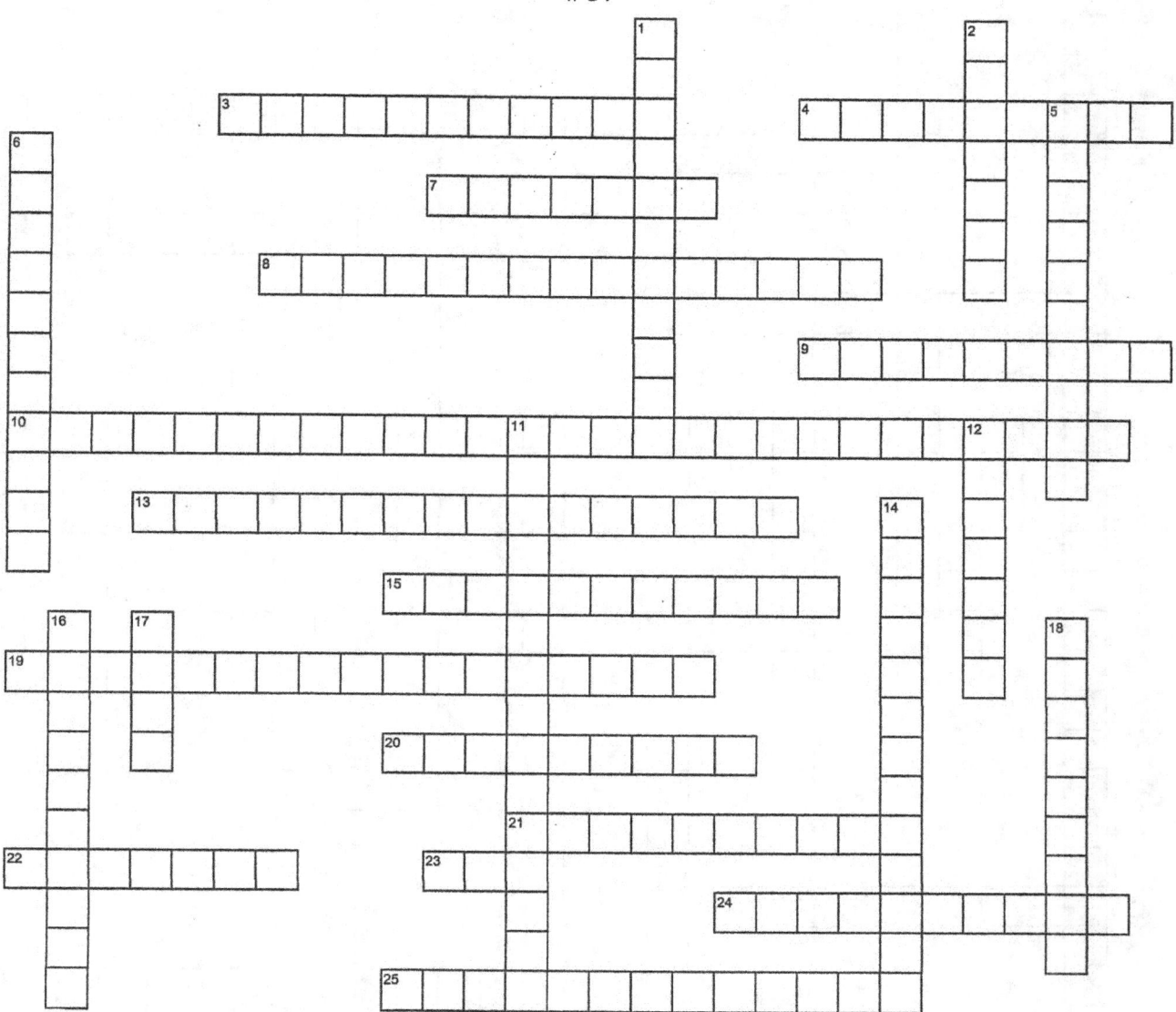

ACROSS

3 Spreading of malignant cells to surrounding tissues and other parts of the body through the blood and lymph.

4 Surgical incision of the amnion to induce labor.

7 Suffix meaning "to suture or sew together".

8 A toothlike formation on the second vertebra upon which the head rotates. (2 wds).

9 Digestive enzyme secreted by the small intestine that converts peptides to amino acids.

10 Psychiatric illness characterized by persistent, uncontrollable thoughts that cause anxiety and compel a person to perform excessive, repetitive activities causing incapacity. (3 wds).

13 Acute spasm and involuntary deviation or fixation of the eyes in an upward gaze. (2 wds).

15 A process wherein a cell engulfs liquid by encircling the substance, forming fluid-filled vesicles.

19 Four congenital heart defects appearing together. (3 wds).

20 Radiographic visualization after injecting a radiopaque contrast dye into the bloodstream, enabling the vessels to be mapped, and identifying areas of narrowing or blockage.

21 Type of anemia where the average size of circulating erythrocytes is smaller than normal.

22 A major protein molecule in the blood produced by the liver.

23 Prefix meaning "up or apart", or "excessive".

24 Presence of abnormal amounts of uric acid in the urine.

25 Hollow space within the uterus. (2 wds).

DOWN

1 Inflammation or infection of the eyelid with redness, exudate, and scales at the bases of the eyelashes.

2 Large bone of the cranium that forms the forehead and superior portions of the orbits.

5 Severe, unrelieved constipation.

6 Intolerance to light.

11 The large, triangular muscle of the chest that flexes the chest and internally rotates the humerus when contracted. (2 wds).

12 Suffix meaning "rupture".

14 The removal of an entire lung.

16 A large brain structure located dorsal to the pons and medulla that functions to maintain balance, ocular movement and posture.

17 True or false: Reduction in vital capacity is a normal physiologic change in an older adult.

18 Pharmacological agents or other substances known to be detrimental or destructive to cells.

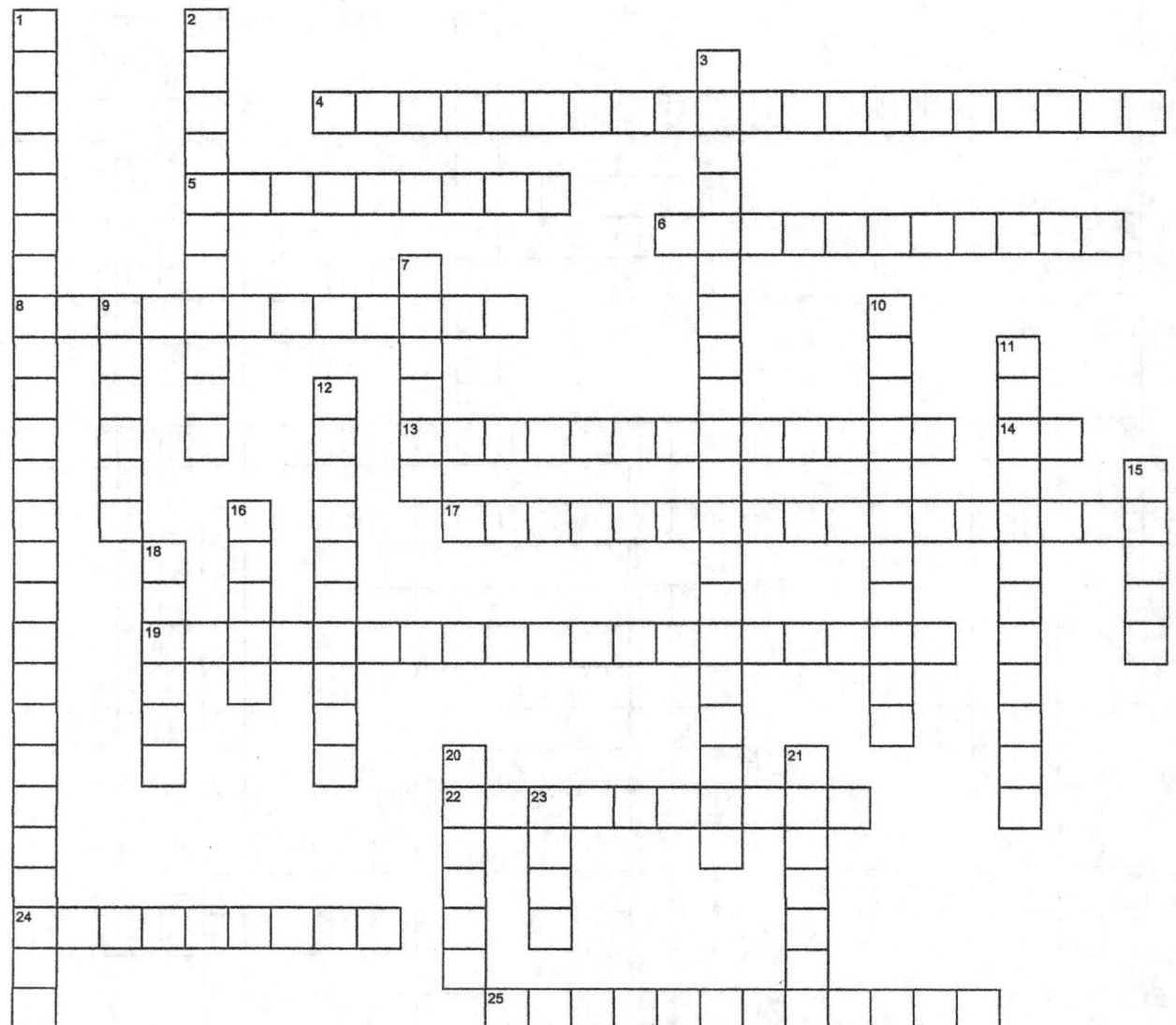

ACROSS

4 This is characterized by lost periods of time. (2 wds).

5 The action of closing off or being closed. Also, the relationship between the upper and lower teeth of the jaw.

6 Passage of multiple minute, non-obstructing calculous particles in teh urine following nephrolithiasis. (2 wds).

8 A superficial blood vessel that returns blood from the dorsal and palmar surfaces of the forearm to the subclavian vein. (2 wds).

13 Skeletal muscle of the upper back that originates at the anfraspinous fossa of the scapula and inserts at the upper edge of the humerus. When contracted, it extends and rotates the arm laterally.

14 Prefix meaning "ovum" or "egg".

17 Surgical removal of an ovarian cyst.

19 Surgical removal of the pylorus and antrum of the stomach with attachment of the stomach to the duodenum. (Also called gastroduodenostomy). (3 wds).

22 Atony of the uterine wall following childbirth.

24 Immobility places a patient at risk for _____ .

25 Malignant tumor of blood vessels.

DOWN

1 Radiographic examination of the bladder before, during and after voiding.

(2 wds).

2 Any reconstructive surgical procedure on the urinary bladder.

3 Surgical removal of the pylorus and antrum with closure of the ends of the stomach and duodenum, followed by attaching the stomach to the jejunum. (Also called gastrojejunostomy). (3 wds).

7 A digestive enzyme from the stomach that breaks down food protein into large protein molecules.

9 A basin-shaped structure that includes the hip, sacrum, and coccyx of the spinal column.

10 Hidden blood in stool that is not visible to the naked eye. (2 wds).

11 A hollow space in the area of the forehead. (2 wds).

12 Five long bones in the foot.

15 Prefix meaning "water" or "fluid".

16 An infant with pyloric stenosis should be weighed _____ .

18 Agoraphobia is characterized by fear of ___ places.

20 Prefix meaning "pertaining to navel".

21 A mood disorder characterized by abnormally high and low moods and severe behavioral disturbance.

23 True or false: A patient should be instructed to drink plenty of fluids the night before a sputum test.

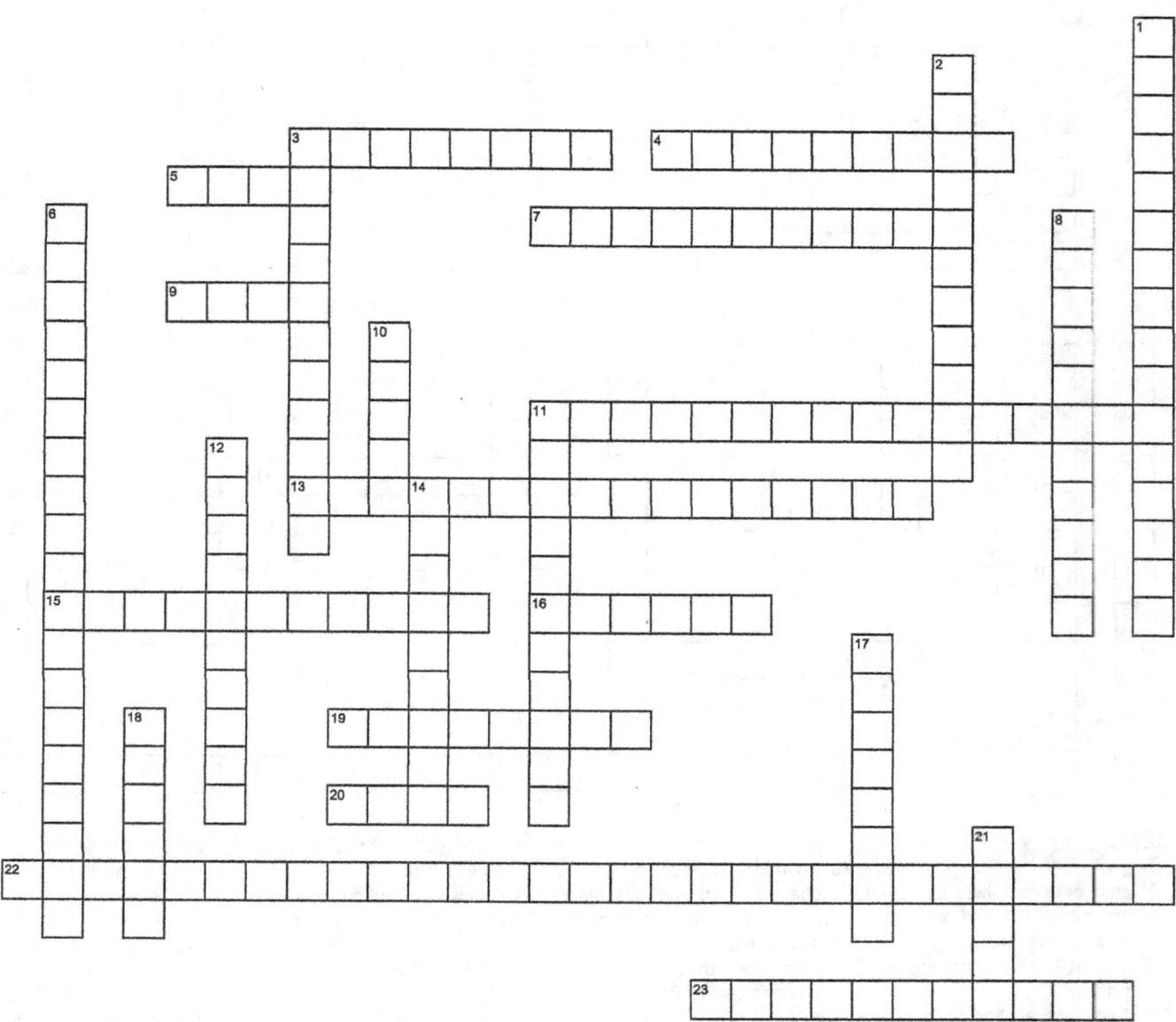

ACROSS

3 The vascular and innermost of the three meninges covering the brain and spinal cord. (2 wds).

4 Structure of respiration located in the right chest and composed of the superior and inferior lobes. (2 wds).

5 Suffix meaning "state of".

7 Abnormal presence of the protein albumin in the urine.

9 Prefix meaning "both" or "two ways".

11 A disorder caused by extra genetic fragments on the X chromosone, resulting in mental retardation, distinctive facial deformity, and macro-orchidism. (3 wds).

13 The percentage of blood emptied from the ventricle during contraction. (The normal value for a healthy heart is between 60-70 percent). (2 wds).

15 Surgical intervention of diseased vessels for recanalization of a blood vessel. Balloon dilation, mechanical stripping, injection of fibrinolytics, or placement of a stint.

16 A thin, transparent, internal fetal membrane that contains the amniotic fluid and fetus during pregnancy.

19 Diversion of urine into a surgically created opening in the abdominal wall so that urine drains continually into an attached appliance or bag.

20 Prefix meaning "starch".

22 Computerized imaging of the vasculature with visualization on a monitor screen following the intravenous injection of iodine through a catheter. (3 wds).

23 Muscle that retracts and tenses scalp.

DOWN

1 Condition that occurs when a blockage of the main bloodstream interferes with tissue perfusion. (May be caused by compression vena cava, pericardial tamponade, or pulmonary embolism). (2 wds).

2 A pinecone-shaped organ in the brain that secretes melatonin. (2 wds).

3 Erosion of the upper gastrointestinal tract caused by excessive secretion of acid. (2 wds).

6 An acute and chronic autoimmune inflammatory disease of connective tissue that affects joints due to antibodies destroying cartilage at the anticular surfaces. (2 wds).

8 Collection of muscles that rotate the arm. (2 wds).

10 Folds and ridges of tissue present in mucous membranes of organs such as the intestine and vagina.

11 The portion of each cerebral hemisphere located anterior to the central sulcus. (2 wds).

12 The third cranial nerve, which functions primarily to send impulses to the muscles of the eyes and eyelids in order to direct movement.

14 Incision into the urinary bladder.

17 Total deafness.

18 Expelled food or chyme. Also, suffix meaning "vomiting".

21 Suffix meaning "discharge".

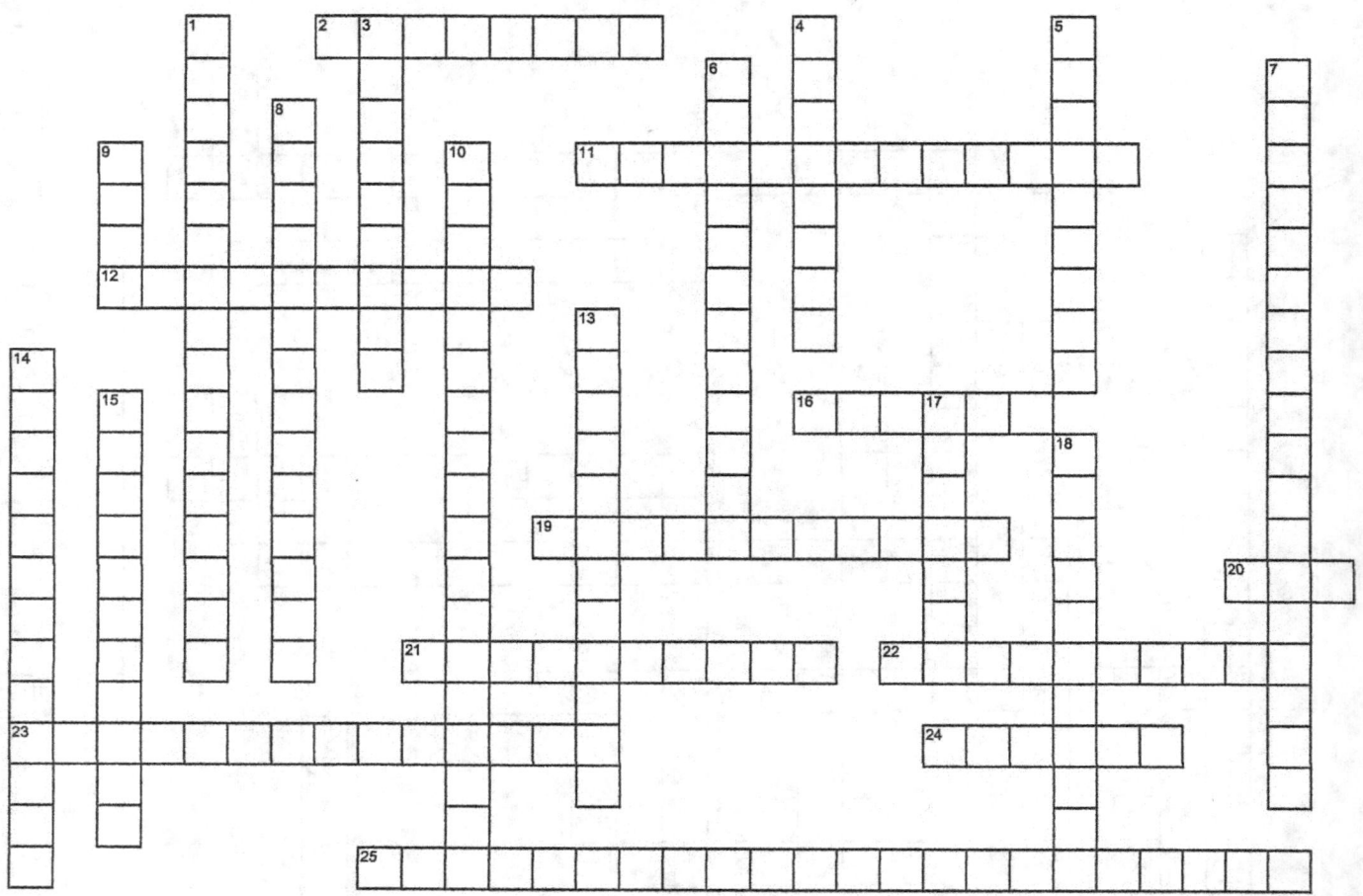

ACROSS

2 Mass of undissolved matter present in the blood or lymphatic vessel brought there by the blood or lymph current.

11 Most distal section of the brain. Where modulation of sounds occurs. (Involved in vision). (2 wds).

12 This regulates muscle synergy.

16 Suffix meaning "enlargement".

19 Upper chamber of the heart that receives deoxygenated blood from the entire body except the lungs. (2 wds).

20 Prefix meaning "within" or "inside".

21 Medical procedure to select the strength of lens that corrects a patient's refractive error and provides 20/20 vision.

22 A benign tumor of the coverings of the brain.

23 An inherited disorder characterized by excessive, thick mucus which causes obstructions in the respiratory and gastrointestinal tract. (2 wds).

24 An agent that causes vomiting.

25 An acute or chronic inflammation of the bile ducts due to cirrhosis or gallstones. (2 wds).

DOWN

1 Efforts by the hypothalamus to maintain body temperature by heat production and heat loss.

3 Condition of the colon with extreme dilation and hypertrophy.

4 Lethargy and depression are early symptoms of _____ disease.

5 Constructive phase of metabolism.

6 Structures leading from the urinary pelvis of the kidney, ureters, and bladder to the urethra. (2 wds).

7 Medical device used to deliver a specific quantity of aerosolized medication to the airway. (3 wds).

8 A walking stance where the legs are spread widely to compensate for disruption of balance and the tendency to fall. (2 wds).

9 Suffix meaning "pertaining to the blood or substance in the blood".

10 Lymphoid tissue located in the groin area. (3 wds).

13 A shallow depression where the head of the humerus joins the scapula to make the shoulder joint. (2 wds).

14 Hair that has been encapsulated in a dermal cyst. (2 wds).

15 A yeast infection that typically occurs as a result of antibiotic use.

17 A person who has lost an extremity or phalange.

18 Process of removal of undigested and residual liquids from the body.

41

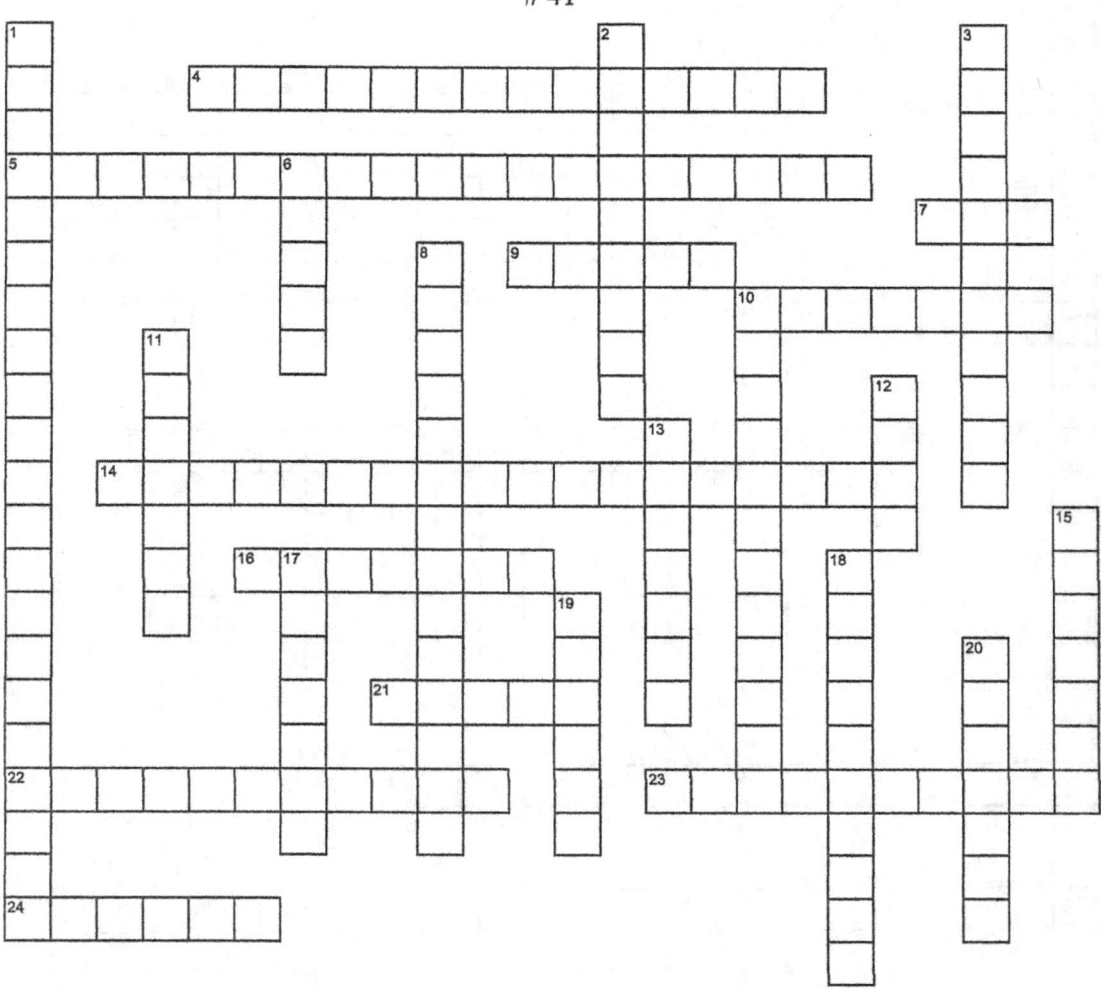

ACROSS

4 An abnormal cardiac sound produced by pumping of blood into the aorta or pulmonary arteries that stops prior to the closure of the aortic or pulmonic valves. (2 wds)

5 Mapping of the cerebral blood vessels using dye and x-rays. (2 wds).

7 Initials for inflammatory bowel disease, a chronic inflammation of various parts of the small and large intestines.

9 Prefix meaning "between".

10 Bone of the heel. (2 wds).

14 Muscle of the hip that extends the hip when contracted. (3 wds).

16 A radioisotope utilized in diagnostic scans for neoplasm, inflammation, and soft-tissue disorders.

21 Suffix meaning "creation of an artificial opening".

22 A circular, membrane-covered opening in the medial wall of the middle ear leading into the cochlea. (2 wds).

23 Process of visual examination of the urinary bladder using a fiberoptic scope.

24 Great toe, which is on the medial side of the foot.

DOWN

1 An instrument used to record the electrical activity of the brain.

2 Rapid growth similar to fungus. It is used to describe some quick-developing tumors.

3 Muscle that raises and adducts the scapula.

6 Prefix meaning "both sides" or "double".

8 Administration of a larger loading dose of digitalis to speed therapeutic response without producing toxic symptoms.

10 Congenital malformations in which intra-abdominal contents protrude through the umbilical cord.

11 Pertaining to bone.

12 Prefix meaning "vinegar", "acid", "sour" or "sharp".

13 Pain in the limbs from neurological sources.

15 Type of vest that vibrates, shaking the chest wall in efforts to break up mucus from lung fields for expectoration or suctioning.

17 Partial or total loss of long-term memory due to trauma or disease of hippocampus.

18 Medical procedure of drawing a sample of venous blood into a vacuum tube.

19 Prefix meaning "pertaining to the vagina".

20 Substance or mass that stops the flow of a vessel.

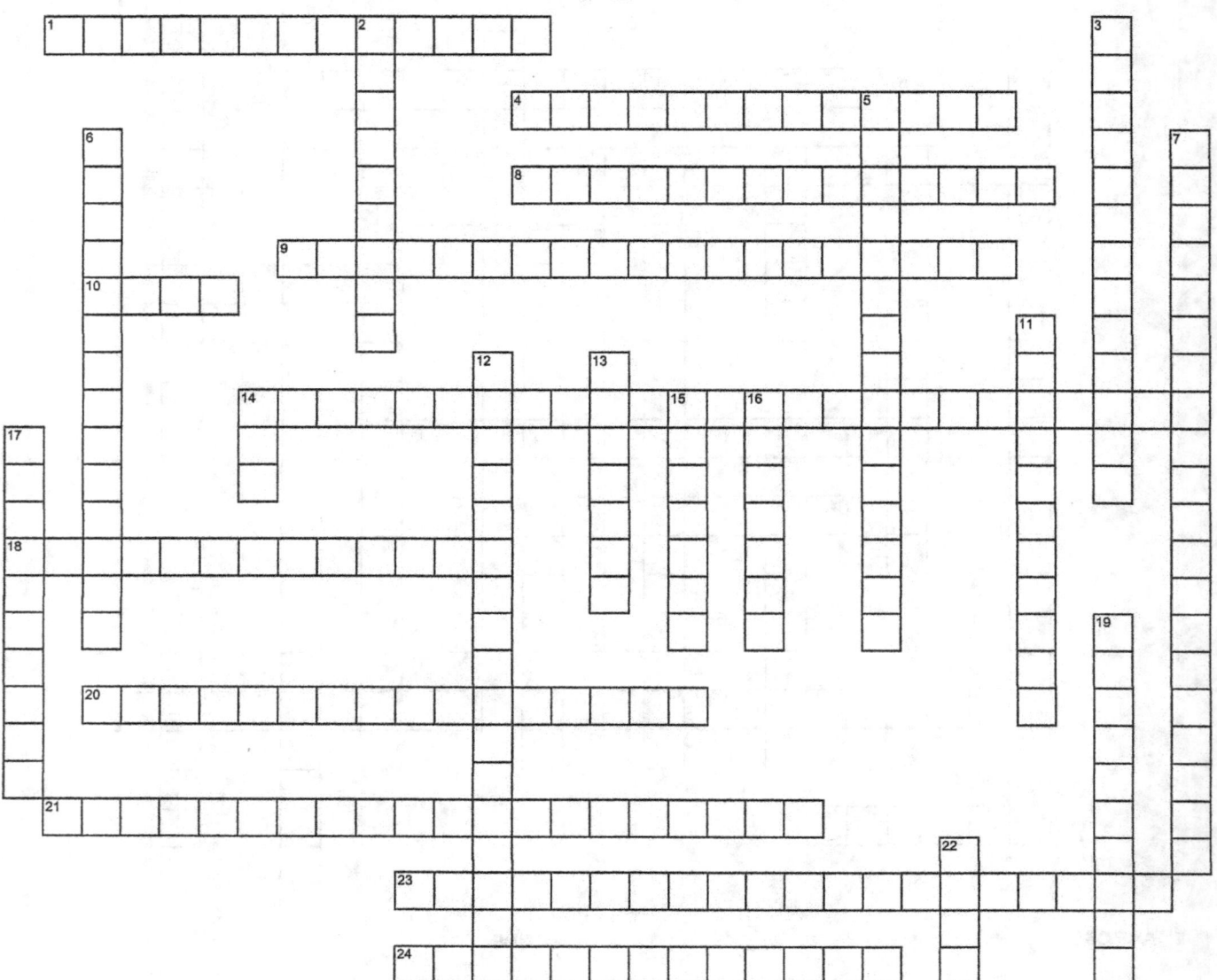

ACROSS

1 Use of a laser light to destroy or cut tissue.

4 A psychological examination through which a patient is shown cards with abstract shapes and asked to describe what the shape of the inkblot represents. (2 wds).

8 Refers to the clarity of liquid excreted by the kidney. (2 wds).

9 Yellowish discoloration of skin and sclera due to a gallstone or other pathology blocking the flow of bile in the bile ducts. (2 wds).

10 True or false: The cause of inflammatory bowel disease (IBD) is not known.

14 Infection of the uterus, fallopian tubes, and adjoining structures caused by infectious agents spreading upward in the female reproductive tract, producing fever, chills, vaginal discharge, dysuria, and dyspareunia. (3 wds).

18 Osseous formation of the posterior base of the cranium. (2 wds).

20 Large blood vessel that receives blood from the lower limbs and the pelvic and abdominal organs. It begins at the fifth lumbar vertebra and continues anterior to the right atrium of the heart. (3 wds).

21 Appearance of any part of the fetal head during vaginal delivery. (2 wds).

23 The rate at which blood is filtered at the glomerulus. (2 wds).

24 Fungal infection of the nail.

DOWN

2 Condition of not experiencing any pain sensation.

3 The artery that supplies blood to the heart tissue. (2 wds).

5 Destruction of the full thickness of the skin and underlying structures due to chemical or thermal exposure. (3 wds).

6 Lower chamber of the heart that receives blood from the right atrium and pumps it out to the lungs by way of the pulmonary artery. (2 wds).

7 Graphic recording of the brain's electrical activity.

11 The red mask appearance of cheeks, nose and skin, typical of rosacea.

12 Procedure to examine the posterior cavity using mydriatic eyedrops to dilate the pupil. (2 wds).

13 Suffix meaning "one who practices a specialty".

14 Percutaneous Endoscopic Gastrostomy. Insertion of a permanent feeding tube through the abdominal wall using visual guidance from an endoscope passed through the mouth into the stomach. (3 initials).

15 Having the characteristic of dark, tarry stools.

16 Any substance that is measured, usually applied to a component of blood or other body fluid. Substance dissolved in a solution.

17 Morbid or excessive fear and sensitivity to pain.

19 Creation of a new opening into the urinary bladder for drainage.

22 Open Reduction and Internal Fixation (4 initials).

43

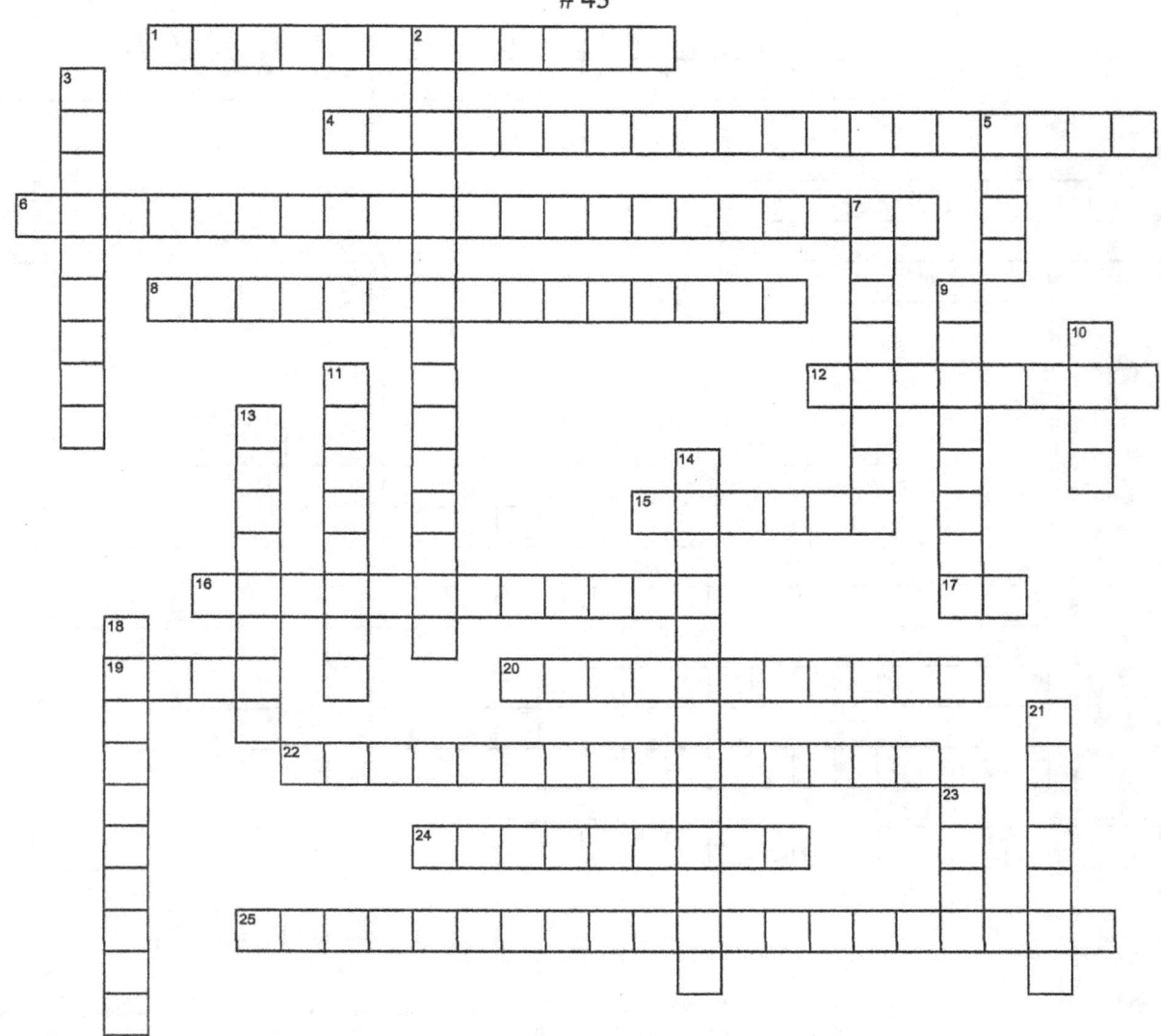

ACROSS

1 Assessing equilibrium by having a patient stand with feet together and eyes closed to check for swaying or falling to one side. It indicates a loss of balance and inner-ear dysfunction. (2 wds).

4 Decrease in appetite due to physical illness. (2 wds).

6 Valve between the right ventricle and the right atrium. Also called the tricuspid valve. (2 wds).

8 Benign muscle tumor of the uterus. (2 wds).

12 Space containing a hair root.

15 Intestinal gas that is the end product of bacteria in the large intestine feeding on undigested food.

16 The autoimmune disease of connective tissue is called _____ erythematosus. (2 wds).

17 Prefix meaning "without" or "not".

19 Prefix meaning "large" or "oversized".

20 The rate at which a drug becomes a solution.

22 A procedure that measures the baldder dysfunction, most commonly urinary incontinence.

24 The dilation of the cervix and scraping of the endometrium is called dilation and _____.

25 Process of recording the electrical activities of the cochlea of the inner ear.

DOWN

2 Hemoglobin A molecule with a glucose group on the N-terminal valine amino acid unit of the beta chain.

3 An instrument used to puncture the amniotic membrane.

5 Prefix meaning "broad" or "thickened".

7 An abnormal increase in hydrogen ion concentration in the body.

9 Malignant tumor of melanocytes.

10 Prefix meaning "bend".

11 A small, fleshy mass.

13 Type of therapy that uses active or passive exercises to improve a patient's range of motion, joint mobility, muscular strength and balance.

14 The application of sutures to the tongue.

18 Normal vision.

21 A general term for spine.

23 Suffix meaning "blood condition".

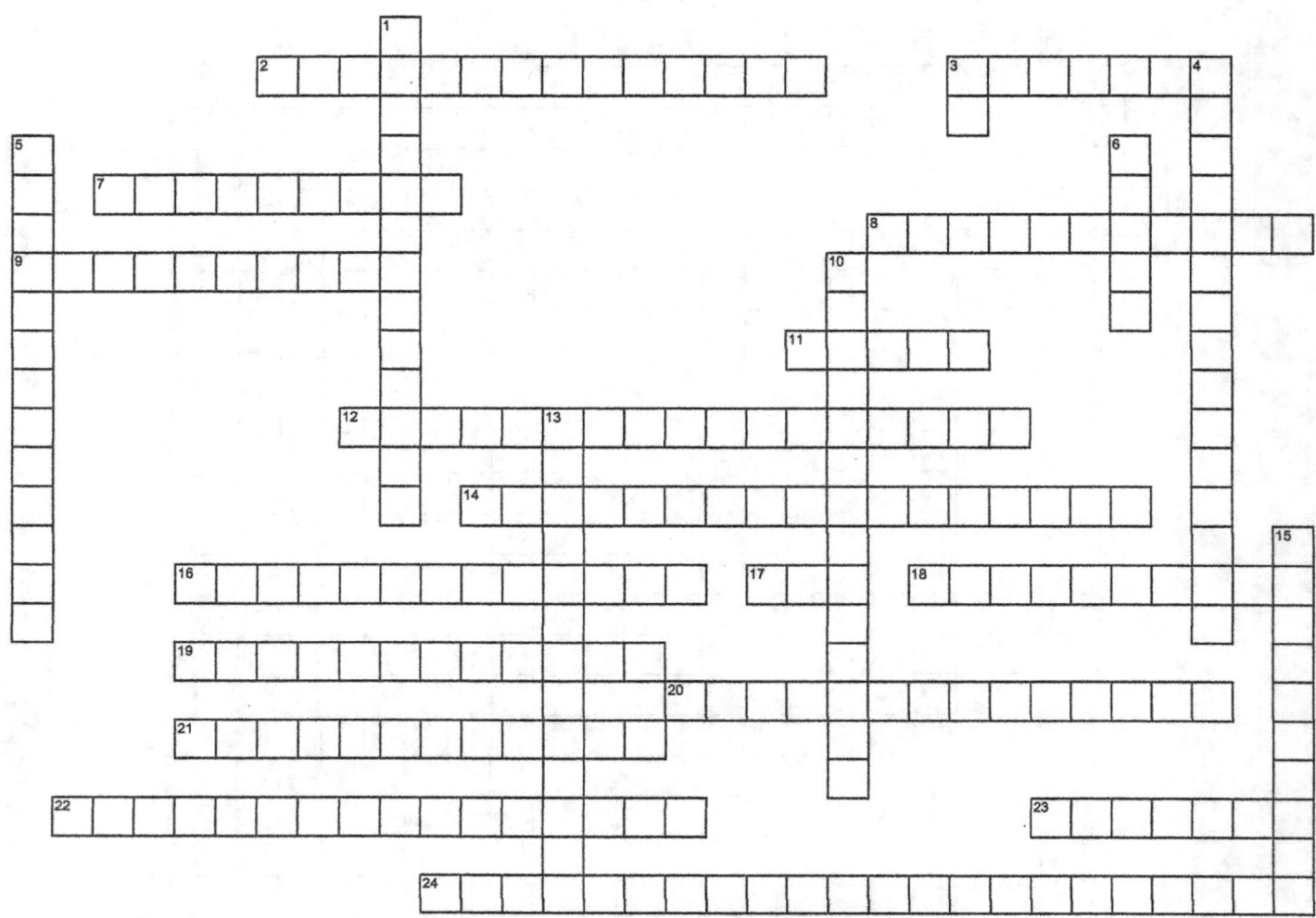

ACROSS

2 Overstraightening, or over-extending beyond normal joint function or near the maximum extension.

3 The inability to produce clear and distinct speech.

7 Infection with Entamoeba histolytica that is spread by ingestion of contaminated food.

8 Middle body cavity, midchest, directly above the diaphragm.

9 Absence of menstruation.

11 A mass of chewed food or medicine that is ready to be swallowed.

12 Record of the electrical forces producing heart contractions.

14 Malabsorption and gastric irritation due to gluten sensitivity. (2 wds).

16 Middle, smaller muscle in the buttock region that extends to the thigh. (2 wds).

17 Suffix meaning "enzyme".

18 The dilation of the cervix and removal of the products of conception is called dilation and _____.

19 Clinical finding indicating appendicitis whereby pressure in the lower left quadrant of the abdomen produces pain in the lower right quadrant. (2 wds).

20 Inflammation of the retina due to prolonged exposure to intense light.

21 Type of test that measures pancreatic urine levels of amylase. (2 wds).

22 Use of electrical stimulation to compete with pain stimuli for transmission to the spinal cord. This may be delivered through the skin, or by an implantable device.

23 Division of a sex cell whereby the nucleus has 23 chromosones.

24 An acute or chronic inflammation of the bile ducts due to cirrhosis or gallstones. (2 wds).

DOWN

1 Abnormal growth extending from membrane of the cervix uteri. (2 wds).

3 Prefix meaning "pertaining to".

4 Acute, life-threatening immunocompromised state characterized by severe depression or complete absence of disease-fighting white blood cells and by leukopenia, resulting in infections of the skin and mucous membranes.

5 A large cell normally found in the bone marrow that gives rise to platelets and has a multilobed nucleus.

6 A muscle protein that is responsible for muscle contraction.

10 Specialized light-sensitive cells of the eye such as rods and cones.

13 Residual structures of the umbilical vein found in the liver. A fibromuscular attachment that attaches to the uterus. (2 wds).

15 Repeated passage of stool into the clothing in a child older than age five in the absence of gastrointestinal illness or disability.

45

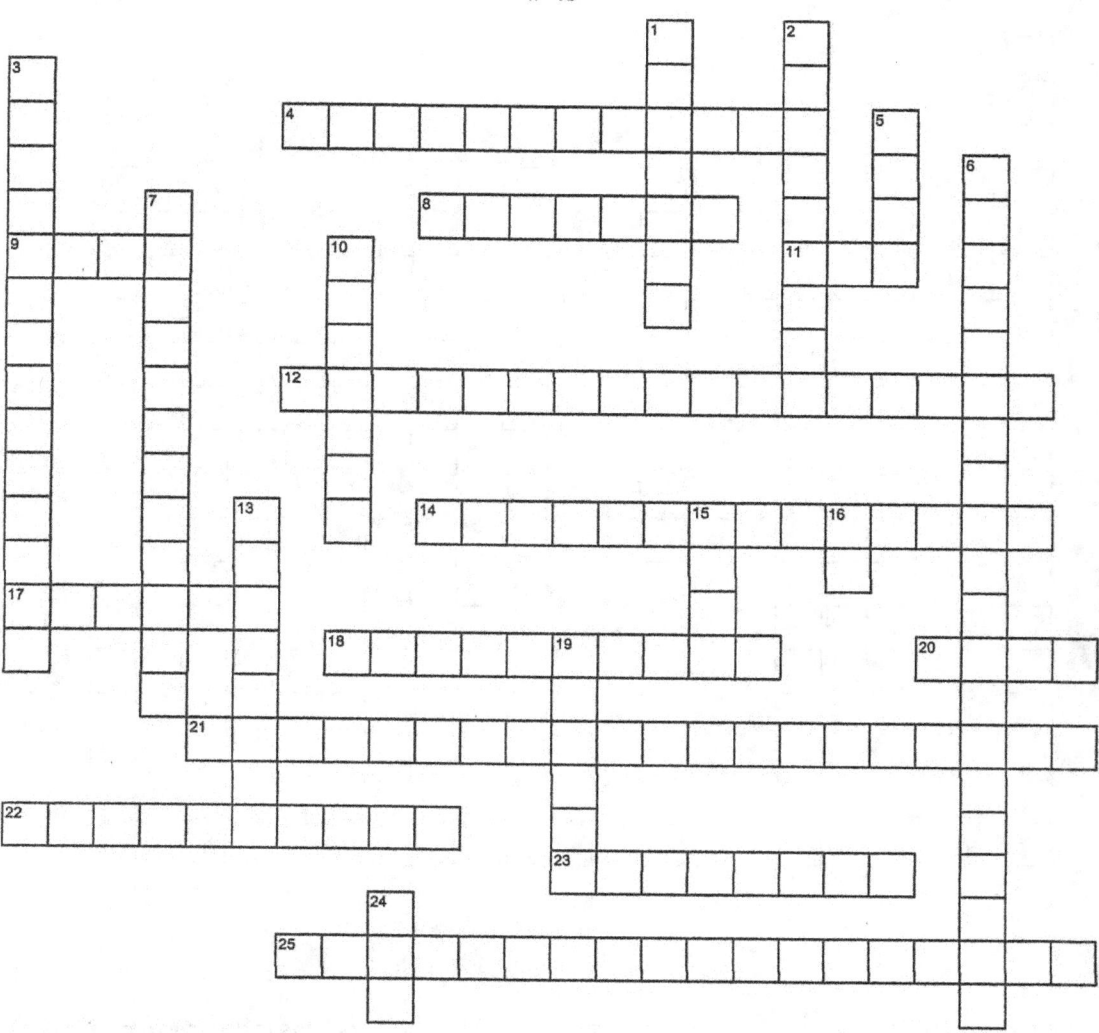

ACROSS

4 Rupture of the amnion.
8 finger- or fringe-shaped projections extending from the distal ends of the fallopian tubes.
9 Prefix meaning "outside".
11 Suffix meaning "pertaining to".
12 Grossly decreased physical height. Disproportion among bodily parts due to inadequate growth hormone levels. (2 wds).
14 The process of breaking down large globules of fat into smaller particles.
17 One of two small tubes that drain urine from the kidneys to the bladder.
18 The destructive phase of metabolism.
20 Suffix meaning "pertaining to urine or urination".
21 Black or dark brown pigment produced by cells called melanocytes. (2 wds).
22 Large hemorrhages or bruises on the skin.
23 An expert who fills prescriptions for eyeglasses and contact lenses.
25 Liver enlargement, fatty deposits, and fibrosis due to chronic ethanol abuse. (2 wds).

DOWN

1 Bending movement of the joint.
2 Abnormal growth and development of tissue.
3 A large muscle forming the buttocks that extends to the thigh. (2 wds).
5 Suffix meaning "to view".
6 A diagnostic study in which the patient is administered 75 g of glucose while fasting, with measurement of blood glucose at regular intervals to determine ability to regulate glucose metabolism. (3 wds).
7 Inflammation of the hair follicles.
10 Photorefractive keratotomy (PRK) is use of an _____ laser to reshape the curvature of the cornea without the creation of a corneal surface flap.
13 Having an undetectable pulse.
15 Prefix meaning a "split" or "cleft".
16 Suffix meaning "toward" or "in the direction of".
19 Prefix meaning "pertaining to the scrotum".
24 Electroconvulsive therapy. The use of electrical current and electrodes on the head to produce seizures while sedated. It alters the brain chemistry to treat severe depression more rapidly than antidepressant drugs. (3 initials).

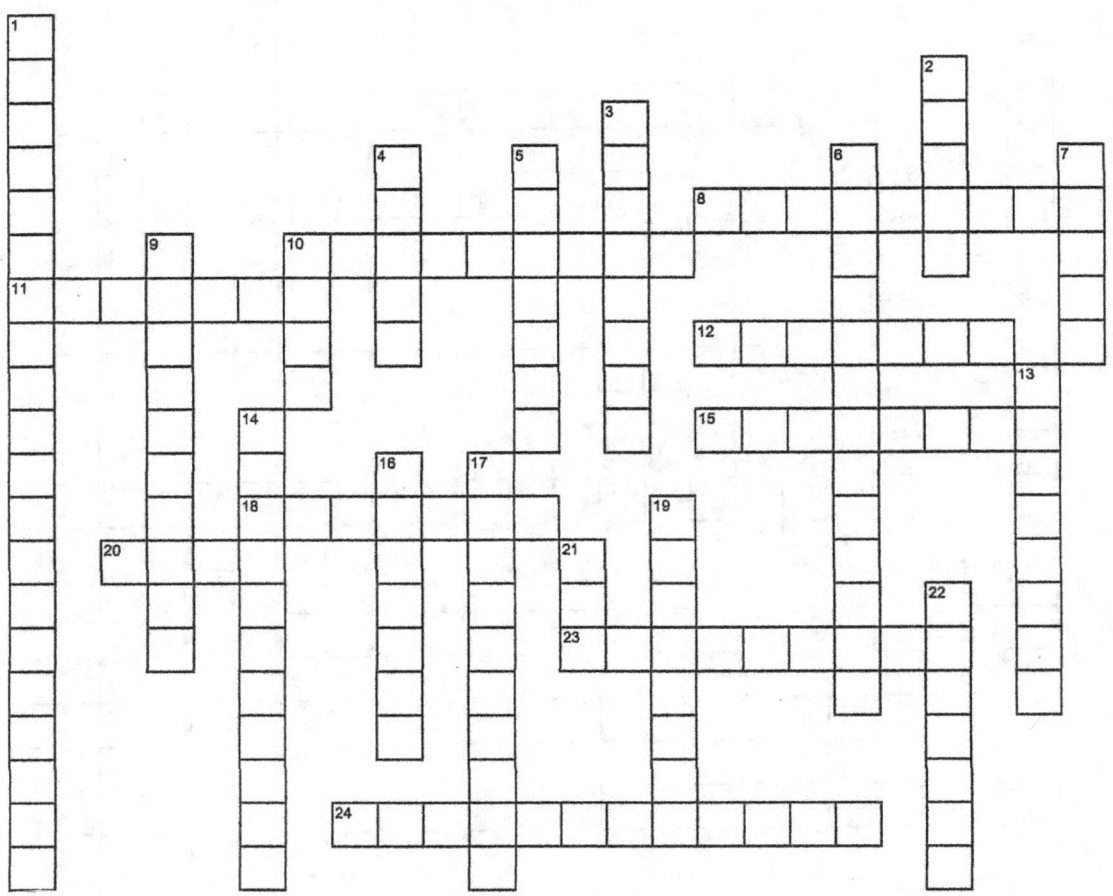

ACROSS

8 Gross, involuntary, jerking tremor of the hand. (also called flapping tremor).

10 Clouding of the lens of the eye, treated by surgical removal and replacement with a prosthetic intraocular lens.

11 The presence of pus in a bodily cavity, used most often in reference to pyothorax.

12 An accumulation of excess fluid in the peritoneal cavity, most commonly caused by cirrhosis of the liver due to alcoholism (but may also be caused by heart failure or kidney disease).

15 The onset of regular menstrual cycle, with usual onset at approximately thirteen years of age.

18 The short vessel used for the purpose of eliminating or passing urine.

20 Prefix meaning "pertaining to odor".

23 Characteristic of body tissues that resonate echoes of sound which are captured under ultrasound examination.

24 The formation and release of a substance to occlude blood vessels in the treatment or prevention of hemorrhaging.

DOWN

1 Analysis of urine to detect androgen metabolites. (3 wds).

2 Round circuit, pertaining to the eye or bony socket in the cranium that surrounds all but the anterior portion of the eye.

3 State of hyper- or hypotonicity of tissue. Most often used to reference muscle tone.

4 Cranial nerve II, which carries nerve impulses of visual images from the rods and cones of the retina to the visual cortex in the brain.

5 Having poor or absent muscle tone.

6 The upper region of the neck consisting of the seven vertebrae. (2 wds).

7 Prefix meaning "pertaining to bone".

9 Experiencing difficulty in performance of voluntary movements.

10 The application of a rigid form around a body part or fracture to stabilize it in a fixed position to facilitate healing.

13 Pain in the limbs from muscular sources.

14 Examination of deep tissues and structures of the body by x-ray using a fluoroscope.

16 Earache.

17 A type of tetanic spasm where the limbs, neck and trunk are held in a rigid, straight line.

19 Suffocation resulting in impaired or absent oxygen exchange.

21 Suffix meaning "small".

22 Suffix meaning "dilation" or "expansion".

ACROSS

1 Hyperbillirubinemia is an abnormally high concentration of billirubin in the circulating blood that results in _____.

4 Hydroxycorticosteroid is the analysis of _____ to detect cortisol byproducts.

5 Skin appears powdery as a result of severe uremia due to dermal deposits of urea and uric acid salt. (2 wds).

7 Prefix meaning "out" or "away from".

8 Bursitis of the Achilles tendon with or without calcification, due to trauma or poorly fitting shoes. (2 wds).

11 Obturating embolism is the complete occlusion of a blood vessel by a clot or _____.

14 Space in the pelvis between the obturator internus muscle and the obturator fascia that the pudendal nerve passes through. (2 wds).

17 Force needed to ensure that adequate oxygen and nutrients are delivered to tissues. (3 wds).

20 Temporary loss of vision in one eye caused by micro-embolism blocking the flow of blood to the carotid system.

21 Excessive gas in the intestinal tract, in either the stomach or intestines.

22 A bacterial infection caused by an unusual strain of E coli bacterium in the large intestine.

23 Chronic, mild to moderate depression.

DOWN

2 Type of fluid secreted by the choroid plexuses of the ventricles of the brain, filling ventricles, subarachnoid spaces, and the spinal cord.

3 Hormone that is formed by the pineal gland and involved in circadian rhythms and bioregulation.

4 Prefix meaning "extreme", "beyond", or "disproportionate".

5 No significance or information worth noting. All findings are normal.

6 Rotator cuff _____ is the inflammation of tendons of the supraspinatus, infraspinatus, teres minor, or subscapular muscles of the shoulder.

9 A soft, infiltrating tumor ot the external layer of cerebellum.

10 Vomitus with presence of blood in stomach contents due to bleeding ulcers.

12 Transabdominal needle aspiration of amniotic fluid from the amniotic sac for diagnostic purposes.

13 Abnormal passage that connects two structures.

15 Initial phase of general adaptation syndrome. A bodily response to stress, by releasing endocrine hormones preparing for fight or flight. (2 wds).

16 Cervical intraepithelial neoplasia is _____ of the squamous epithelium of the uterine cervix that may extend into deeper layers.

18 The study of the origin and development of a fetus from fertilization up to the time of birth.

19 Surgical incision into bone.

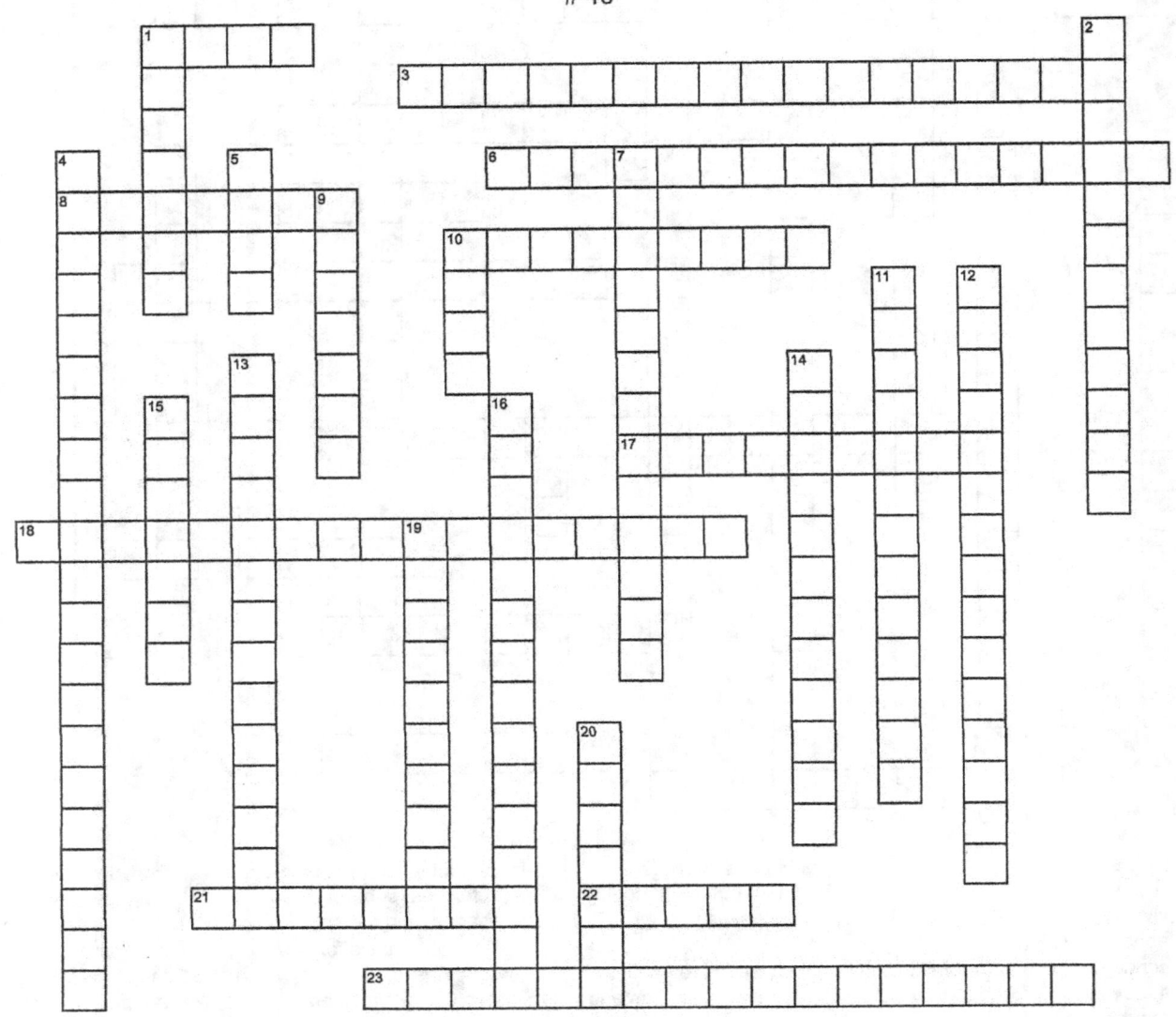

ACROSS

1 Prefix meaning "to burn".
3 The seven vertebral segments forming the cervical column in the region of the neck. (2 wds).
6 Section of the brain stem that is continuous with the spinal cord. (2 wds).
8 Malplacement of an organ or an object.
10 A whiplike structure that propels sperm.
17 Hyperaldosteronism is excessive production of aldosterone altering the regulation of _____ and sodium exchange in the distal renal tubule.
18 A degenerative brain disorder that causes dementia and physical deterioration with typical onset late in life. It disrupts brain function by formation of amyloid plaques, neurofibrillary tangles, and cerebral atrophy. (2 wds).
21 Impaired speech and reasoning due to a mental disorder.
22 Pertaining to vision or the orbit.
23 Enteral or parenteral infusion of a solution containing complete nutritional requirements for normal growth, development and tissue repair.

DOWN

1 Inflammation of the vena cava.
2 Cervix uteri is the neck of the uterus through which _____ and the fetus pass. This structure is subject to tears during delivery of a fetus. (2 wds).
4 Use of artifically supplied respirations using an automated respirator. (2 wds).
5 Suffix meaning "condition of vision".
7 Surgical procedure that involves plastic surgery to reposition the urethra. It is used to correct congenital hypospadias and epispadias.
9 Cytophotocoagulation is the destruction of a portion of the _____ body using an intense beam of light from a laser.
10 Suffix meaning "flow".
11 Roux-en-Y gastric bypass is a surgical treatment of _____ by attaching the jejunum to a surgically reduced stomach pouch and connecting the bypassed duodenum to the pylorus, resulting in decreased gastric capacity and reduced absorption of food. (2 wds).
12 A beta-group herpes virus that may be transmitted through sexual or intimate contact that may cause permanent disability, including hearing loss and mental retardation for infants, and blindness and mental disorders for adults.
13 Surgical repair of a cleft palate.
14 Alanine aminotransferase test is a blood enzyme test to evaluate _____. (2 wds).
15 The obturator foramen is a large opening in the _____ that is covered by a fibrous membrane and is a point of attachment for some muscles of the hip.
16 A rare condition of the inner ear characterized by progressive hearing loss, sensation of pressure in the ear, tinnitus and vertigo. (2 wds).
19 Mendelsohn maneuver is a technique of _____ that maintains voluntary muscular contraction for a few seconds at the highest position.
20 A benign tumor of the bone.

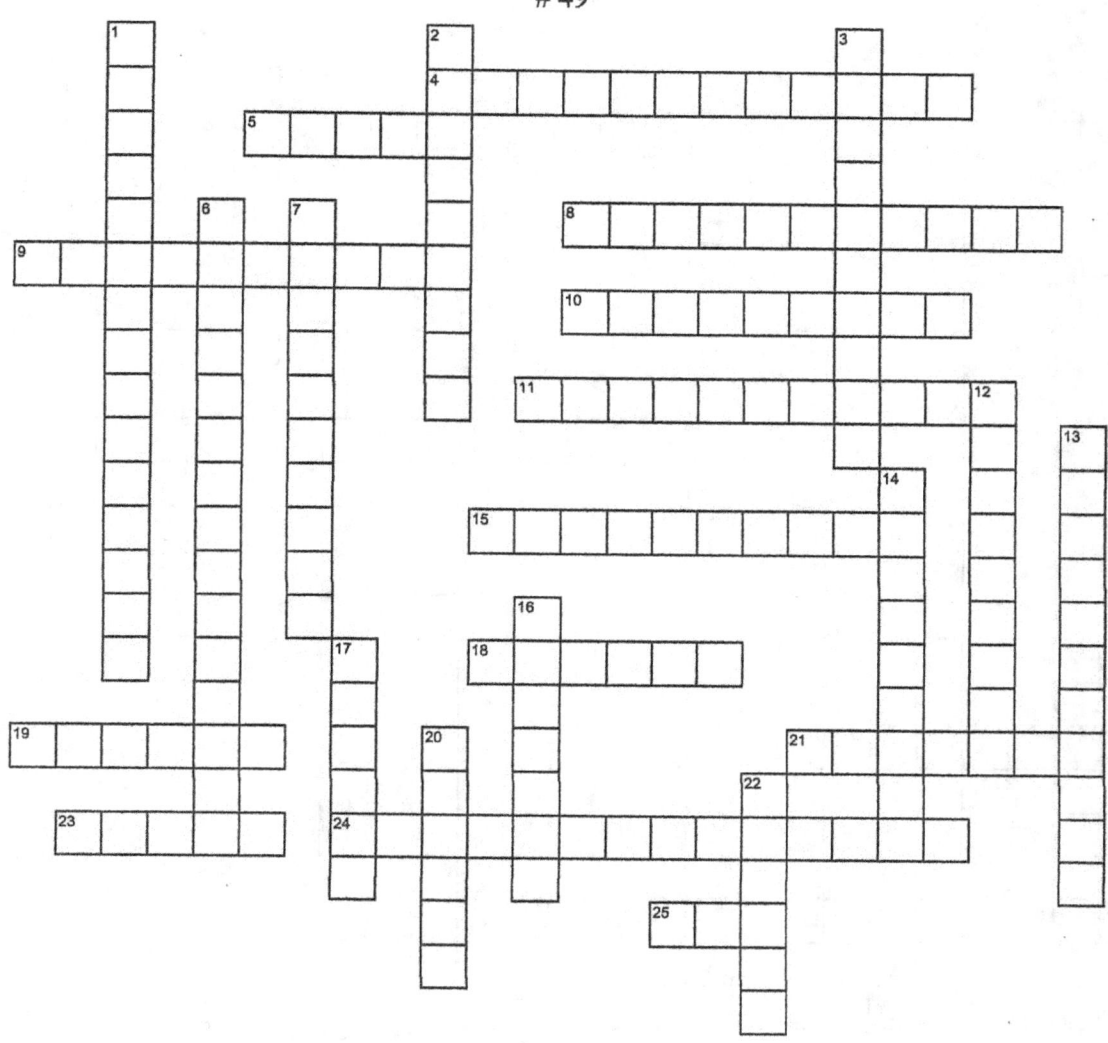

ACROSS

4 Inflammation of the hair follicle and associated sebaceous glands. (2 wds).

5 Condition in which the hind foot turns inward, usually associated with club foot.

8 Administration or absorption of a drug through intact skin.

9 Alteration in the position of the metacarpophalangeal joints, where the fingers curve toward the ulnar bone of the forearm. (Caused by rheumatoid arthritis). (2 wds).

10 Referring to a leg, arm, or phalange.

11 Area in the brain where parts of the right and left optic nerves cross and join the other optic nerve. (2 wds).

15 Breakdown or separation of the prickle-cell layer of the epidermis leading to cellular degeneration.

18 A single finger or toe.

19 Fibrous connective tissue that covers, supports and separates muscles.

21 Difficulty breathing or shortness of breath.

23 Vessels that carry blood toward the heart.

24 The segment of the bowel that extends upward on the right side of the abdomen, joining the transverse colon. (2 wds).

25 Prefix meaning "loosen" or "dissolve".

DOWN

1 Bundle of autonomic nerves located in the submucosa of the small intestine. (2 wds).

2 A surgical procedure involving bilateral surgical removal of part of the vas deferens for the purpose of sterilization.

3 Inflammation of the ureter.

6 Implantation of a living body part, organ or tissue graft from a donor.

7 Region of the throat located between the soft palate and the epiglottis.

12 Type of sebaceous glands at the edges of the eyelids that secrete sebum from their ducts.

13 Overproduction of fibrous tissue.

14 Prefix meaning "pertaining to odor or sense of smell".

16 Ions with positive charge.

17 General directional term pertaining to the tail-end or distal portion of any structure.

20 A small, circumscribed, discolored skin lesion.

22 Suffix meaning "to cut", "to excise" or "to remove".

50

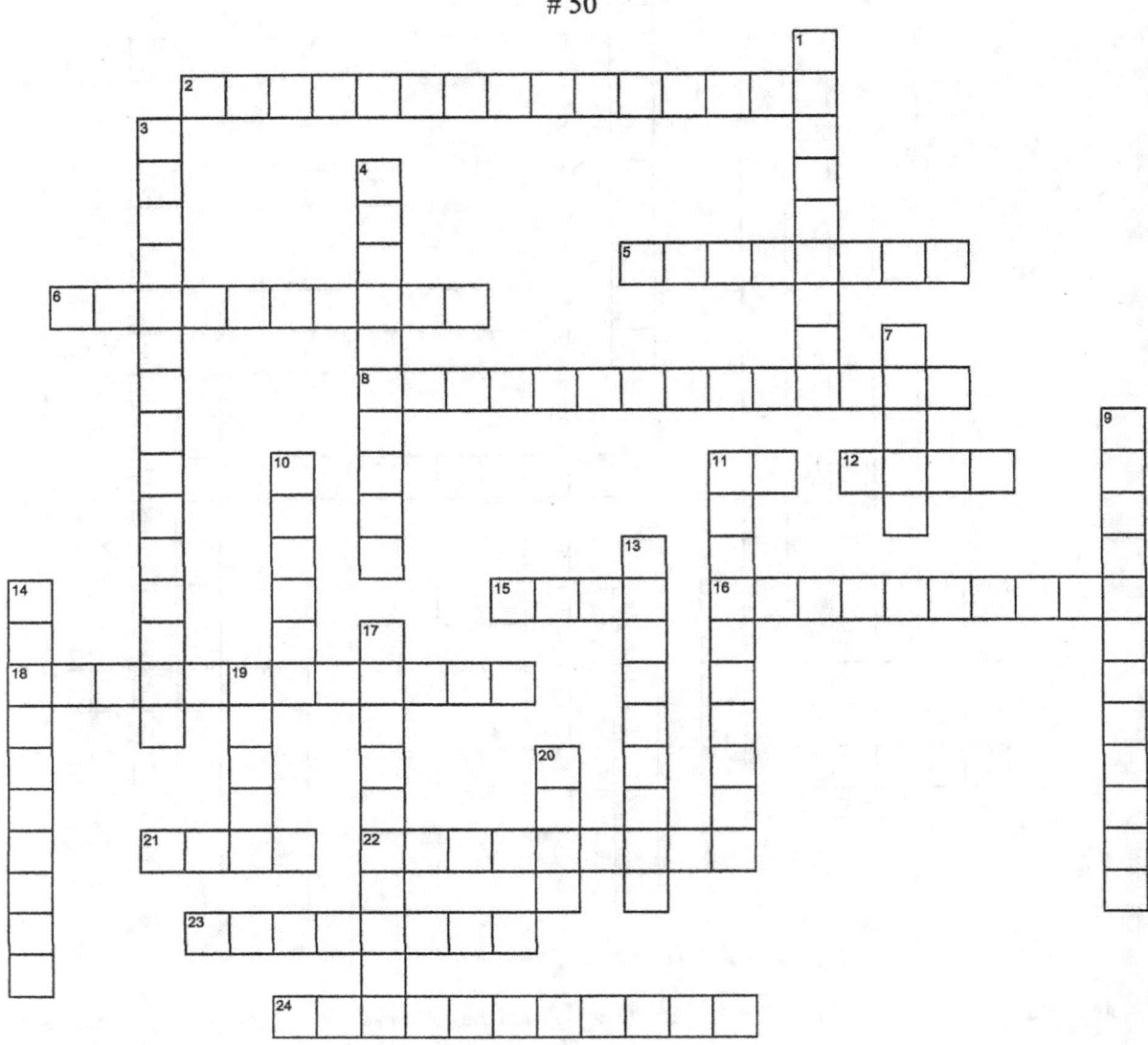

ACROSS

2 The long cavity in the center of a long bone that contains yellow bone marrow. (2 wds).

5 In pressure ulcers, _____ tissue develops because the vascular supply to the area is diminished.

6 Conditions produced from sources outside of the body.

8 Surgical repair of the Achilles tendon by suturing.

11 Prefix meaning "toward midline"

12 Prefix meaning "burning".

15 Forearm bone located along the little-finger side of the lower arm.

16 A woman who is pregnant for the first time.

18 If the right atrium and right ventricle are damaged, right-sided _____ would result. (2 wds).

21 A closed sac in or under the skin that contains fluid or semisolid material.

22 A bruise on the brain's surface.

23 The third stage of labor extends from birth of the neonate to expulsion of the _____, and lasts from five to thirty minutes.

24 Any disease of a joint, including inflammatory and hereditary disorders.

DOWN

1 Generally unhappy mood, depression, and anxiety.

3 Damage to the epidermal layer. Burned-tissue reaction as a result of thermal, radioactive, chemical or electrical insult. (3 wds).

4 Total concentration of dissolved substances in a solution.

7 A raised, reddish area that's commonly itchy and lasts no more than twenty-four hours.

9 The muscle that moves the eye toward the midline. (2 wds).

10 An ophthalmoscope is an instrument used to examine the _____ and interior structures of the eye.

11 Removal of an extremity due to trauma or circulatory disease. It is classified as either traumatic or surgical, depending on the circumstances in which removal occurred.

13 Pharmacological agents that stimulate peristalsis and evacuation of the bowel.

14 Bronchial breath sounds are discontinuous and are loudest during _____.

17 Condition where three or more consecutive ribs have fractured in close proximity. It creates instability of the wall of the thorax, moving opposite to the normal direction during respiratory movements. (2 wds).

19 The end product of digestion composed of undigested fibers and liquid. (also called stool).

20 True or false: A patient with expressive aphasia can comprehend written or verbal communication.

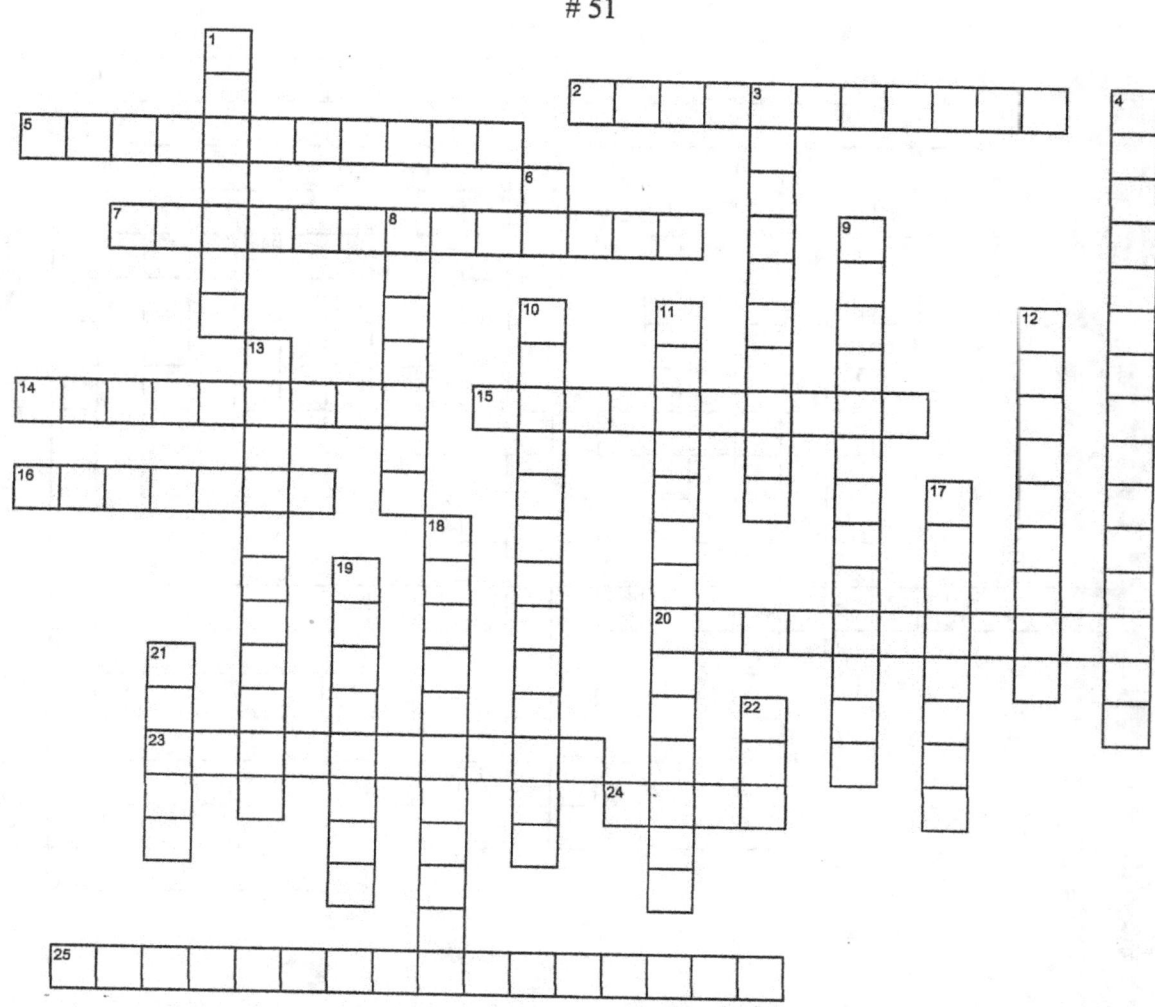

ACROSS

2 Paralysis of the soft palate of the mouth.
5 Specialist in the testing of visual function and in the diagnosis and nonsurgical treatment of eye conditions.
7 Pertaining to the cartilage.
14 Chronic and irreversible damage to alveoli characterized by trapped air in the lung. Often due to smoking or pollution.
15 Inflammation of the urethra caused by infection or mechanical irritation associated with a stone.
16 A ureterocystostomy is a surgical connection made between the ureter and the _____.
20 Painful sexual intercourse.
23 Confined to one side.
24 True or false: When peroxide is applied full-strength to halo vest pin sites, it can disrupt the healing process and normal flora.
25 Injection of a local analgesic agent into the epidural space of the sacrum. (2 wds).

DOWN

1 Suppressor T cells reduce the _____ response.
3 The mouth, inclusive of the teeth, mucosa and lips. (2 wds).

4 Chronic adrenocortical insufficiency possibly due to autoimmune disease, adrenal tumors, or tuberculosis. (2 wds).
6 Prefix meaning "in".
8 An enzyme that breaks down starch into smaller carbohydrates. It begins the process of digestion. Found in starch and pancreatic juice.
9 Surgical reconstruction of a testicle.
10 An upper gastrointestinal series is the study of the esophagus, stomach, and sometimes small bowel after swallowing _____. (2 wds).
11 Image of the heart produced by ultrasound.
12 The medullary rhythmicity area is the brain region that regulates _____ patterns.
13 Surgical fracture or breaking of a bone.
17 Mediastinal nodes are lymph tissue in the ____ chest.
18 The use of finger pressure applied to specific nerve junctions on the body to promote healing.
19 Non-ossified membrane covering the anterior portion of the skull of a fetus. Commonly known as the "soft spot".
21 Meckel's diverticulum is a blind ___ that results when the omphalomesenteric duct, which connects the gut to the yolk sac during embryonic development, fails to atrophy.
22 Suffix meaning "action" or "process".

52

ACROSS

2 Hardened feces that become a stonelike mass, occurring most often in the appendix or a diverticulum.

3 Use of sound waves to assess the body structures and create computerized images for study.

6 Suffix meaning "to loosen", "to dissolve" or "to relieve".

7 Prefix meaning "reversal of" or "absence".

9 Magnetic resonance imaging (MRI) is diagnostic imaging by use of electromagnetic _____ to visualize soft tissues of the body.

15 The diamond-shaped anterior fontanel normally closes between ages ____ and eighteen months.

16 These destroy bacteria and viruses, s are evacuated.

18 Impaired vision that is unrelated to an ocular lesion and cannot be fully corrected with glasses.

19 Mesodermal cells capable of producing new bone tissue.

20 A dressing applied to stasis ulcers of the lower leg using layers of gauze and a mixture of zinc oxide in a glycogelatin base. (2 wds).

21 Airway inflammation and edema in asthma increase ____ production.

22 Breast enlargement, decrease in prostate size, and flushing are expected effects of _____.

23 Movement of fluid from a vessel wall into a body cavity or adjacent tissue.

24 A transient episode of extreme muscular weakness, triggered by extreme emotional states such as fear, anger, or surprise.

DOWN

1 Bent section of the lumbosacral region of an embryo. (2 wds).

2 To strain or separate by passing liquid through a device to separate wanted from unwanted substances, as in dialysis.

4 Prefix meaning "across" or "through".

5 Fine motor skills such as purposeful grasps occur at age _____ months.

8 Pubic bone. One of three bones that fuse together to form the hip bone. (2 wds).

10 Perception of an irritating sensation in response to normal stimuli due to nerve dysfunction.

11 A buildup of nitrogenous waste products in the blood, which indicates impaired renal function.

12 A small circular portion of the retina where the optic nerve passes through and does not have visual capacity. (2 wds).

13 Chemical involved in nerve impulse transmission.

14 Veins that are knotted or swollen, often occurring in the lower legs and esophagus due to defective vein valves.

17 Difficult childbirth due to large fetal size, small pelvic outlet, or malpositioning of the fetus, such as breech presentation.

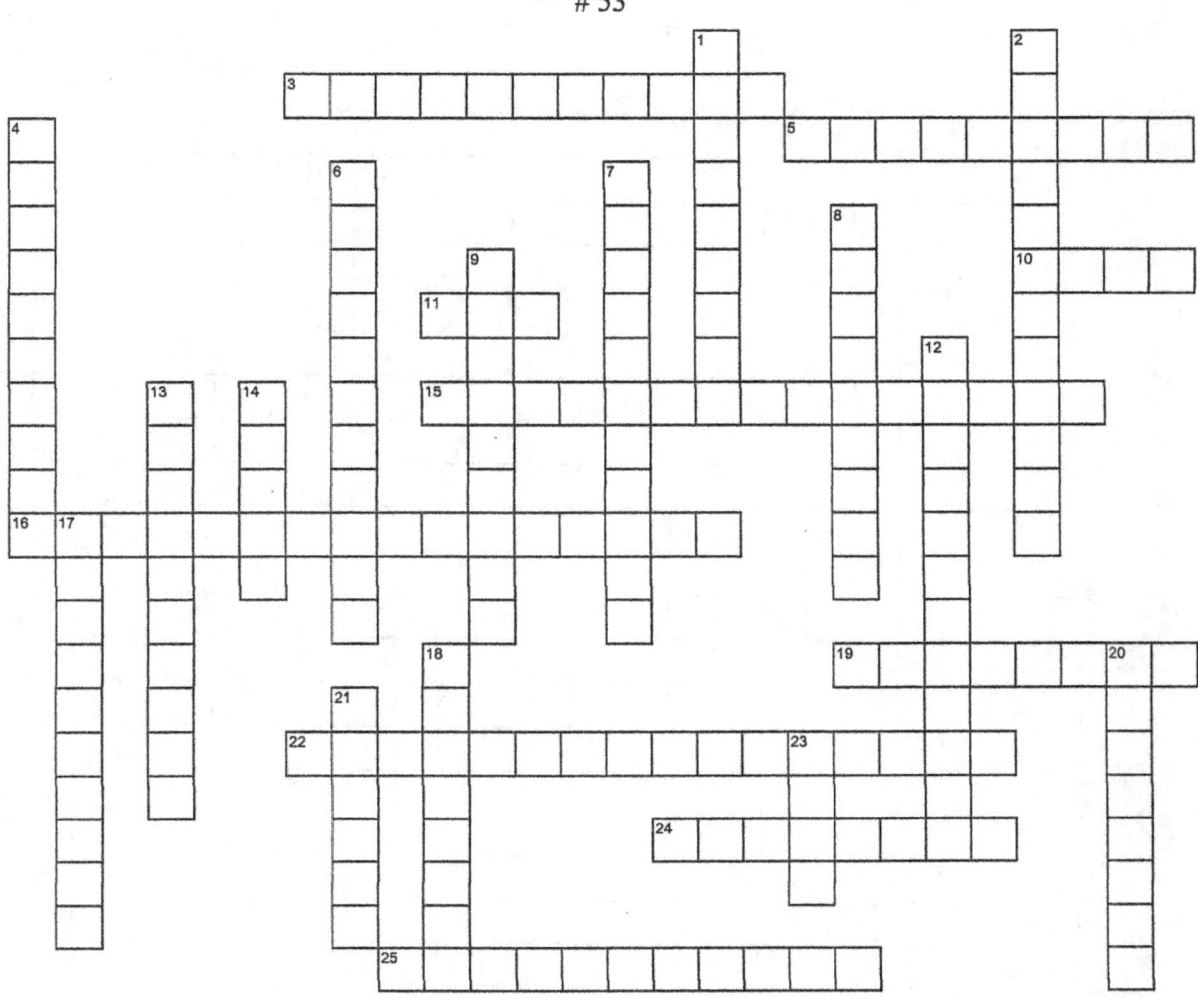

ACROSS

3 A fetus's head is considered to be engaged when the biparietal diameter passes the ___. (2 wds).

5 A classic sign of systemic lupus erythematosus (SLE) is a ____ rash, which presents as superficial lesions over the cheeks and nose.

10 True or false: After amniotomy, contractions may intensify.

11 Prefix meaning "bad" or "inadequate".

15 Part of the blood pressure that is due to plasma proteins. (2 wds).

16 Record of muscular activity for diagnostic purposes using electrodes.

19 The process of putting a limb, bone or group of muscles under tension by means of weights and pulleys to align or immobilize the part to reduce muscle spasm or to relieve pressure.

22 Defective, poor, or absent muscle control caused by a nerve lesion. (2 wds).

24 Cutis marmorata is bluish ____ of the skin.

25 The body of the uterus has three layers: _____, myometrium, and endometrium.

DOWN

1 Hypothyroidism slows the _____ rate and mental responses, causing edema, decreased body temperature, and slower respiratory and heart rates.

2 Treatment of anemia by administration of iron compounds.

4 A horizontal plane that divides the body into two sections... upper and lower.

6 Irregular heart rhythm, rate or sequence of cardiac activation.

7 Port-wine stains found on the face or extremities may be associated with soft tissue and bone _____.

8 Indigestion or epigastric pain that may be accompanied by gas or nausea.

9 A severe sensation of burning pain, often in an extremity.

12 A process that occurs during childhood, until cartilaginous tissue is gradually replaced by bony tissue.

13 Excessive leanness earned by muscle wasting.

14 The clitoris consists of the glans, the body, and two ____.

17 These tissues filter out bacteria and other foreign cells, and are grouped by region. (2 wds).

18 Studies show this to be the most severe form of muscular dystrophy.

20 Orthopedic device such as a brace, splint, or collar used to immobilize or correct an orthopedic problem.

21 Type of muscle that bends or flexes a limb or part.

23 Suffix meaning "dissolved substance".

54

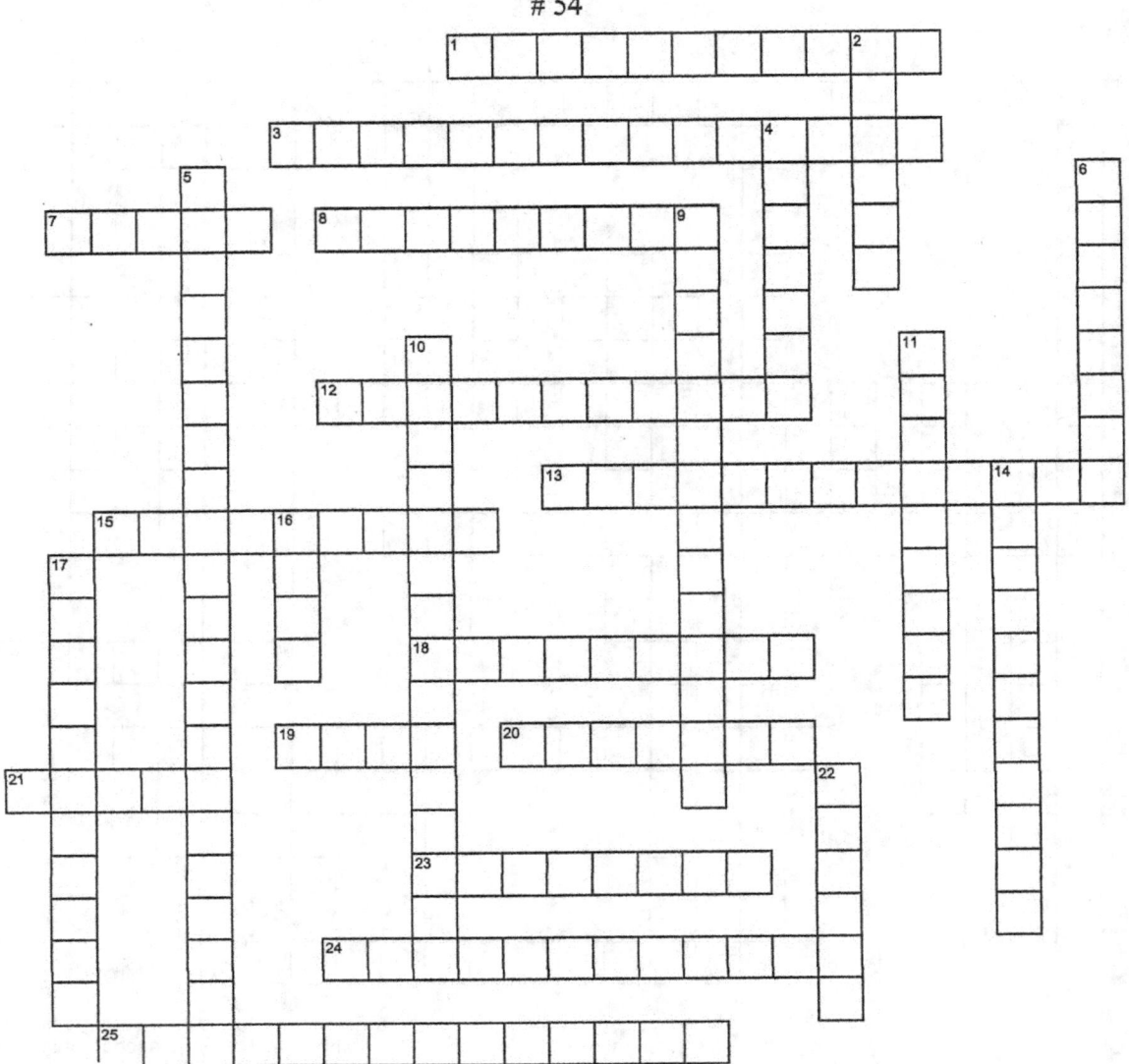

ACROSS

1 Removal of a clot from a blood vessel by surgical or enzymatic methods.
3 Malignant masses on the surface of the liver. (2 wds).
7 Thighbone extending from the hip to the knee.
8 Capillary network of a nephron in the kidney. (2 wds).
12 The bundle of spinal nerves arising from the lumbosacral and lumbar region. (2 wds).
13 Chronic muscle inflammation with hyperplasia of the connective tissue.
15 Depressed point on the surface of the abdomen where the umbilical cord was formerly attached.
18 When a lobe of the lung is removed.
19 True or false: A pericardial friction rub has a scratchy, rubbing quality.
20 Dark green, leafy vegetables are the best non-dairy sources of _____.
21 Patients over the age of ____ should be screened for glaucoma.
23 A long, bladelike spine along the upper half of the scapula bone.
24 Motor movement is regulated by the ____, which consists of the caudate nucleas, putamen, and globus pallidus. (2 wds).
25 The best time to teach a patient postoperative care is _____.

DOWN

2 Multiple sclerosis is caused by loss of the ____ sheath.
4 Presence of any type of cells in the urine.
5 A postviral illness characterized by ascending paralysis. (3 wds).
6 Three tiny bones in each ear. (The malleus, incus, and stapes).
9 A slightly moveable joint where the surfaces of the opposing bones are connected by cartilage.
10 A regular, alternating pattern of weak and strong pulses and is associated with left-sided heart failure. (2 wds).
11 Who should explain a surgical procedure to a patient?
14 Blood chemistry test to determine the total iron-binding capacity of the blood.
16 The ____ lung is smaller than the other, and only has an upper and lower lobe.
17 Anatomical region immediately adjacent to or near the outside surface of the eye.
22 Dyspnea, cough, and palpitations occur with ___ insufficiency.

55

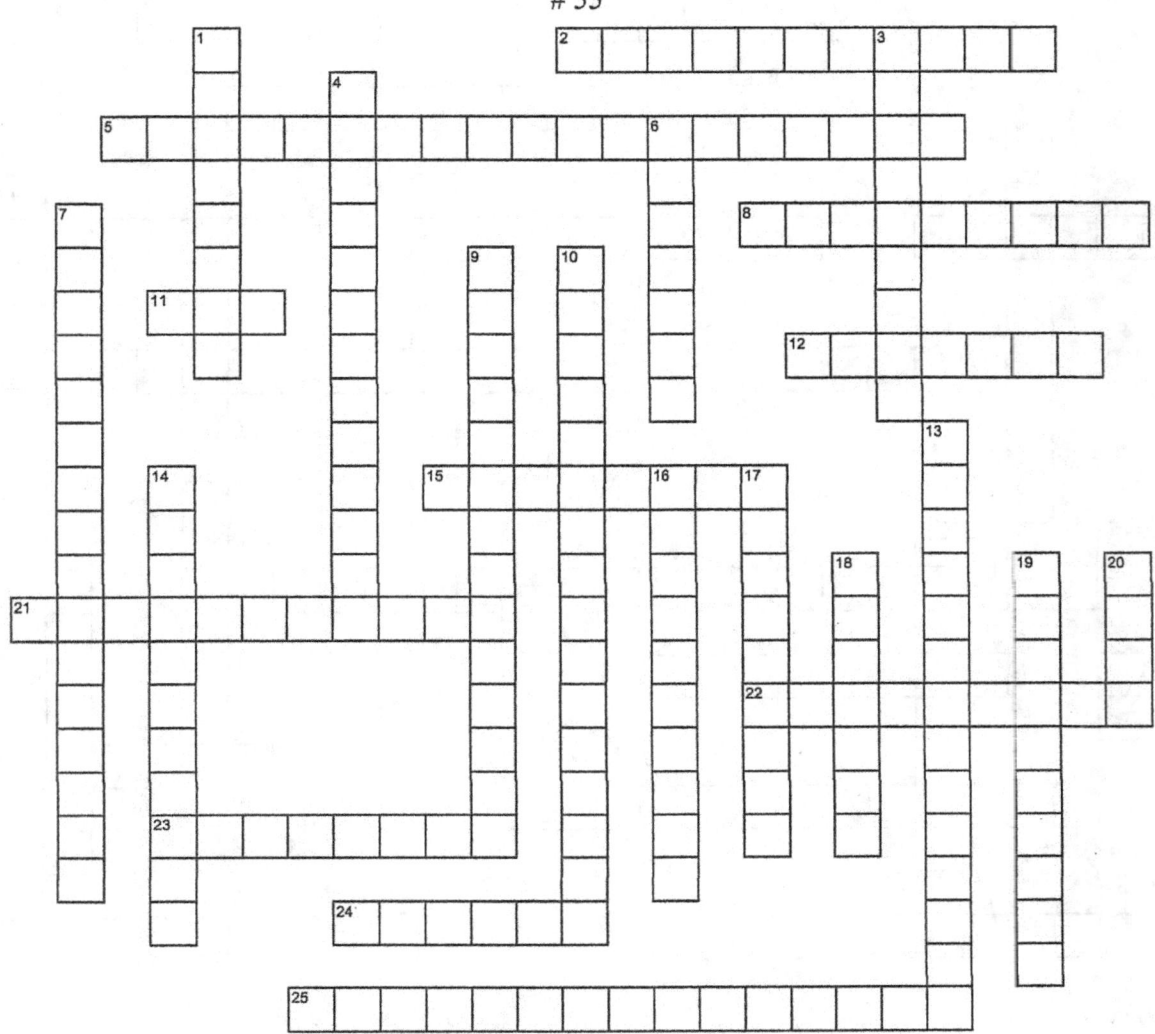

ACROSS

2 A physician who diagnoses and treats patients with skeletal and muscular disorders.

5 A process of converting glucose into energy in the absence of oxygen. (2 wds).

8 Suffix meaning "rupture".

11 Prefix meaning "cold".

12 Fat.

15 A small opening to relieve pressure. Microscopic openings in capillaries for the purpose of filtration within the glomerular capillaries of the kidneys.

21 Excessive flow of tears.

22 Substance that leaks into or out of tissues.

23 Neoplasm of lymph tissue.

24 Hard coverings that result when exudate on the skin dries.

25 Skin lesions due to prolonged pressure. (2 wds).

DOWN

1 Universal precautions are _____ measures to prevent exposure to blood-borne pathogens.

3 Difficulty producing speech with regard to sound quality and pronunciation.

4 A urethrally inserted urine drainage tube with an inflatable retaining balloon. (2 wds).

6 An inability to stand or maintain erect posture due to muscular incoordination.

7 Condition of having numerous elongated cone-shaped keratinic projections on the dorsal surface of the tongue. (2 wds).

9 Degeneration of elastic and connective tissues in the trachea.

10 Muscle of the hand that pulls the thumb across the palm to enable a pinch-type grip. (2 wds).

13 Pooling of blood in the periphery. (2 wds).

14 Type of muscle that controls the movement of the eyes.

16 The fifth cranial nerve is a _____ nerve which stimulates the face and upper neck.

17 Clinical finding of dissimilar proportion in two normally similar body parts.

18 Pain during urination, often caused by infection, irritation or obstruction of the urinary tract.

19 Having the appearance of being pitted or indented.

20 Suffix meaning "pertaining to small size".

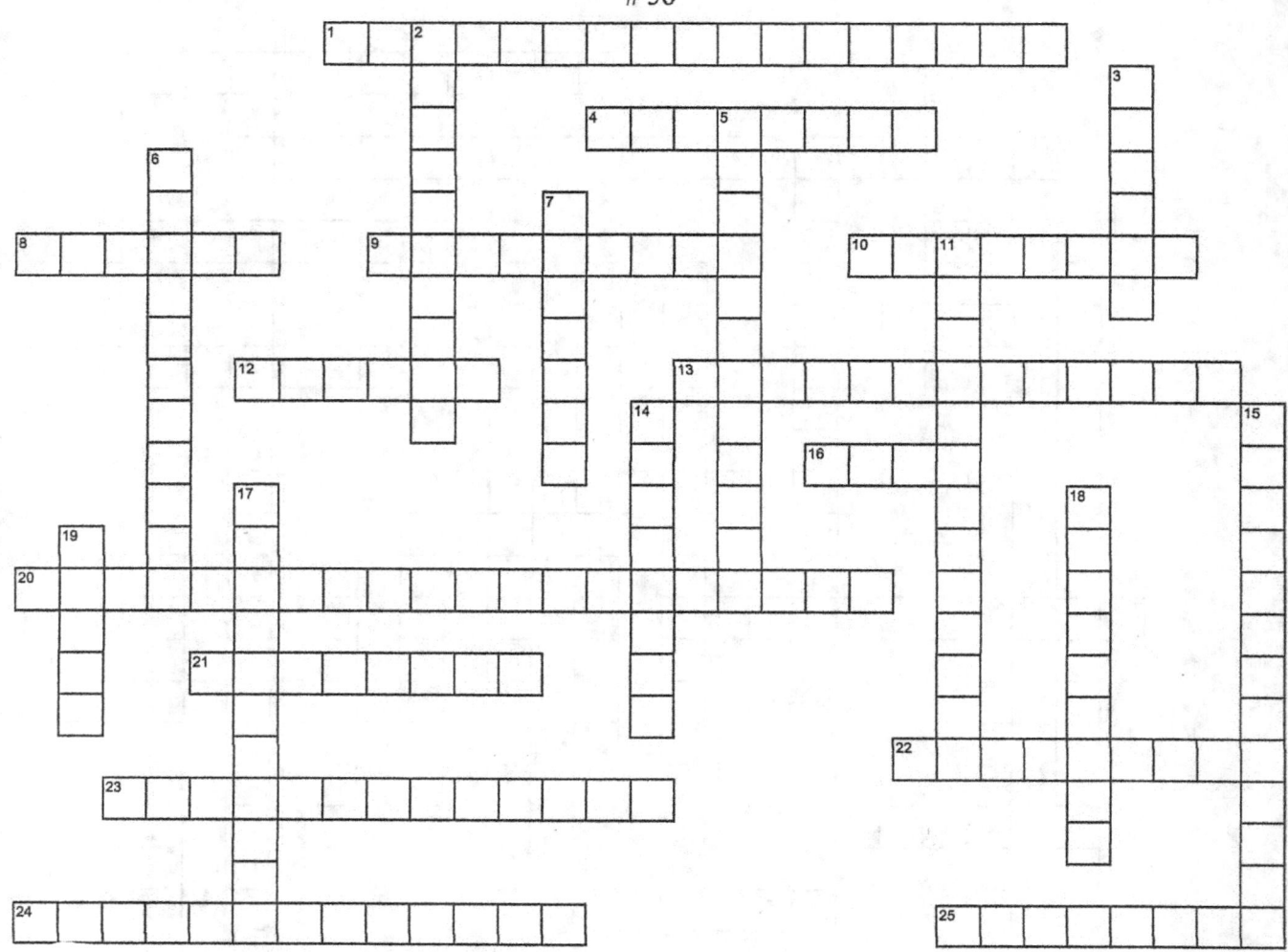

ACROSS

1 Amyotrophic lateral sclerosis (ALS), an idiopathic degenerative disease of upper and lower motor neurons that causes motor weakness and spastic limbs, is also known as _____. (3 wds).
4 Loss of cognitive and intellectual functioning due to a variety of brain disorders.
8 A thick scar that forms over a healed burn.
9 A surgical tool used to cut bone.
10 Inflammation of a gland or lymph node.
12 An amygdaloid body is an _____-shaped area of grey, unmyelinated nerve tissue located in each temporal lobe that plays a major role in processing memory and sensing dangerous situations.
13 Dilation of a heart valve to relieve stenosis by balloon dilatation during cardiac catheterization or surgery.
16 Prefix meaning "within" or "inside".
20 Repair of a septal defect using a septal occluder or Rashkind device during cardiac catherization. (2 wds).
21 Clumps of gel or cellular debris within the vitreous; small specks seen moving across the visual field.
22 An antibody or other substance that attacks the cells, preventing their normal function and/or destroying them.
23 Documentation method using a columnar format to chart data, action and response. (2 wds).
24 Involuntary contraction of muscles of teh eyelid.
25 Increase or abnormal growth of fibrous or connective tissue in reparative or reactive processes.

DOWN

2 A noninvasive procedure that generates images via computer analysis to assess blood-flow velocity, direction, and occlusions. It uses a transducer, which is placed over the blood vessel, and a computer, which analyzes the echoes for aberrations.
3 One of the seven bones of the ankle.
5 Inflammation of the brain due to bacterial or viral infection.
6 When a body has a water deficit.
7 Formation of attachment between parent and child. Also means the adhesion of one substance to another.
11 Intentional obstruction of the lumen of a blood vessel by injection of a solution or dislodgement of thrombus or plaque.
14 An illness acquired by ingesting improperly cooked or canned food containing Clostridium botulinum. It causes paralysis, and may be fatal.
15 Circulation of lymph through the lymphatic vessels and lymph nodes.
17 A yellow-colored spot visible on the retina near the optic nerve of the retina that contains the fovea centralis, which is the point of greatest visual focus. (2 wds).
18 Estimation of the size, age, and growth of a fetus using ultrasonography.
19 Laryngotracheobronchitis in infants and young children caused by bacterial or viral infection of the pharynx. Characterized by difficult and noisy respiration and a hoarse cough.

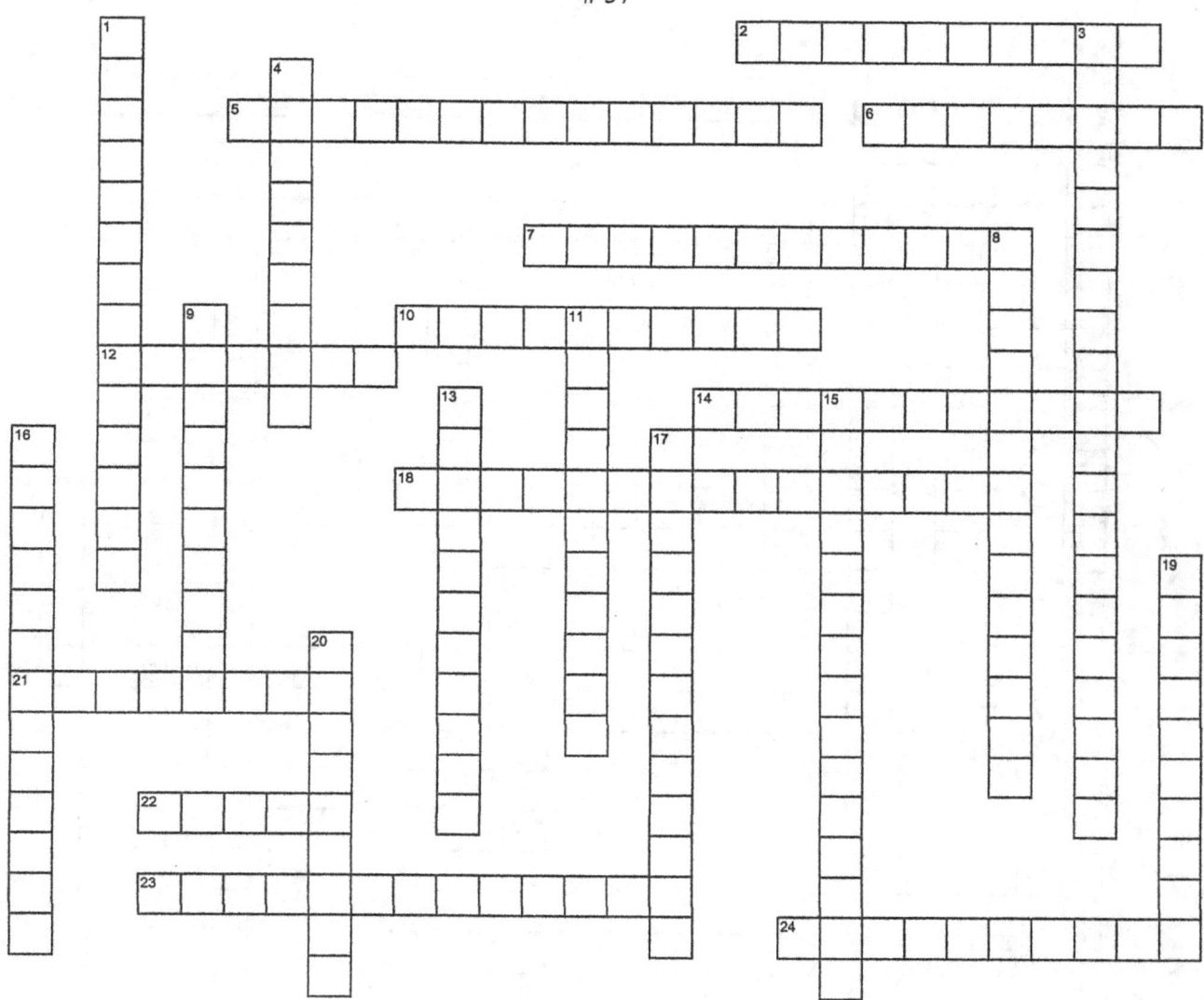

ACROSS

2 A vascular channel that transports lymph.
5 Outside the body.
6 Blood chemistry test used to diagnose iron deficiency anemia, that indirectly measures the amount of iron stored in the body by measuring the small amount that is always present in the blood.
7 Progressive destruction of cells due to disease or aging process.
10 Process of elimination of end products of digestion by bowel movement.
12 Pertaining to the skull or head.
14 Wave pattern on an electroencephalogram typical of deep sleep. (2 wds).
18 Insertion of a flexible tube into a body cavity for the instillation or withdrawal of fluid.
21 Suffix meaning "weakness", or "decreased strength".
22 Suffix meaning "secretion of a substance".
23 Uncontrollable, localized contraction of a single muscle group that is visible through the skin.
24 Surgical removal or extensive incision.

DOWN

1 Cancer tumor, mass gland.

3 Disorganized or agitated behavior commonly associated with dementia when the individual faces overwhelming or threatening situations that are beyond his or her coping ability. (2 wds).
4 Type of asthma caused by an environmental allergen.
8 Developmental stage that occurs during the first two-eight weeks after fertilization of a human egg. (2 wds).
9 Monocyte cells that have migrated from circulation into tissues and are responsible for immune response by engulfing and ingesting foreign antigens.
11 Bluish discoloration around the umbilicus in postoperative clients. It can indicate intra-abdominal or perineal bleeding. (2 wds).
13 Injection of solutions, blood, and/or chemotherapeutic agents into a vein for therapeutic purposes.
15 Narrowing of the lumen of the trachea.
16 Intravascular insertion of a tubular meshwork to keep an artery open. (2 wds).
17 Surgical removal of a vein after ligation of varicose veins. (2 wds).
19 Component of cognitive development that refers to the changes that occur as a result of assimilation and accommodation. An ongoing process by which an individual adjusts to stressors in order to achieve homeostasis.
20 The five lower costal bones on either side of the chest that do not attach directly to the sternum. (2 wds).

58

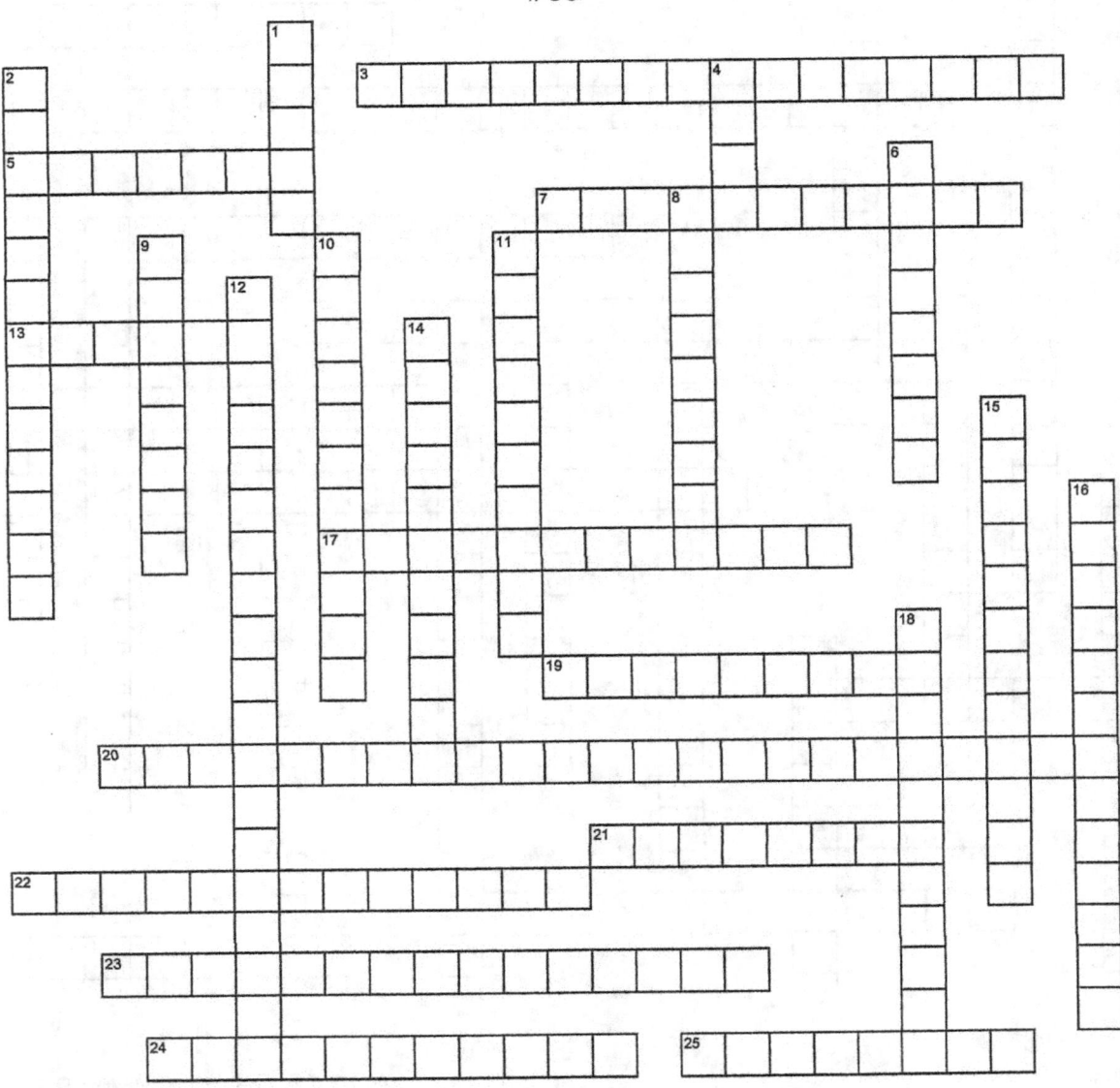

ACROSS

3 Pharmacological agent used to decrease blood glucose levels. (2 wds).
5 Bony structure that contains the brain.
7 Localized freezing of diseased tissues for surgical removal.
13 Connecting parts of a structure.
17 Surgical replacement of a joint.
19 Burning tissue with thermal heat using electricity, steam, laser, or dry ice, often to destroy diseased tissue or coagulate blood vessels.
20 Temporary interference with blood supply to the brain by small clots, causing no permanent brain damage. (3 wds).
21 A fixed false belief that is sustained even when provided evidence to the contrary, due to psychosis or delirium.
22 Blood vessel of the medial aspect of the thigh that carries oxygenated blood. It originates at the external iliac artery and terminates at the popliteal artery behind the knee. (2 wds).
23 Surgical excision of the scrotal sac and dilated veins.
24 Condition of fixed resistance to the passive stretch of a muscle, associated with paralysis or lack of use of a muscle group.
25 Lacking strength. Weakness.

DOWN

1 Suffix meaning "skin".

2 Protrusion or herniation of the brain and meninges.
4 A toothlike projection from the second cervical vertebra (C2), upon which the head rotates.
6 Distention of the colon with gas.
8 Lung disease that causes the patient to assume an upright or semi-upright position in order to breathe and sleep comfortably.
9 Lymphatic tissue on the back of the nasopharynx.
10 Cells that break down areas of old or damaged bone.
11 Tissue in the central cavity of long bones that functions to store fat or produce red blood cells. (2 wds).
12 Loss of central vision due to disruption of the integrity of the retina. (2 wds).
14 The process of swallowing and/or passing food, liquid or air.
15 Abnormally slow speech.
16 Factors or body actions that contribute to lymph circulation. Includes arterial pulses, passive compression of soft body tissues, postural changes, and skeletal muscle contractions.
18 To increase in speed or rate.

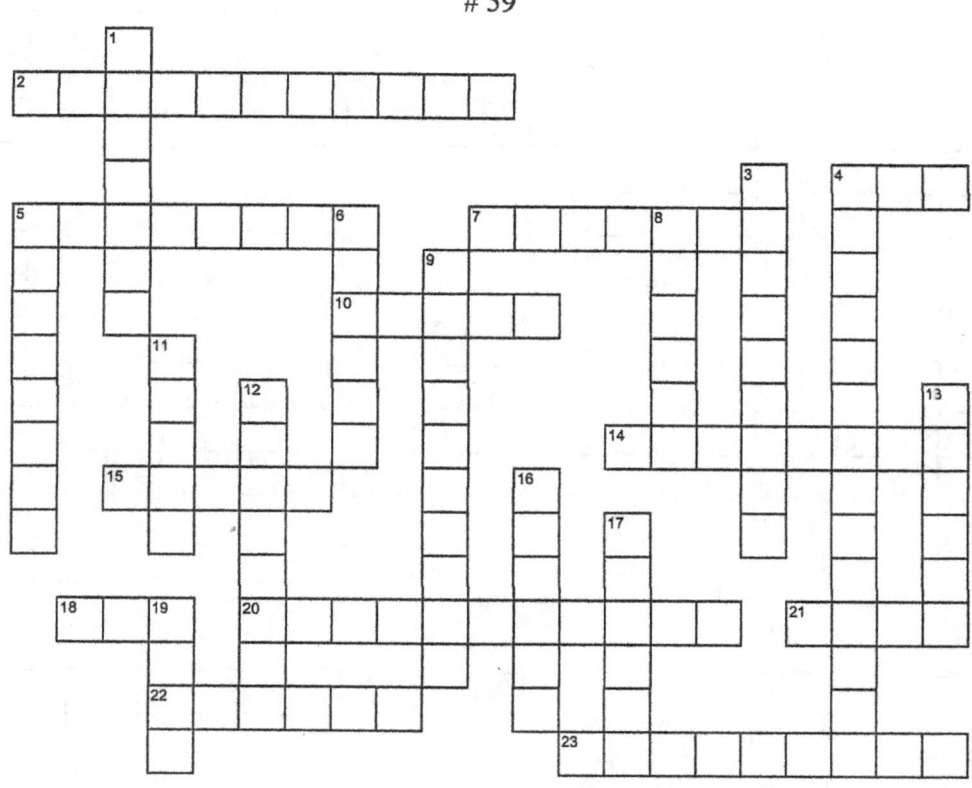

ACROSS

2 The process of exchanging oxygen and carbon dioxide in the body. Breathing movements.

4 Prefix meaning "before".

5 Front of the body.

7 Bone of the upper jaw.

10 A cup-shaped structure within an organ, such as the kidney.

14 An enzyme that splits organic compounds such as fats.

15 Soft blowing sound heard on auscultation, caused by turbulent blood flow.

18 Suffix meaning "small".

20 To gasp. Sudden or temporary loss of breath. (2 wds).

21 The crystalline structure of the eye.

22 In a contained or localized position, not extending beyond the point of origin. (2 wds).

23 The appearance of being without jaundice.

DOWN

1 Inflammation and pain in the loins originating from the psoas muscle.

3 The largest bone of the foot, also called the heel.

4 Type of muscle that flexes a joint. (2 wds).

5 Agents used to neutralize acids, most commonly in the stomach.

6 A short, straight segment of bowel connecting the sigmoid colon to the outside of the body.

8 Transitional area of cornea where the cornea is overlapped by the sclera.

9 Brain waves typical of a person who is awake and at rest. (2 wds).

11 Prefix meaning "behind" or "backward".

12 Female external genitalia.

13 An opening or tunnel that connects internal and external surfaces.

16 Washing out of a hollow organ using a flow of liquid.

17 Disorder of the foot associated with swelling and inflammation of the great toe.

19 Suffix meaning "condition or state of being".

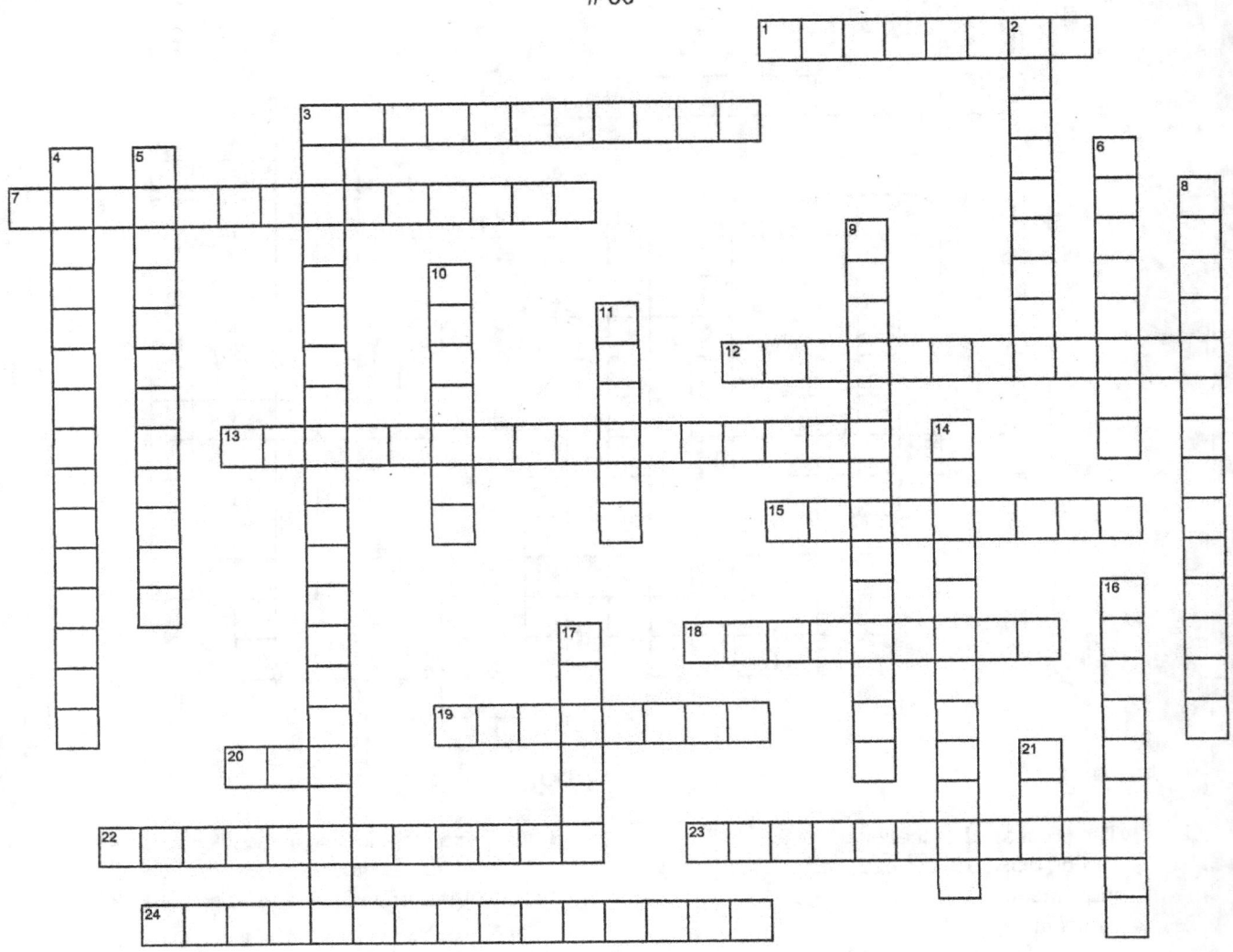

ACROSS

1 Pertaining to the duodenum.
3 Use of cold in the treatment of a disease or injury.
7 Narrowing of the lacrimal duct due to cysts, tumors, or stone formation.
12 Inability to discern an object by touch alone.
13 Softening of the brain due to ischemia or infarction.
15 Patient with asthma.
18 Wedge-shaped bones of the hand.
19 Increased urine formation and secretion.
20 Prefix meaning "through", "throughout" or "completely".
22 _____ defiant disorder is a persistent, aggressive behavior, defiance of and refusal to obey rules, disrespect for authority figures, with anger, stubbornness, and touchiness.
23 An inability to choose words that accurately reflect thoughts and/or to speak correct words due to a cerebral lesion.
24 Vestibular folds in the larynx that do not produce sounds. (3 wds).

DOWN

2 Discomfort identified by sudden onset and relatively short duration, mild to severe intensity, and a steady decrease in intensity over several days or weeks. (2 wds).
3 Concept that states that clinicians should act only if the action is based on a principle that is universal. (2 wds).
4 Development of new blood vessels in tissue such as the myocardium.
5 The long, spiral-shaped structure that extends along the floor of the cochlear duct and is stimulated by sound waves. (3 wds).
6 The smooth muscle of the bladder wall.
8 A person's belief that he or she has been assigned the wrong gender identity, and needs to change his or her outward appearance to the opposite sex.
9 Degenerative joint disease characterized by deterioration of articular cartilage and bone hypertrophy.
10 A transurethral resection is the surgical removal of a structure performed through the _____.
11 Layer of skin below the epidermis.
14 A diagnostic study in which an isotope is injected into the patient's blood, taken up by the lymphatic system, and visualized through radiographic pictures.
16 Premature upstroke of the initial polarization of the heart. A complex of an electrocardiogram finding associated with an atrioventricular bypass tract. (2 wds).
17 Pertaining to the back part.
21 Prefix meaning "faulty", "painful", "difficult" or "abnormal".

61

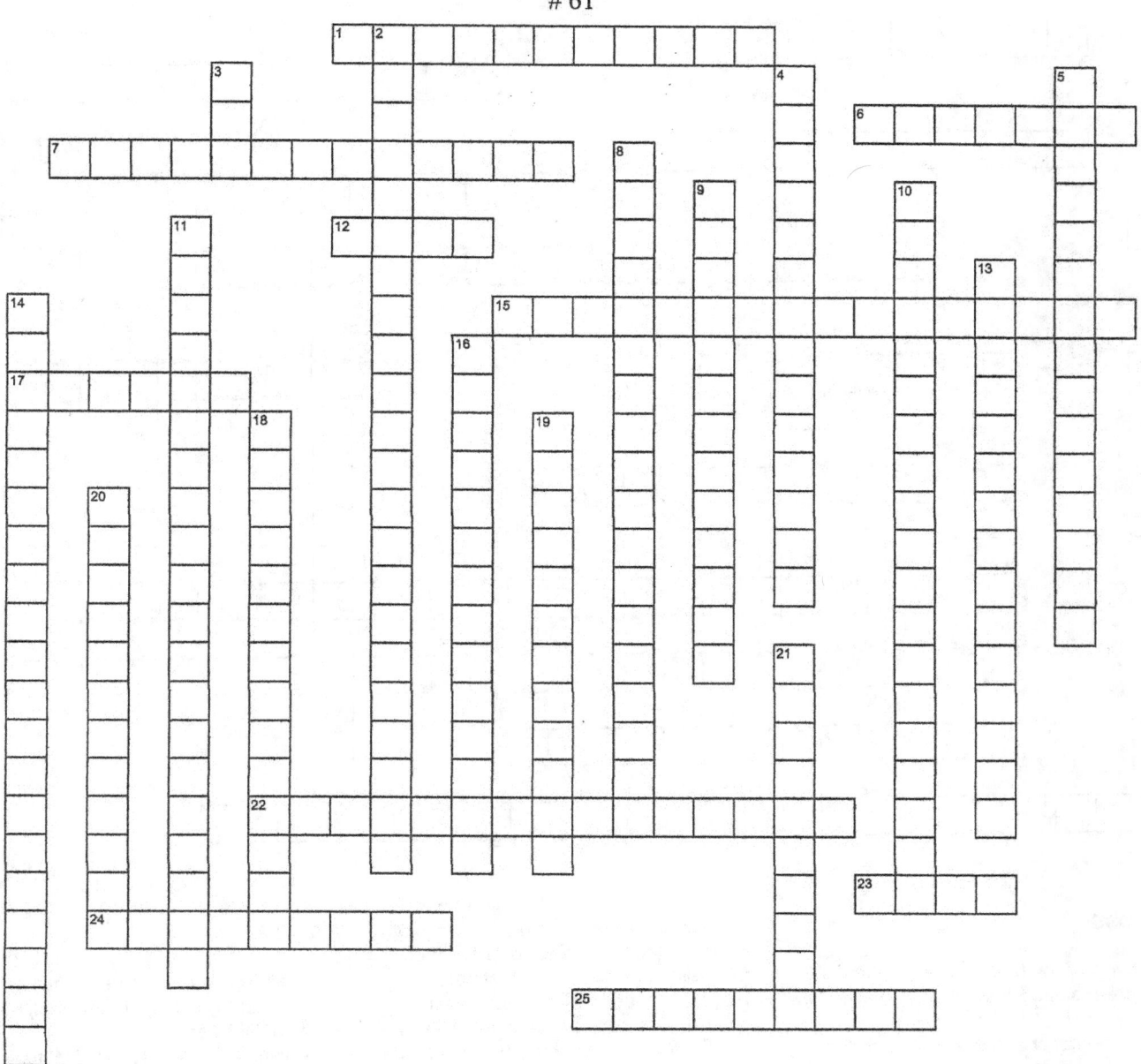

ACROSS

1 Severe state of disorganization that occurs when the individual's usual coping mechanisms, physical or emotional, are no longer effective. (2 wds).
6 The intensity of a sound or tone. Measurement noted on audiograms and other assessments of hearing.
7 Damage to tissue of the vein and surrounding structures when a chemotherapeutic drug leaks into the soft tissue surrounding the infusion site.
12 Suffix meaning "measured quantity or amount".
15 Sac-shaped outward bulge on an artery. (2 wds).
17 Outward display on the face.
22 The change in electrical charge within a nerve or muscle when stimulated. (2 wds).
23 A pair, or two people in an interaction, often used to describe a mother and newborn.

24 The degree of compliance or continuance of a therapeutic action.
25 Pharmacological agents that increase urinary output.

DOWN

2 Psychiatric disorder characterized by marked disturbance in thought process, stupor, negativism, and rigidity alternating with periods of great excitement. (2 wds).
3 Transposition of the great arteries. (3 initials).
4 Failure of one or both testicles to descend.
5 An abnormal, excessive C or S shaped lateral curvature of the spine.
8 The smooth, nonvascular, dense connective tissue that covers the end surfaces of bones forming synovial joints. (2 wds).
9 The clumping together of cells as a result of interaction with specific antibodies called agglutinins.

10 Disease that affects both the brain and spinal cord.
11 Radiological procedure that uses orally ingested tablets of radiopaque contrast dye. (2 wds).
13 The muscle that compresses the lips. (2 wds).
14 The inverted treelike structure of the trachea, main stem bronchi, and bronchioles. (2 wds).
16 Injection of a hypertonic solution, causing the vein to harden and eventually atrophy. (2 wds).
18 A medical device that delivers an electric shock to the atria or ventricles of the heart to restore normal heart rhythm.
19 Exceedingly rapid contractions or twitching of muscular fibrils, but not of the muscle as a whole.
20 Tumor made up of lymph vessels.
21 Sensory nerve fibers of the spinal cord. (2 wds).

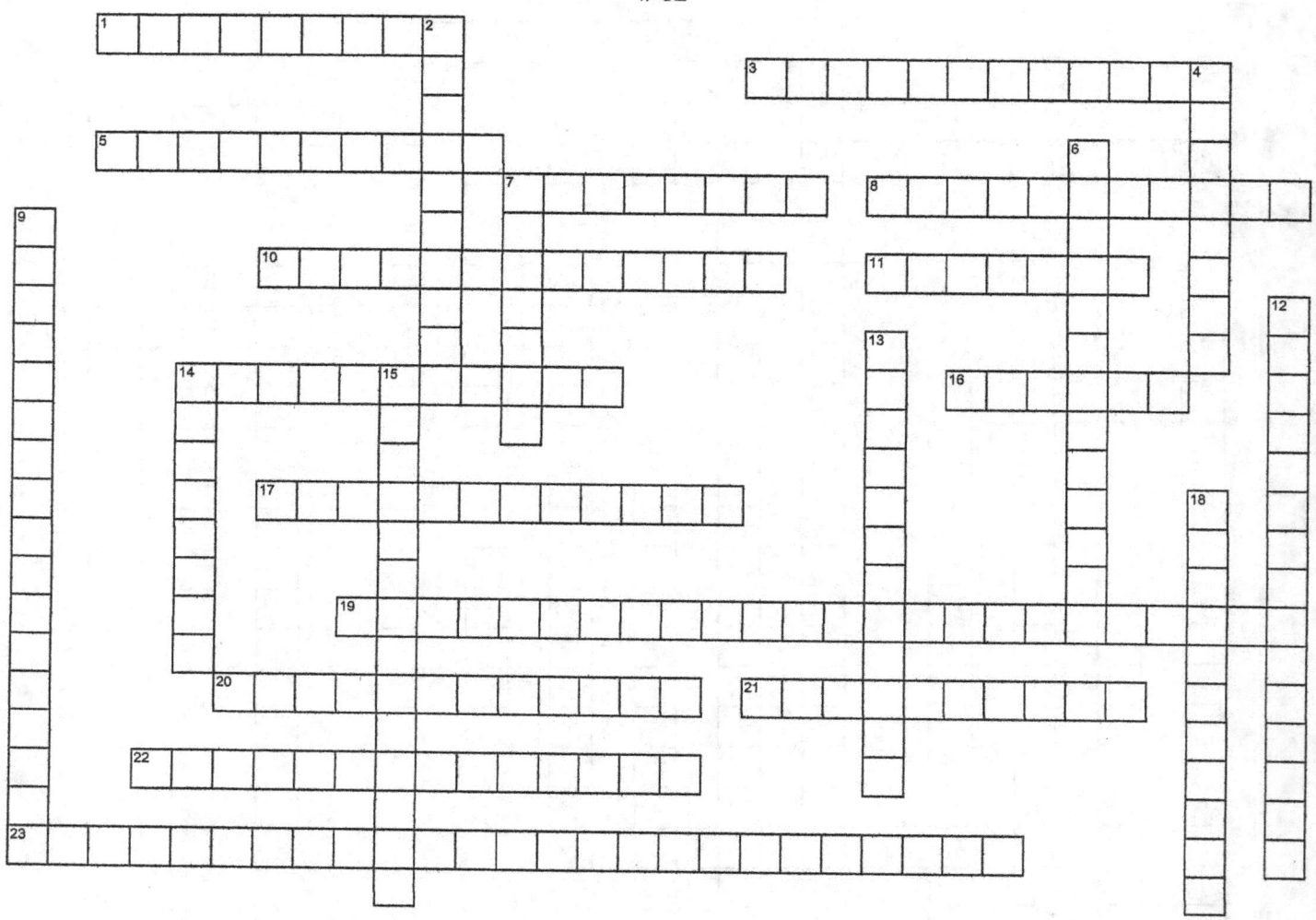

ACROSS

1 Deformity of the angle of the femoral neck resulting in outward displacement. (2 wds)

3 Not demonstrating external signs or complaints of a disease.

5 A substance in urine that is found in elevated quantities in patients with muscular dystrophy and other pathologies.

7 To transport or carry toward the center. Nerves that return impulses to the central nervous system.

8 Leukocytes found in lymphatic tissue.

10 Union of the sperm and egg that develops into an embryo.

11 Determination of blood flow. Velocity, direction, and possible occlusion using a transducer placed over the blood vessel.

14 Cauda equina syndrome is the _____ of nerve roots of the sacral and coccygeal nerves resulting in numbness in the buttocks, genitalia, or thigh along with disturbed bowel and bladder function.

16 Away from the center or point of origin.

17 Malignant bone tumor that occurs predominantly in adolescents and is usually located at the metaphysis of the distal femur, proximal tibia or proximal humerus.

19 Surgical procedure that is an alternative to a total knee replacement. Used to treat middle-age adults with degenerative joint disease of the knee to delay the need for total knee replacement surgery. (2 wds).

20 Widespread muscle and joint pain of unknown origin.

21 Excessive secretion of the growth hormone somatotropin that produces enlargement of head, face, hands and feet.

22 Turbulent blood flow due to incomplete closure of the heart. (2 wds).

23 Loss of control of urine flow caused when the sphincter mechanism has been bypassed. (2 wds).

DOWN

2 A large group of viruses causing common colds and upper respiratory tract infections.

4 Hydrocortisone secreted by the adrenal cortex.

6 Procedure of using bone taken from the patient's own body to use to stabilize and fuse with bony structures. (2 wds).

7 A lack of normal thirst.

9 Inability to control defecation. (2 wds).

12 Degeneration and necrosis of the growth center of bones.

13 An incision into the trachea creating a permanent opening to allow for a patent or open airway.

14 Crunching or grinding sounds produced in certain pathological states such as severe arthritis or pneumonia.

15 Cerebral dysfunction due to an insult to the brain such as a toxin, injury, inflammation or anoxic event.

18 Muscle that closes the eyelid.

63

ACROSS

2 Administration of electrical shock to restore cardiac muscle conduction and contractions.

6 Physical and/or psychological symptoms that are consciously fabricated by the patient. Pretending to be sick, often with symptoms that are difficult to evaluate. (2 wds).

8 Formation of bone fragments in the joint due to inflammation.

9 Pertaining to the esophagus.

14 Infection with the protozoa from the genus Cryptosporidium that is transmitted through exposure to contaminated food or may be sexually transmitted. (symptoms include diarrhea and abdominal cramps).

19 Treatment of skin disorders using rays such as ultraviolet radiation.

20 Suffix meaning "the branched portion of a nerve cell that receives an impulse".

22 A potent vasodilator used to perform cardiovascular perfusion studies without having the client exercise.

24 Surgical procedure that uses a fiberoptic scope to visualize a joint and remove tissues such as damaged cartilage or bone spurs.

25 A plasma coagulation factor syntehsized in the liver.

DOWN

1 Suffix meaning "pertaining or related to".

3 Decrease in the diameter of a blood vessel.

4 Fetal development which is impaired by maternal consumption of alcohol. (3 wds).

5 Muscle that circles the eye. (2 wds).

7 Dermatological procedure that mechanically scrapes away skin layers.

10 Muscle of the thigh and one of five medial femoral muscles. It functions to adduct and flex the thigh. (2 wds).

11 Establishment of artificial lymph ducts to bypass areas of blocked lymphatic circulation.

12 Any measure or action taken to prevent disease.

13 Hardening of the brain, especially the cerebrum, due to plaque formation or hypertension.

15 Congenital disorder characterized by mental retardation, small head, small stature, generalized failure to thrive, and hirsutism. (3 wds).

16 Structure of respiration located in the left chest, composed of the superior, middle and inferior lobes. (2 wds).

17 Loss of the sense of smell.

18 Formation of firm, densely fibrous, benign tumors in glandular tissue, frequently observed in a breast.

21 Prefix meaning "left".

23 Transmyocardial revascularization is the use of a _____ to open small channels in the heart muscle to restore blood flow in patients with angina associated with advanced coronary artery disease. This is done when other surgical interventions are not viable.

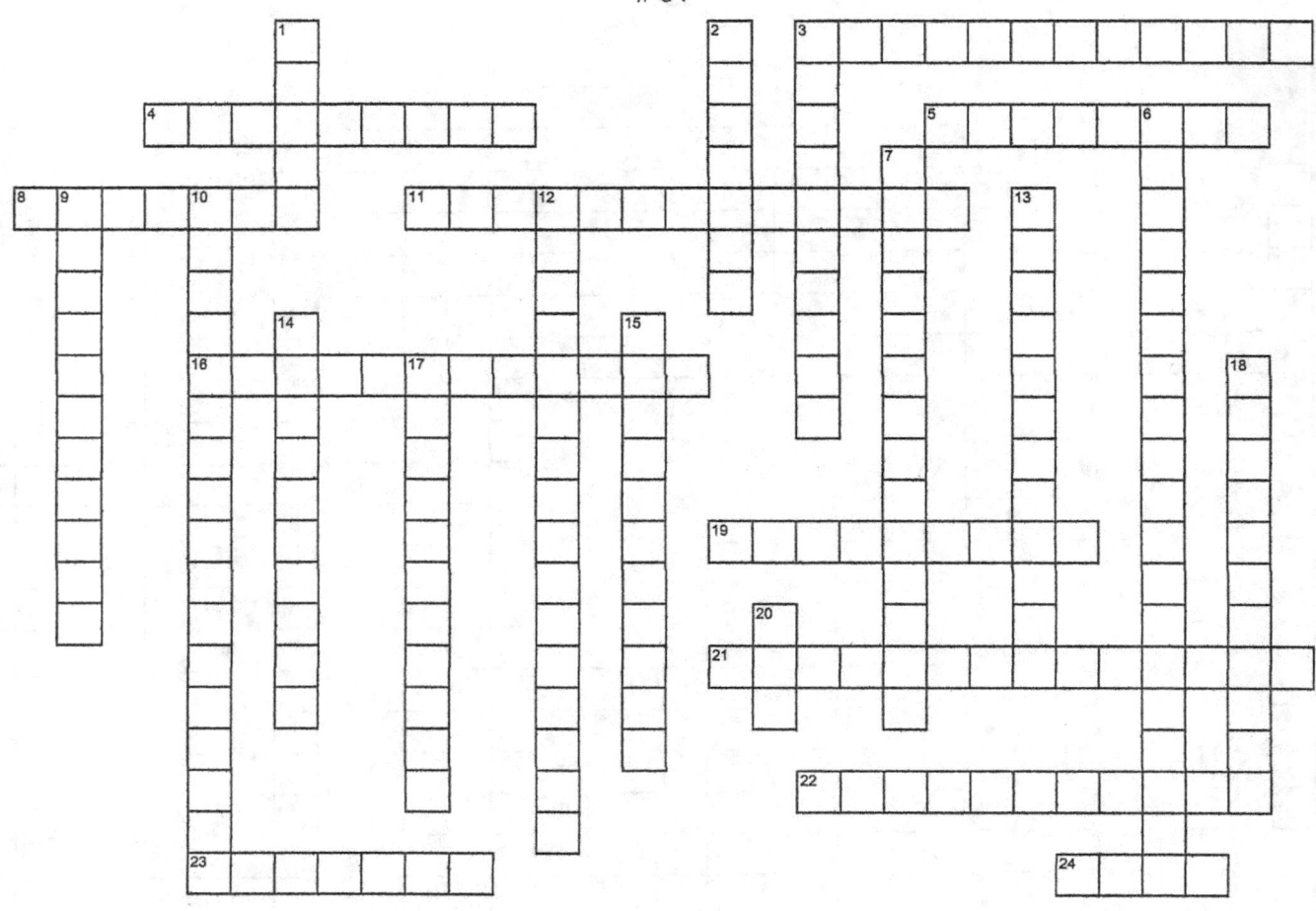

ACROSS

3 Pertaining to muscles in spaces between the ribs.

4 A fibro-optical device used for direct visualization of an embryo.

5 Strong, fibrous bands of connective tissue that function to hold the two bone ends to a muscle or organ.

8 Enzyme that converts maltose to glucose.

11 Surgical puncture to remove fluid from the cul-de-sac of Douglas.

16 Drugs that widen blood vessels, decreasing blood pressure.

19 Hormone produced by the anterior pituitary gland that stimulates breast development and lactation during pregnancy.

21 Generalized skeletal dysplasia with prominent forehead and small mandible. Irregular ribbon-like constrictions of the ribs and tubular bones demonstrated on x-rays.

22 Blood vessel of the thigh that returns blood from the lower leg, starting at the popliteal vein and ending at the iliac vein. (2 wds).

23 Adjective form referring to the tongue.

24 Transcutaneous electrical nerve stimulation. The application of mild electrical current to the skin over a painful region, providing pain relief by interfering with transmission of pain signals. (4 initials).

DOWN

1 Suffix meaning "running".

2 Pertaining to a daily occurrence of body rhythms, such as circadian rhythm.

3 Visual observation of external surfaces or internal body cavities.

6 The paired, bilateral blood vessels of the neck that return blood from the head and neck to the heart. (3 wds)

7 Loss of information as to person, date, time, surroundings, and situation, caused by acute illness or dementia.

9 Malignant tumor of the brain or spinal cord composed of astrocytes, with typical onset in the fifth decade of life.

10 An agent given by mouth or nasogastric tube to absorb toxic substances in the stomach. (2 wds).

12 Neurological response to percussion of tendons which produces muscular contraction as demonstrated by the patellar and Achilles reflexes. (3 wds).

13 Inflammation of the lymph vessels.

14 Removal of fluid or accumulation from the body by suction. Also, inhalation of a substance or object into the airway, such as food or drink.

15 Surgical procedure of opening the skull and removing a portion of the bone.

17 Collective group of multifunctional cytokines.

18 The process of chewing.

20 Prefix meaning "same" or "equal".

65

ACROSS

2 To warm or to make hot, as in applying a hot compress.

6 Liquid in the body that is outside the cells. (2 wds).

9 Loss of bone structure when the rate of resorption exceeds new bone formation. It results in demineralized bone that is at risk for fractures.

10 Suffix meaning "seizure".

14 A muscle of the pelvic floor that supports the pelvic organs. (2 wds).

16 A slender, elongated pocket of synovial membrane that contains synovial fluid and acts as a cushion to reduce friction in areas where a tendon rubs against a bone.

17 Congenital hypothyroidism that can cause mental retardation if left untreated.

19 To cut across a plane to study tissue or cells. (2 wds).

21 Abnormal fibrous bands of tissue that form after abdominal or other surgeries.

22 Large furuncle.

23 Physical sign of pathology in the corticospinal tracts characterized by flexion of the arms and legs. (2 wds).

24 Defective use of the insulin that is produced. (2 wds).

25 Plastic surgery performed to correct drooping breasts to improve their look and form.

DOWN

1 Actions causing injury, harm, or destruction to a patient.

3 Large muscle mass of the upper leg composed of four smaller muscles which work together to extend the leg and are often referred to as quadriceps. (3 wds).

4 The left lower chamber of the heart that receives blood from the left atrium and pumps it out to the body through the aorta. (2 wds).

5 Process of taking deliberate action that will hasten the client's death. (2 wds).

7 The efferent passage for lymph. (2 wds).

8 Electrical stimulation of the heart that sets a rate that is independent of the heart's own pacemakers. (2 wds).

11 Suffix meaning "indicating frenzy or a hyperexcited state".

12 Softening of the bone due to vitamin D deficiency in adults.

13 The largest muscle of the anterior lateral aspect of the femoral shaft that extends the lower leg. (2 wds).

15 Extrapyramidal side effects. An untoward effect of neuroleptic medications with distressing symptoms including tremors, bradykinesia, dystonia, and restless movements of the mouth, legs and hands. (3 initials).

18 The muscle that abducts the upper arm.

20 Malignant, carcinoma.

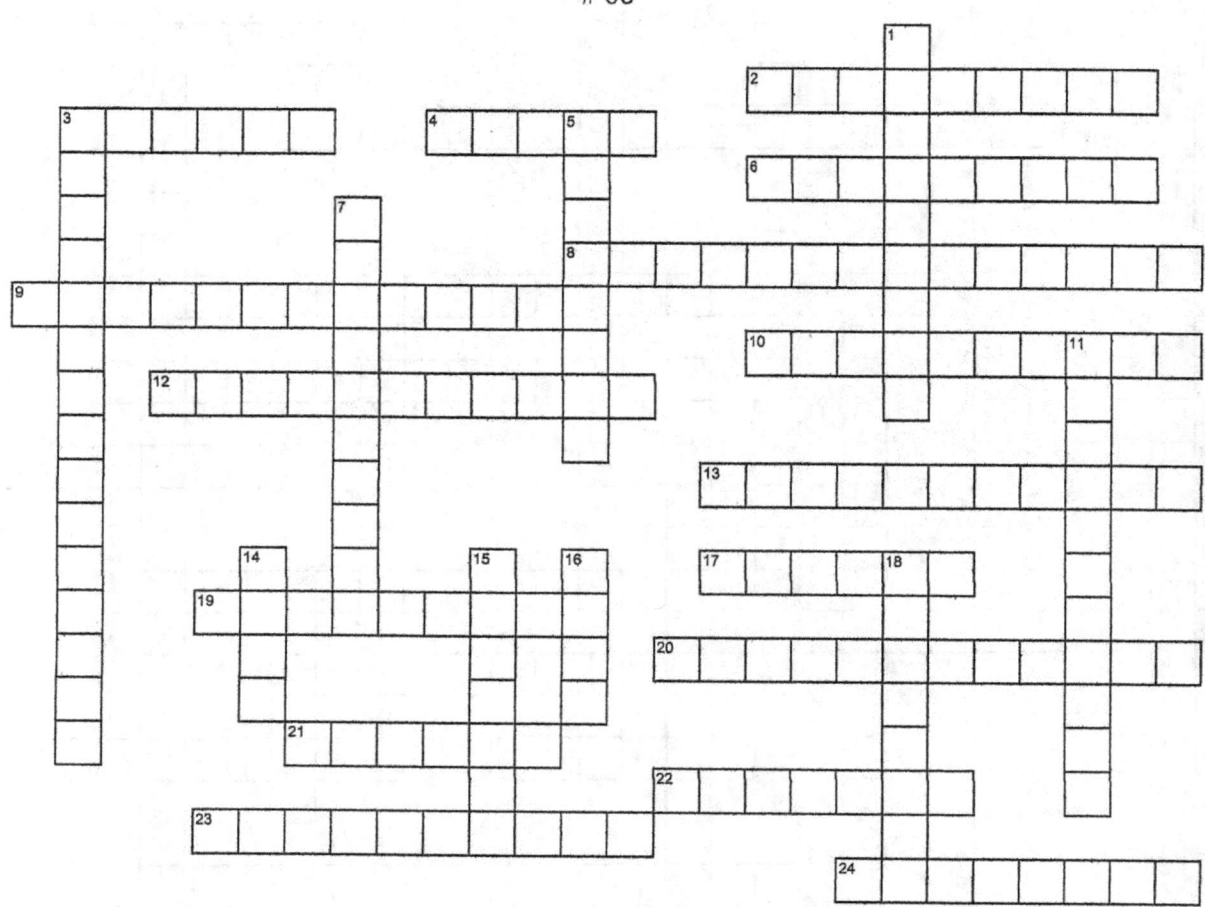

ACROSS

2 The moving back or shortening of, for example, a muscle.
3 Ions with a negative charge.
4 Suffix meaning "to cut or incise".
6 A naturally occurring estrogen that is formed by the ovary, placenta, testes, and adrenal cortex.
8 Main blood vessel bringing blood to the arm, branching off the subclavian artery and terminating at the cubital fossa of the elbow. (2 wds).
9 A nerve cell that senses change in position or location of body parts.
10 The fibrous sheath that surrounds each bundle of skeletal muscle fibers.
12 The inability to perceive neurological deficits such as paralysis or loss of vision.
13 Paired blood vessels of the kidneys that supply oxygenated blood to the kidneys, suprarenal glands, and ureters. (2 wds).
17 Pertaining to the area of the lower back between the ribs and pelvis.
19 To cut out and remove.
20 Psychiatric condition where the patient has signs and symptoms of pregnancy including lack of menses, morning sickness, and weight gain, but is not pregnant.

21 Suffix meaning "specialist in study or treatment of a clinical area".
22 The fallopian tube.
23 To move backward to a previous state of events, previous development, or primitive behavior.
24 Lymphatic capillaries in the small intestine that absorb and transport fatty acids and other fat soluble substances through the lymphatic system.

DOWN

1 Severe pain along the course of a nerve.
3 Drug effect contrary to what is therapeutically intended. (2 wds).
5 The middle region of the brain stem responsible for auditory and visual reflex centers.
7 Instrument used to visualize the rectum.
11 Muscle group that contracts and relaxes the rib cage during respiration.
14 Prefix meaning "around".
15 The division of cells in the body in which the 46 chromosomes in the nucleus duplicate and then split, creating two identical cells, each with 46 chromosomes.
16 Prefix meaning "before".
18 Partial or complete lack of hair.

67

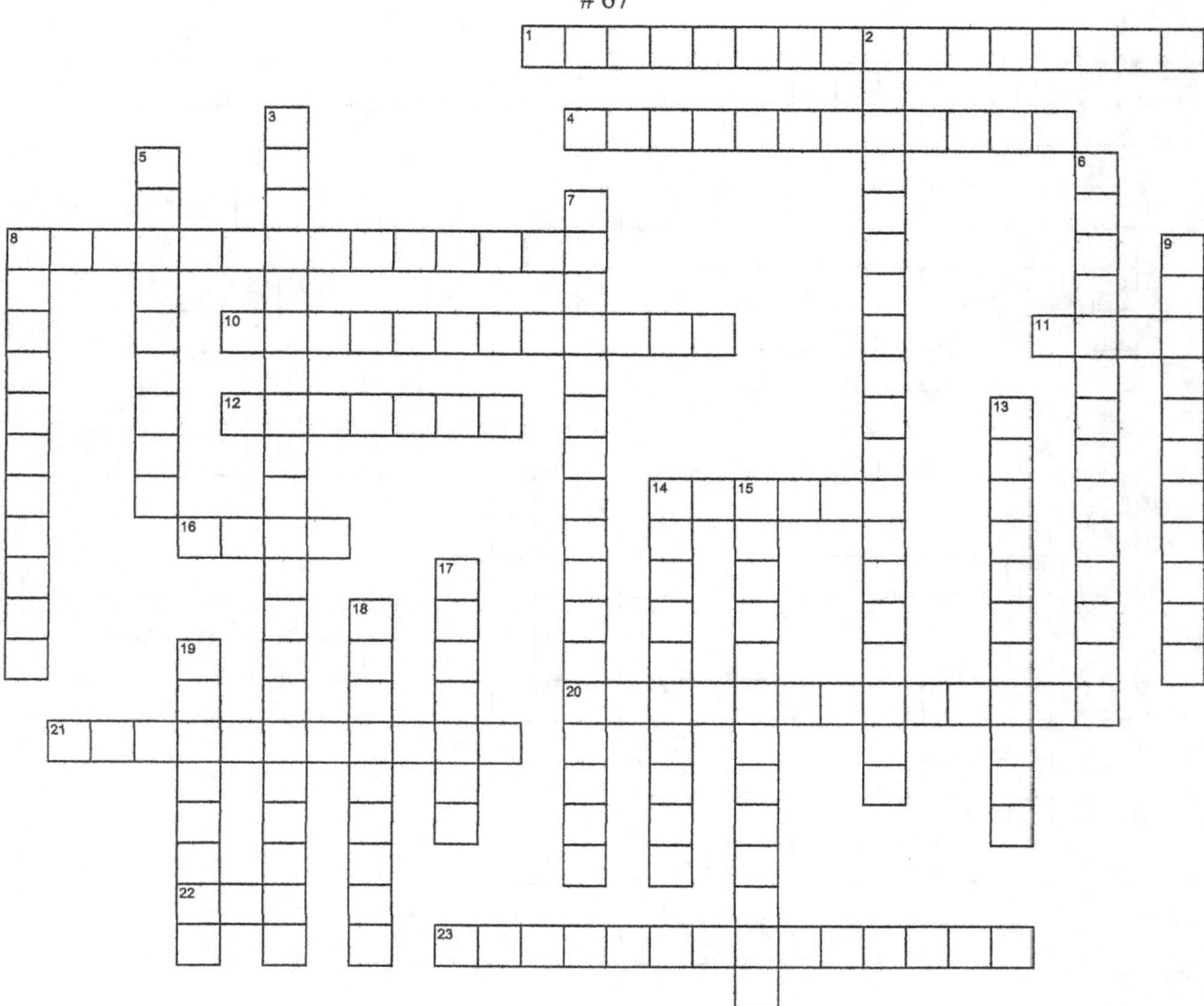

ACROSS

1 Localized thickening and scaling of the outer layers of the skin as a result of prolonged exposure to the sun. (2 wds).

4 Increase in the actual number of leukocytes in the blood.

8 Channels that collect lymph from organs and regions of the body. (2 wds).

10 Abnormally slow movement.

11 Extremely enlarged, tender lymph node of the groin that may be associated with syphilis, chancroid, or lymphogranuloma venarum.

12 A febrile illness with malaise, headache, fatigue, and muscular aches due to infection by protozoa from the genus Plasmodium.

14 A small area of the stomach at the point nearest the heart where the esophagus joins the stomach.

16 Prefix meaning "same" or "like self".

20 Inflammation of the bone and bone marrow.

21 Rotation of an organ or structure in such a manner as to cut off function and/or blood supply.

22 Suffix meaning "person or category of agent".

23 The reduction of the membrane potential in nerve or muscle cells to a less negative value.

DOWN

2 The large, more superficial division of the common iliac artery that extends down into the thigh and becomes the femoral artery. (3 wds).

3 A laboratory test that utilizes a swab of material from a body part or wound to grow bacteria in culture medium in a Petri dish to identify the infectious agent, then determine which antibiotics are capable of impeding their growth. (3 wds).

5 Small blood vessel connecting arteries to veins.

6 Muscle of the anterior thigh situated on the interior aspect of the femoral shaft that extends the lower leg. (2 wds).

7 A developmental disorder characterized by poor social skills, repetitive behaviors, and focused interest in an esoteric topic that limits social and occupational functioning. (2 wds).

8 Dacryocystorhinostomy is a surgical procedure that creates a new opening between the _____ and the nose. (2 wds).

9 Habitually swallowing of food without completely chewing.

13 Use of external pressure to compress the bladder and express urine when nervous impulses are interrupted. (2 wds).

14 A thyroid hormone that lowers plasma calcium and phosphate ion levels by inhibiting bone resorption. Increases renal excretion.

15 A split or tear in the retina of the eye.

17 Adenosine monophosphate is a _____ secreted by the parafocicular cells of the thyroid gland to regulate the level of blood calcium.

18 Any method of restricting movement with cloth, belts, and other devices to prevent harm to the patient and others.

19 Abnormal, excessive, anterior curvature of the lumbar spine.

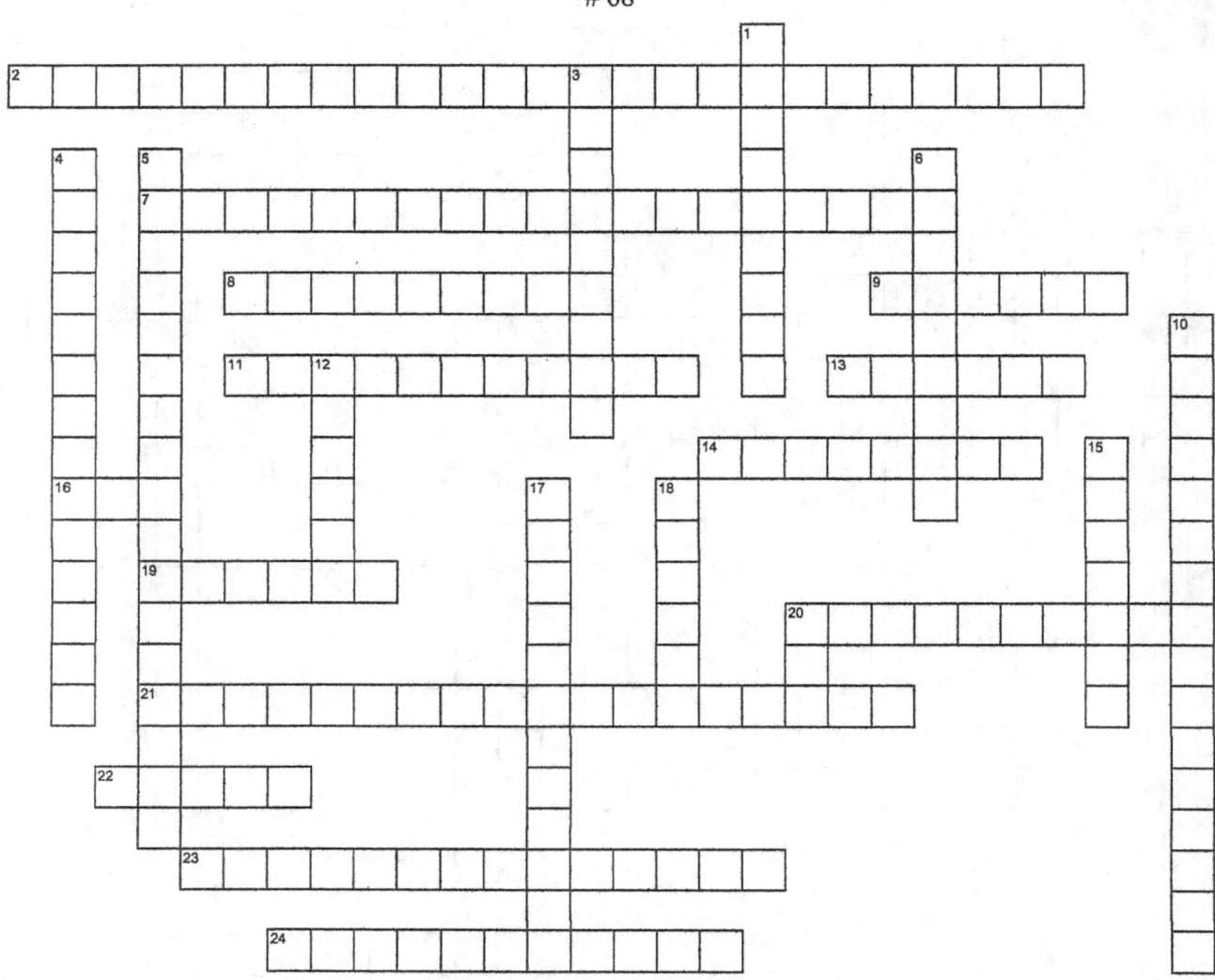

ACROSS

2 A therapeutic procedure in which shock waves are transmitted to the kidneys to break apart renal calculi. (2 wds).

7 Lung infection caused by foreign material entering the lung. (2 wds).

8 Cancerous cells. A tumor or abnormal cells composed of anaplastic or abnormally shaped epithelial cells.

9 Blister.

11 Demonstrating factitious medical or psychiatric symptoms in order to get a tangible reward, such as narcotic drugs or disability payments.

13 Inflammation of nasal passages associated with profuse nasal discharge, as seen with the common cold.

14 Structure of respiration located in the left chest, composed of the superior, middle, and inferior lobes. (2 wds).

16 Prefix meaning "apart" or "excessive".

19 Membrane lining the posterior cavity of the eye that contains rods and cones.

20 A system of ethical decision making that considers the intrinsic moral significance of an action as the basis of decisions.

21 A psychotic state wherein the patient experiences continued false beliefs despite the efforts of others to persuade, or evidence showing otherwise. (2 wds).

22 Cheek.

23 Space between the sclera and cornea of the eye that drains aqueous humor from the eye. (3 wds).

24 Whitening of the epithelium.

DOWN

1 Lymphogranuloma venereum is a sexually transmitted disease caused by the _____ species that causes reddened, painless erosions of the genitals and rectum, followed by lymph node enlargement and fistulous tracts, obstructions, and infection of the perirectal lymph nodes.

3 The system that is composed of the main lymphatic duct, draining lymph from the upper right body quadrant and returning it to the bloodstream via the right subclavian vein.

4 Major conductive pathways of the heart involved in coordination of the heart muscle. (2 wds).

5 A muscle of the anterior thigh covering the femoral shaft, situated between the vastus lateralis and vastus medialis. Its purpose is to extend the lower leg. (2 wds).

6 A triangular bone located at the most superior part of the sternum.

10 Premature closing of the cranial sutures during the first eighteen months of life.

12 Structural or functional alterations.

15 Acute respiratory distress syndrome describes massive damage to _____ due to injury to lungs from burns, aspiration of vomitus, or infection which renders lungs incapable of making surfactant required to keep lung tissue open.

17 Creutzfeldt-Jakob disease is a progressive fatal _____ disorder caused by an infectious protein particle contracted from cows infected with bovine spongiform encephalopathy.

18 Inflammatory bowel disease that can involve any part of the digestive tract. It is most often found in the ileum, resulting in obstruction of the intestine.

20 Degenerative joint disease. A loss of articular cartilage due to aging and cumulative injury to a joint. (3 initials).

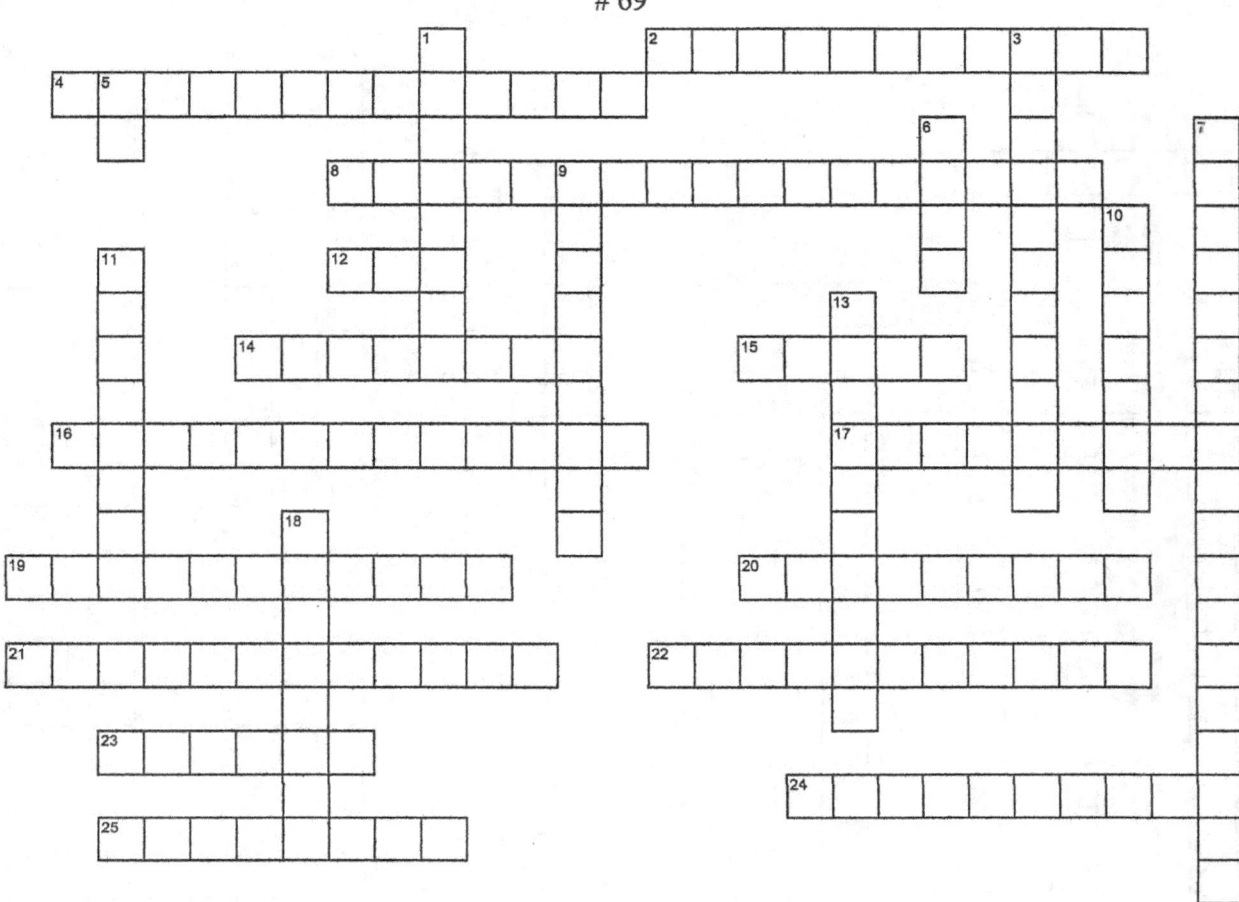

ACROSS

2 Bending forward a part of an organ.
4 The reflux of small amounts of food and acid back into the mouth.
8 A group of nerve cells in the pons and medulla that control breathing. (2 wds).
12 Aspartate aminotransferase test. Intracellular enzyme test to detect tissue damage in the liver, brain, and muscles. (3 initials).
14 A type of stress that results in positive change or growth.
15 A muscle of the internal aspect of the hip that extends from the lumbar vertebrae to the lesser trochanter of the femur. Contraction causes flexion and lateral movement of the spine.
16 Spinal curves toward the patient's left.
17 The ability to recall. Also, the inability to defecate, urinate, or expel other bodily substances normally.
19 Abnormally slowed heart rate, with less than sixty beats per minute in an adult patient.
20 Enlargement of a passageway or channel by making an incision.
21 Assist-control ventilation is _____ supported breathing where the patient is permitted to initiate breathing but the ventilator delivers a preset volume of air and will initiate breathing if the patient's breathing slows or stops.
22 Procedure to remove an embedded kidney stone through a percutaneous incision.
23 Pertaining to the inside of the cheek.
24 An acute or chronic inflammation of the bronchial tubes.
25 Class of enzymes that breaks down protein.

DOWN

1 The muscle that closes the jaw and is used for chewing.
3 (IFN's) Antimicrobial glycoproteins produced in response to viral invasion. Their presence stimulates cytotoxic T-cell activity and amplifies macrophage action.
5 Prefix meaning "out or away from", or "external".
6 Prefix meaning "opposed" or "against".
7 Blood-clot formation in a deep vein, occurring most frequently in the iliac and femoral veins. (3 wds).
9 A period of time when symptoms of a disease are absent or greatly diminished.
10 Disorder characterized by episodes of self-induced purging after binging.
11 Loss of appetite.
13 A facial muscle that draws the eyebrows together to frown.
18 Bone of the hand. Used to describe rounded shape of structures.

#70

ACROSS

2 Teeth clenching or grinding, usually while asleep.
7 Abnormal presence of protein in the urine.
11 Normal labor.
12 A circular tissue of the eye whose color is genetically determined.
17 Physical presentation of rigid extension of the trunk, arms, hands, legs and feet. Associated with lesions of the brain stem. (2 wds).
20 Abbreviated as "a.c." when written in medical instructions or physician orders, this indicates that medication or treatment is administered before meals. (2 wds).
22 Turning of the hand or other body part downward.
24 Sudden stoppage of the heartbeat. (2 wds).
25 Any disorder that causes destruction or disruption of the function of the retina.

DOWN

1 Instrument that generates sound waves to break up a stone in the body.
3 Suffix meaning "having the nature or characteristic of".
4 Thrush. An oral infection caused by the fungus Candida albicans, often due to immunosuppression.
5 An unconscious defense mechanism that pushes painful, traumatic events, anxiety, or guilt-producing knowledge into the subconscious, where it is dormant but able to resurface.
6 Infection of the airway including the bronchi, bronchioles, and lung tissue.
8 A bilateral muscle of the lateral chest that begins at the fifth ribs and inserts into the anterior iliac crest, serving the function of compressing the abdomen and maintaining an upright posture. (2 wds).
9 Rounded distal projections of the distal tibia and fibula that compose the ankle.
10 Hormones secreted by the placenta, and in small amounts by the adrenal cortex. It is responsible for many female reproductive functions, including secondary female characteristics.
13 Disruption of the cranium where bone is pushed inward toward the brain. (2 wds).
14 Vessels transporting blood from the lungs to the heart. (3 wds).
15 A complex of symptoms following the administration of aspirin for fever in children, characterized by liver damage, brain dysfunction, fever, and vomiting. (2 wds).
16 Kidney drop resulting from loss of supporting adipose tissue. (2 wds).
18 A reactive, obstructive lung disease caused by the inhalation of foreign material such as mold, fungus, and bacteria associated with exposure to unprocessed cotton, flax, or hemp fibers.
19 Abnormally slow respiratory rate.
21 Pertaining to breast tissue or ducts.
23 Adenosine triphosphate. A molecular substance that supplies the energy for muscle fiber contraction. (3 initials).

71

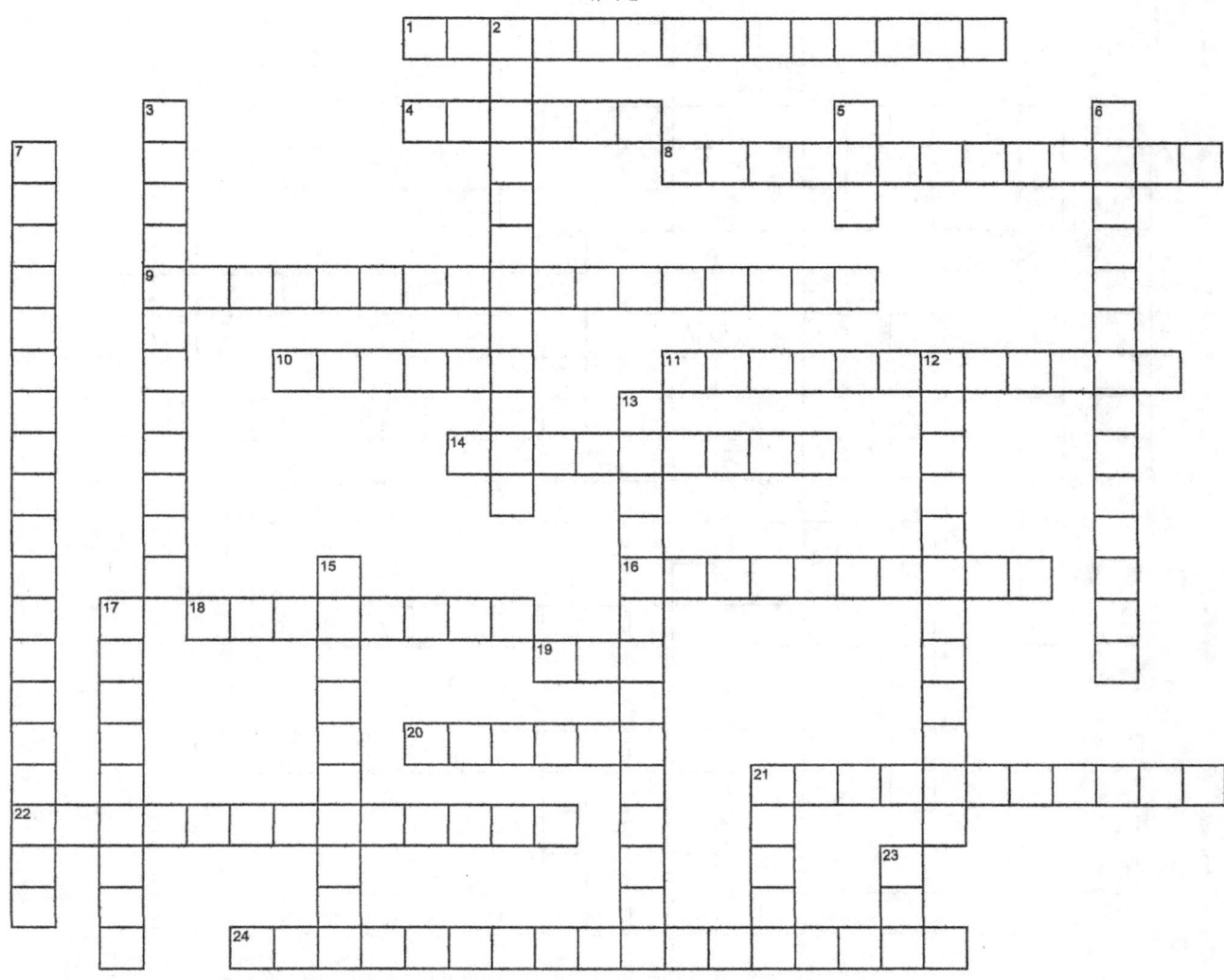

ACROSS

1 Muscle of the medial aspect of the thigh which acts to adduct the thigh. The proximal portion acts to rotate the thigh medially and to flex it on the hip. (2 wds).

4 Abnormal construction of the iris muscle to decrease the size of the pupil and limit the amount of light entering the eye.

8 Surgical excision of all or portions of the prostate gland, often by a perineal incision.

9 Processing of nutrients in the presence of oxygen. A metabolic pathway that uses oxygen to convert glucose into cellular energy. (2 wds).

10 Mucous membrane.

11 Innermost surface of the facial cheek. (2 wds).

14 White blood cells including the five subtypes (lymphocytes, monocytes, neutrophils, basophils, and eosinophils).

16 Epinephrine. A hormone secreted by the adrenal medulla.

18 Inflammation of a fluid-filled synovial sac located over a bony prominence or point of

articulation between tendon and bone.

19 Irritable bowel syndrome. A disorder that consists of severe spasms of cramping, abdominal pain, diarrhea, and bloating, alternating with constipation, and excessive secretion of mucus from the colon. (3 initials).

20 Breathing with normal depth and rate.

21 Nearly translucent band of fibrous tissue and fascia that holds the extensor and flexor tendons that cross the wrist and ankle.

22 Liquid that has the same concentration as normal body fluid. (2 wds).

24 Lack of the ability to recall events that occurred before the onset of amnesia. (2 wds).

DOWN

2 Without sufficient oxygen.

3 The layer of the eye containing the retina. (2 wds).

5 Suffix meaning "condition or state of excess".

6 A genetically transmitted rhythm disturbance that places children at risk for ventricular fibrillation and sudden death. (3 wds).

7 Particular body position caused by a lesion of the upper brain stem. It is characterized by rigid extension of limbs, internal rotation of the arms, and notable plantar flexion of the feet. (2 wds).

12 Arrangement of bone fragments after a fracture such that they do not heal properly.

13 A cup-shaped structure that encloses the glomerulus in the renal tubule or nephron. (2 wds).

15 A formation that appears to be a cyst but lacks the internal fluid-filled nature of an actual cyst.

17 Turning inward of the eyeball.

21 Enzyme released by the juxtaglomerular cells when there is a drop in renal blood flow that converts angiotensin to constrict blood vessels and maintain blood pressure.

23 Suffix meaning "throw".

72

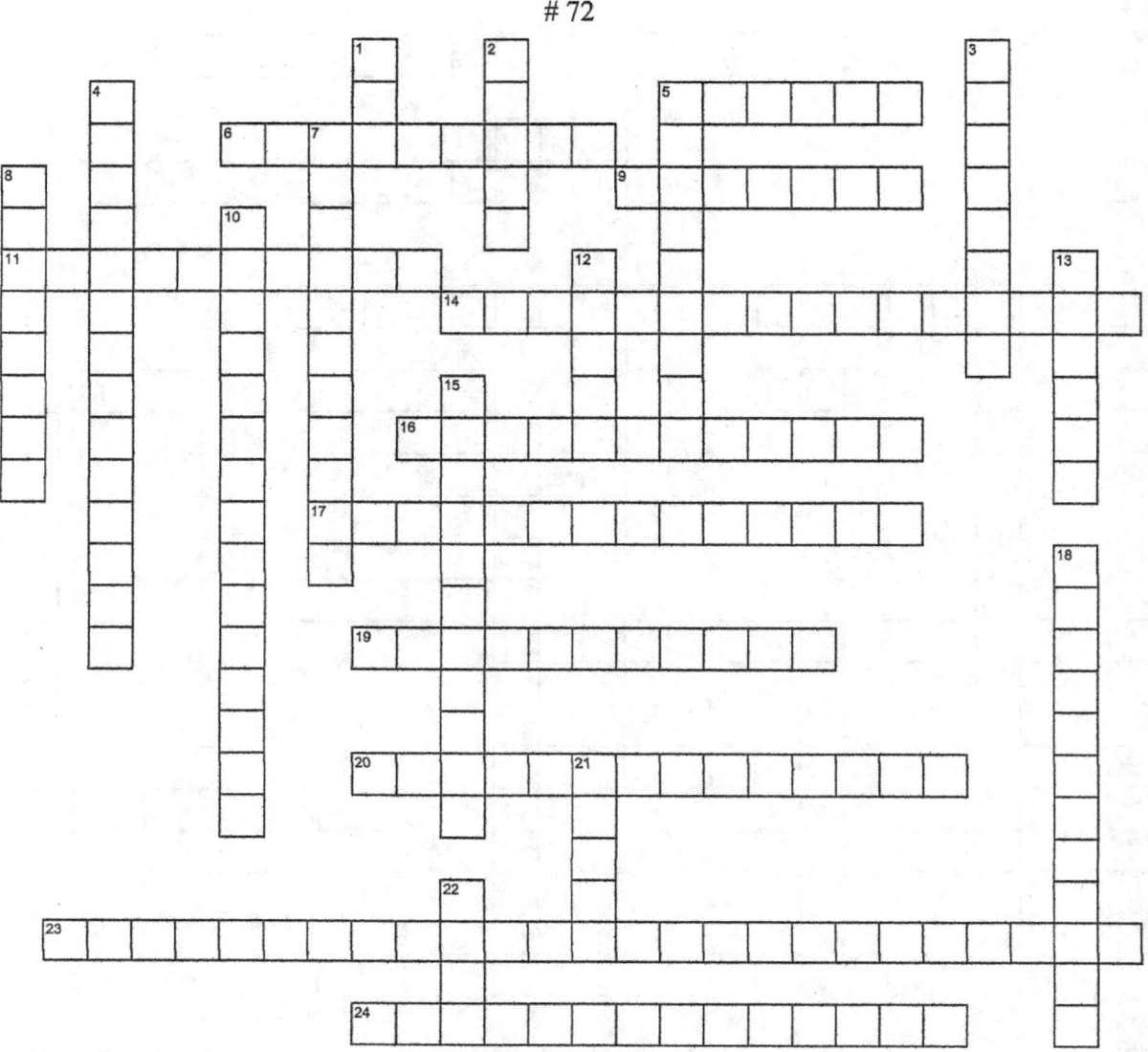

ACROSS

5 The outermost layer of any organ such as a lymph node, kidney, ovary, thymus or cerebrum.
6 Fat cells.
9 Portion of the temporal bone of the skull located just behind and inferior to the ear.
11 Loss of melanin as a result of disease.
14 Reduction of minerals such as calcium in body tissues, particularly related to bone.
16 Moveable or downward displacement of the kidney.
17 Diminished blood supply to a particular area due to an embolism or thrombosis. (2 wds).
19 Making an identical duplicate of DNA during the early stages of mitosis or meiosis.
20 Restoration of an individual to the highest level possible following an injury, functional loss, addiction, or incarceration.
23 Shunting of blood outside the body to a device that performs a body function. Blood is then returned to the patient's circulatory system. (2 wds).
24 Production of red blood cells.

DOWN

1 Prefix meaning "new".
2 Prefix meaning "outside of".

3 A round gland surrounding the neck of the bladder and urethra, producing fluid that becomes part of semen.
4 Lymphatic tissue located on both sides of the base of the tongue in the hypopharynx. (2 wds).
5 Seborrheic dermatitis in infants. (2 wds).
7 Ulcerative skin lesions occurring as a result of scabies.
8 Acute confusion, disorientation, and agitation due to toxic levels of body chemicals, drugs, or alcohol in the blood that affect the brain.
10 Anterior pituitary gland that produces hormones.
12 The largest solid organ of the body, located in the upper right abdominal area, that contains four lobes and is responsible for metabolic, excretory, and detoxification functions.
13 A small lymph node. A small circumscribed swelling.
15 Kidney disease.
18 Severe hypoglycemia produced by excess insulin and inadequate food intake. It is characterized by diaphoresis, tremors, restlessness, confusion, diplopia, delirium, convulsions, and circulatory collapse. (2 wds).
21 Prefix meaning "within".
22 Suffix meaning "thing" or "structure".

73

ACROSS

1 Impulsive flight from one's life and familiar surroundings following a traumatic event. The patient begins a new life, and functions normally without recall of the past. (2 wds).
3 Any position of the fetus in the pelvis other than head first. (2 wds).
5 Turning a body part outward.
7 Hemoglobin that is lacking oxygen.
9 A crescent-shaped bone located in the proximal row of the carpus.
10 Cysts containing fluid within a fibrous capsule attached to a tendon sheath of the hands, wrists, or feet.
14 Acute inflammation of the bronchioles and alveoli that produces congestion. (2 wds).
16 Contagious skin condition caused by streptococci or staphylococci bacteria.
19 Unnatural lightness in color of skin due to lack of blood supply to tissue.
20 Enzyme excreted by the villi within the small intestine to break down the sugar lactose found in milk.
22 Layer of fibrocartilage surrounding each intervertebral disc. (2 wds).
23 Protrusion of the wall of the rectum that pushes on the adjacent wall of the vagina, causing it to collapse and partially block the vaginal canal.
25 Suffix meaning "cessation".

DOWN

2 Sudden, involuntary and often painful contraction of the muscles of the esophagus.
4 A self-limiting condition occurring in children ages two through twelve in which there is a necrosis of the ossification centers of bone followed by regeneration and recalcification. (3 wds).
6 Prefix meaning "not".
8 A procedure for making a person insensitive to an antigen. Desensitization.
11 Separation of the retina from the choroid layer of the eye due to trauma, aging or diabetes, causing the blood vessels to become increasingly fragile. (2 wds).
12 A U-shaped segment of the renal tubule, composed of the thin descending limb and thick ascending limb. (3 wds).
13 Neurotransmitter in the brain.
15 Underlying cause of a disorder.
17 Surgical correction of deformities of the external ear.
18 Degenerative renal condition characterized by damage to the renal tubules without inflammation.
21 An involuntary movement or action due to a particular stimulus.
24 Prefix meaning "referring to oxygen".

74

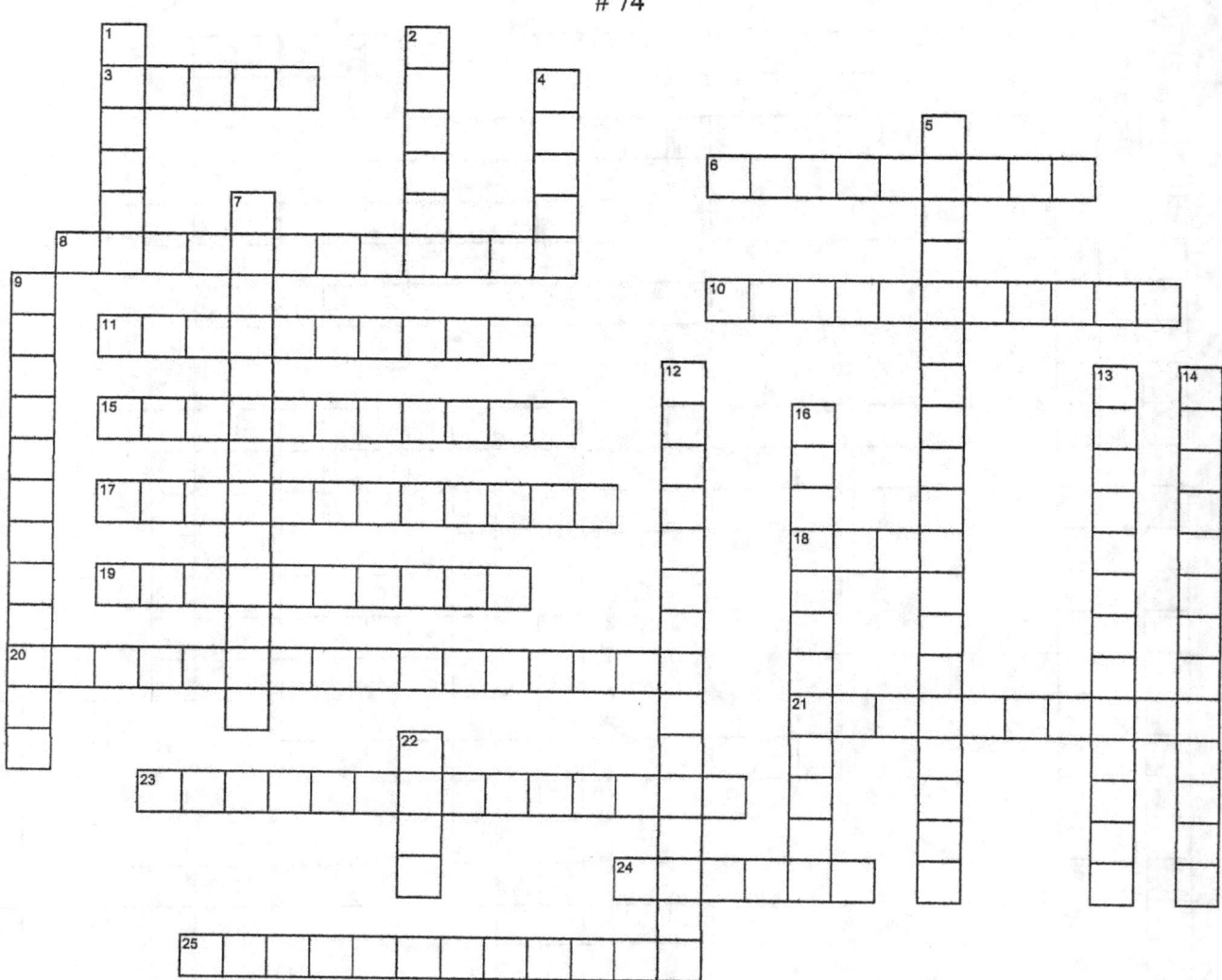

ACROSS

3 Space inside the tubular artery, or tube. A standardized unit of light measurement called international candles.

6 The inability to achieve or maintain an erection.

8 Substance, agent, or conditions that produce malignant cells.

10 Method of calculating the age of a human embryo in days. Calculated by taking the square root of the length from vertex to breech in centimeters, then multiplying by 100. (2 wds).

11 To remove by the process of absorption.

15 Surgical removal of a kidney.

17 A small-diameter fiberoptic instrument used to visualize and biopsy the upper airway and lung tissue.

18 Suffix meaning "small".

19 Movement opposite of the normal pattern, moving backward to a less developed or well state.

20 Cognitive deterioration with rapid decline, delusions, and agitation. (3 wds).

21 Unequal sizes of the pupils, often caused by glaucoma, head trauma, stroke, or a tumor that causes the iris to dilate and constrict.

23 Formation of a stone in an organ or blood vessel.

24 Region of the throat starting at the base of the tongue and ending at the upper trachea encircled by nine musculocartilaginous rings.

25 Limited ability to dorsiflex the foot. (Associated with club foot). (2 wds).

DOWN

1 Suffix meaning "paralysis".

2 Lipid deposition on the arterial wall of a vessel or structure.

4 Pertaining to the hip bone.

5 A severe bacterial infection with early presentation of fever and body aches. It progresses to liver and kidney damage, and possibly death. (2 wds).

7 A rod or oval-shaped cytoplasmic organelle that produces energy within the cell by the production of adenosine triphosphate (ATP).

9 Areas of lymphocyte formation within the lymph nodes. (2 wds).

12 A gram-positive yeast organism that causes infections of the mouth, skin, and vagina. (2 wds).

13 A series of osseous chambers located within the temporal bone. Essential to hearing. (2 wds).

14 Pertaining to the maxilla and upper face region.

16 Memory encoding or learning in the central nervous system.

22 Prefix meaning "single".

75

ACROSS

1 Supportive, non-nerve tissues of the peripheral and central nervous system.
4 One who suffers from a medical condition requiring treatment by a clinician.
7 Suffix meaning "possessing" or "full of".
12 A small canal between the inner ear and throat that allows air pressure in the middle ear to equalize with air pressure in the mouth and outside the body. (2 wds).
14 The broad, splaying portion of the hip bone which joins the pubis and the ischium, forming the acetabulum.
18 Disorder characterized by not eating due to a morbid fear of weight gain, resulting in severe emaciation. (2 wds).
20 Anatomical landmark of the lung where the lung tissue indents to allow for the physical presence of the heart. (2 wds).
22 Inflammation of the middle ear. (2 wds).
24 An increase in variation of the size of cells, frequently used in reference to red blood cells.
25 Labor and delivery of a fetus.

DOWN

2 Pertaining to the area of the larynx.
3 Surgical procedure to remove the prominent part of a metatarsal bone that is causing a bunion.
5 New growth of cells that may be malignant or benign.
6 A sensory nerve ending that receives a chemical message by linking or binding to a specific factor, drug, hormone, antigen, or neurotransmitter.
8 Chronic inflammation of the esophagus. It can progress to esophageal ulcers or cancer.
9 A medical tool used to dilate a body part, such as the urethra.
10 Infestation with a parasitic hookworm.
11 Suffix meaning "condition of speech".
13 Condition of wide dispersement throughout a tissue , organ or body part.
15 Ringlike muscle around the mouth used in smiling, compression of the cheeks, and chewing food.
16 Membrane forming the myelin sheath.
17 Unable to be resolved by treatment.
19 Suffix meaning "pertaining to".
21 Prefix meaning "all".
23 Prefix meaning "injury" or "experiencing or producing pain".

PUZZLE

SOLUTIONS

Solution:

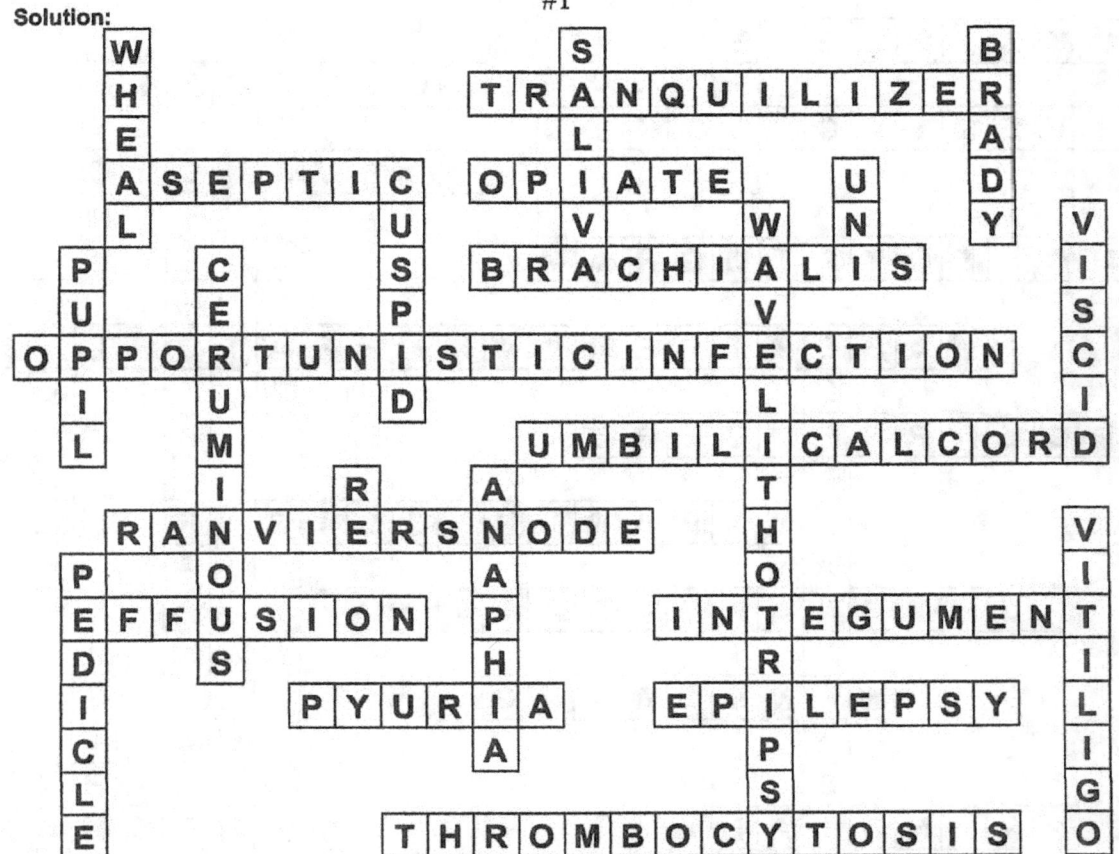

Solution:

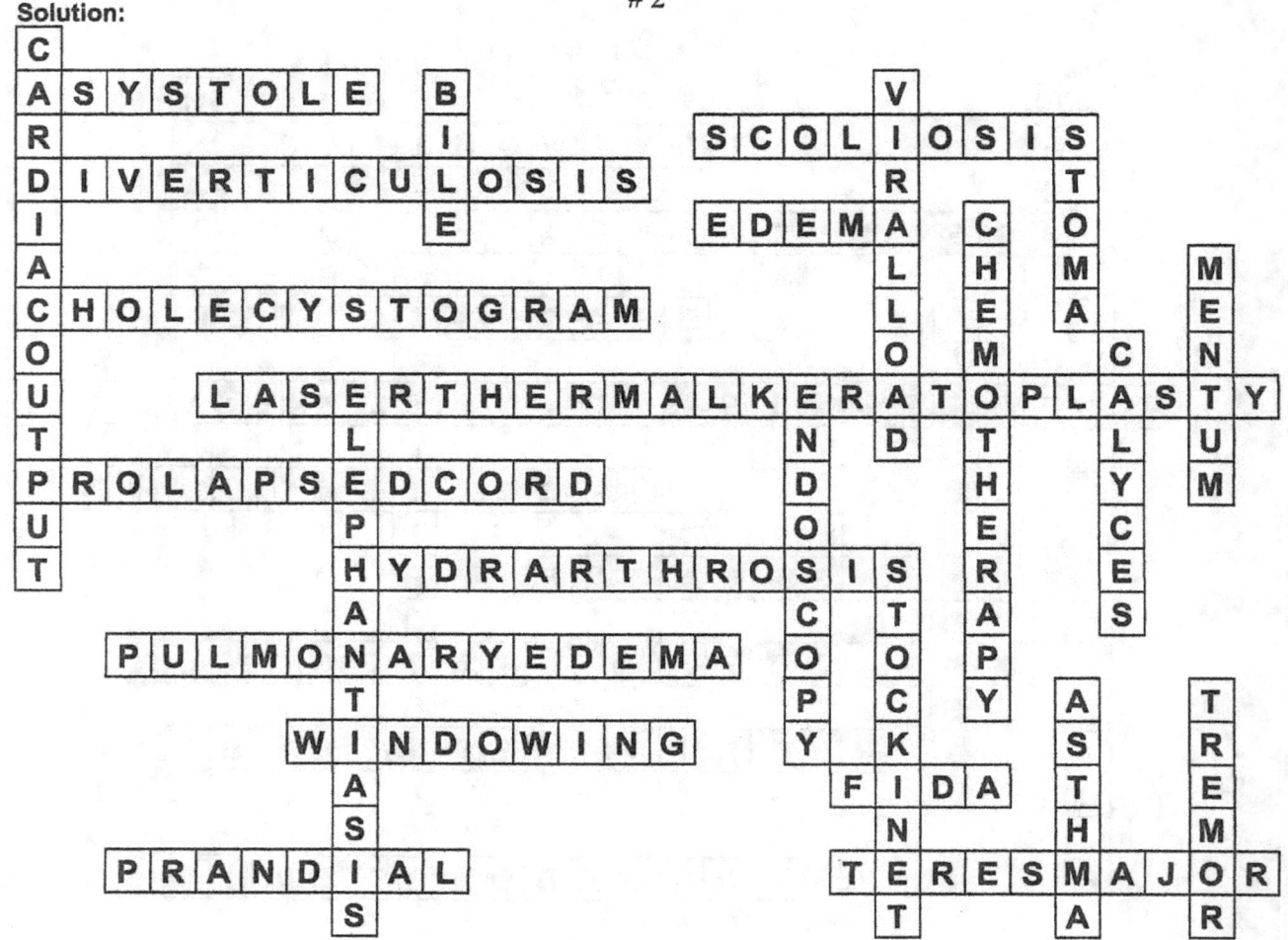

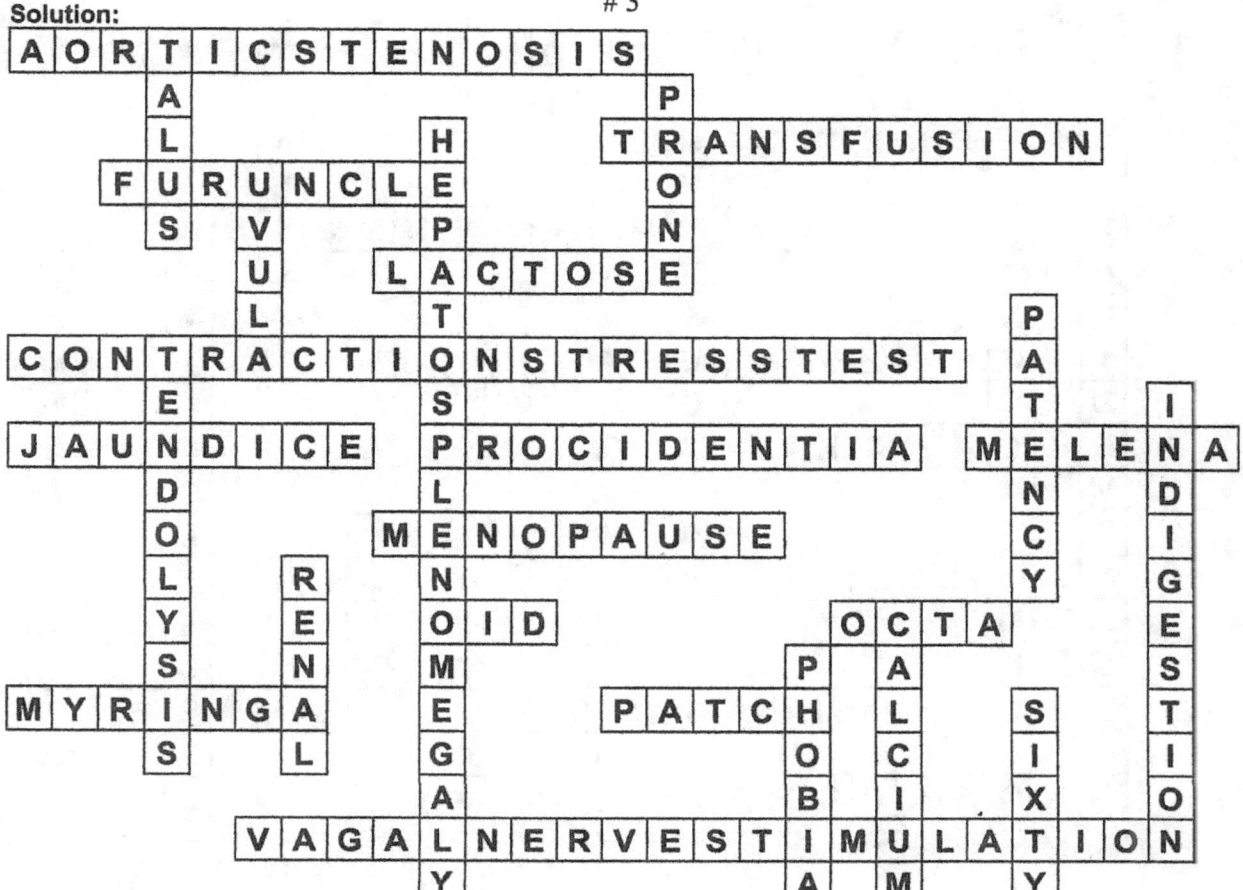

Solution:

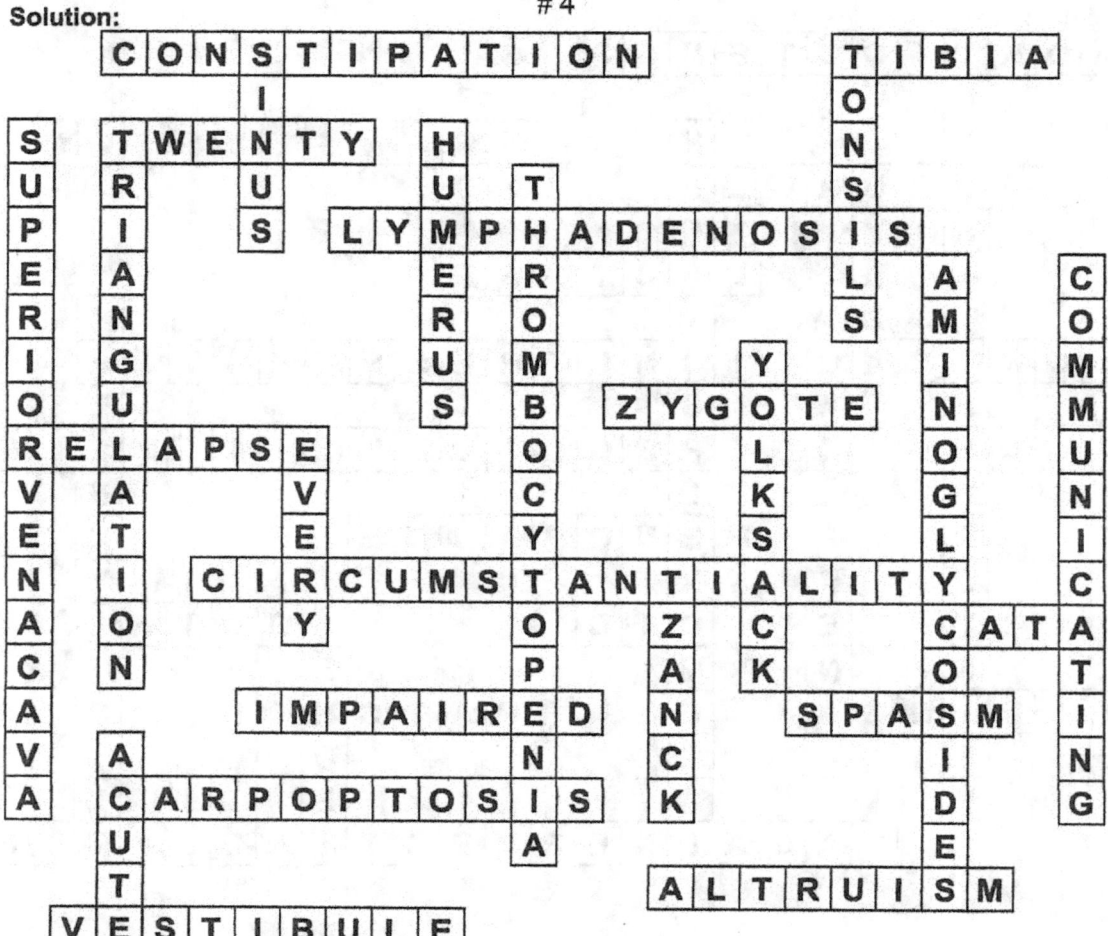

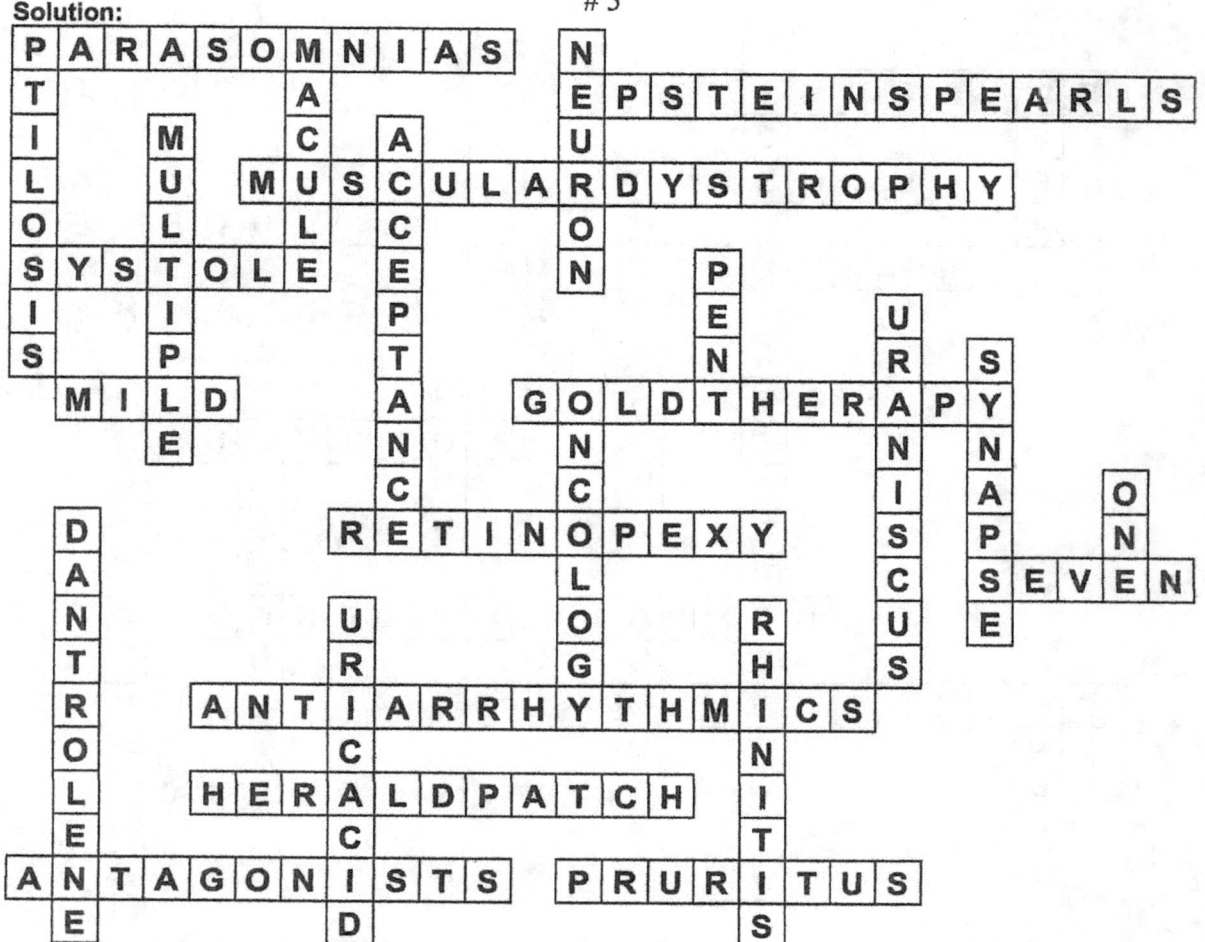

Solution:

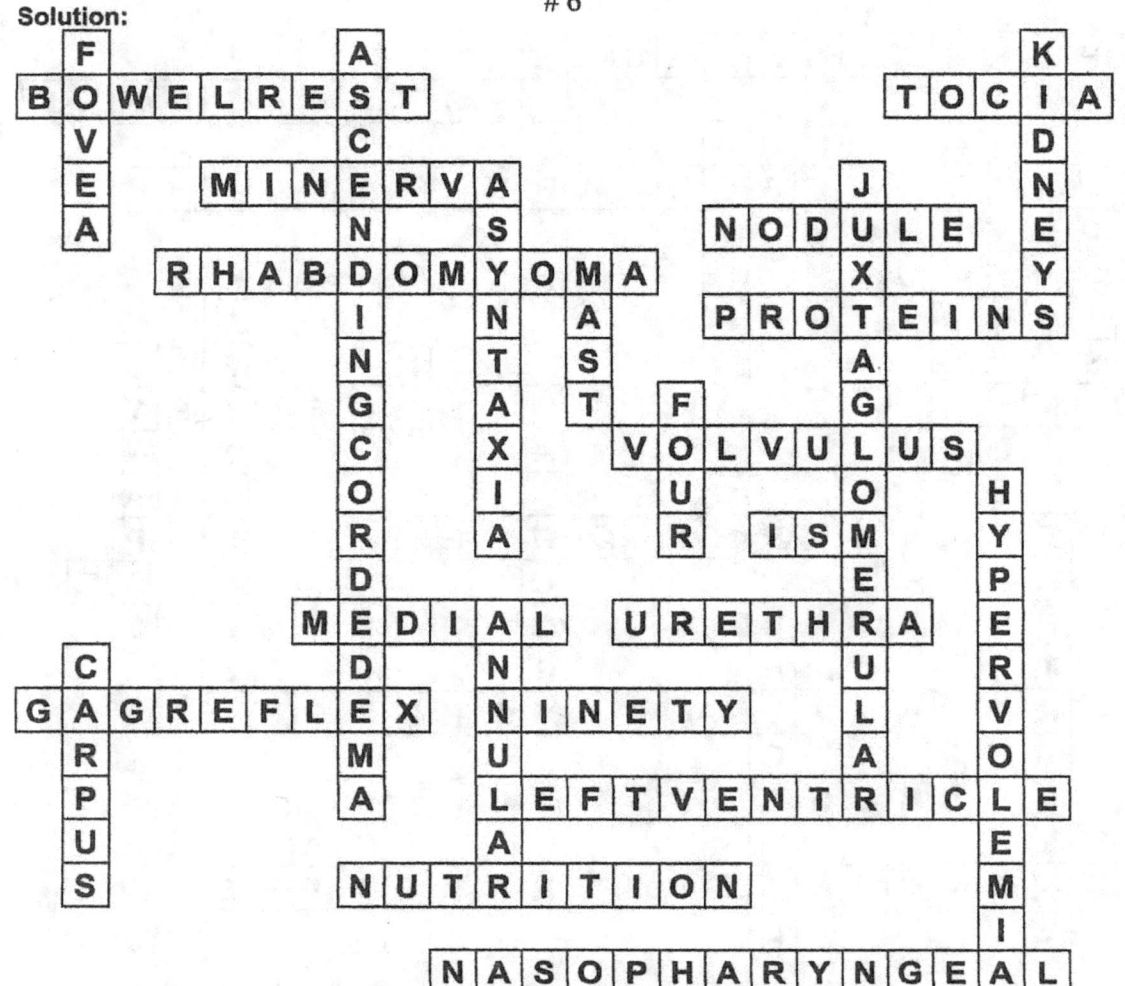

Solution:

A crossword puzzle solution with the following words:

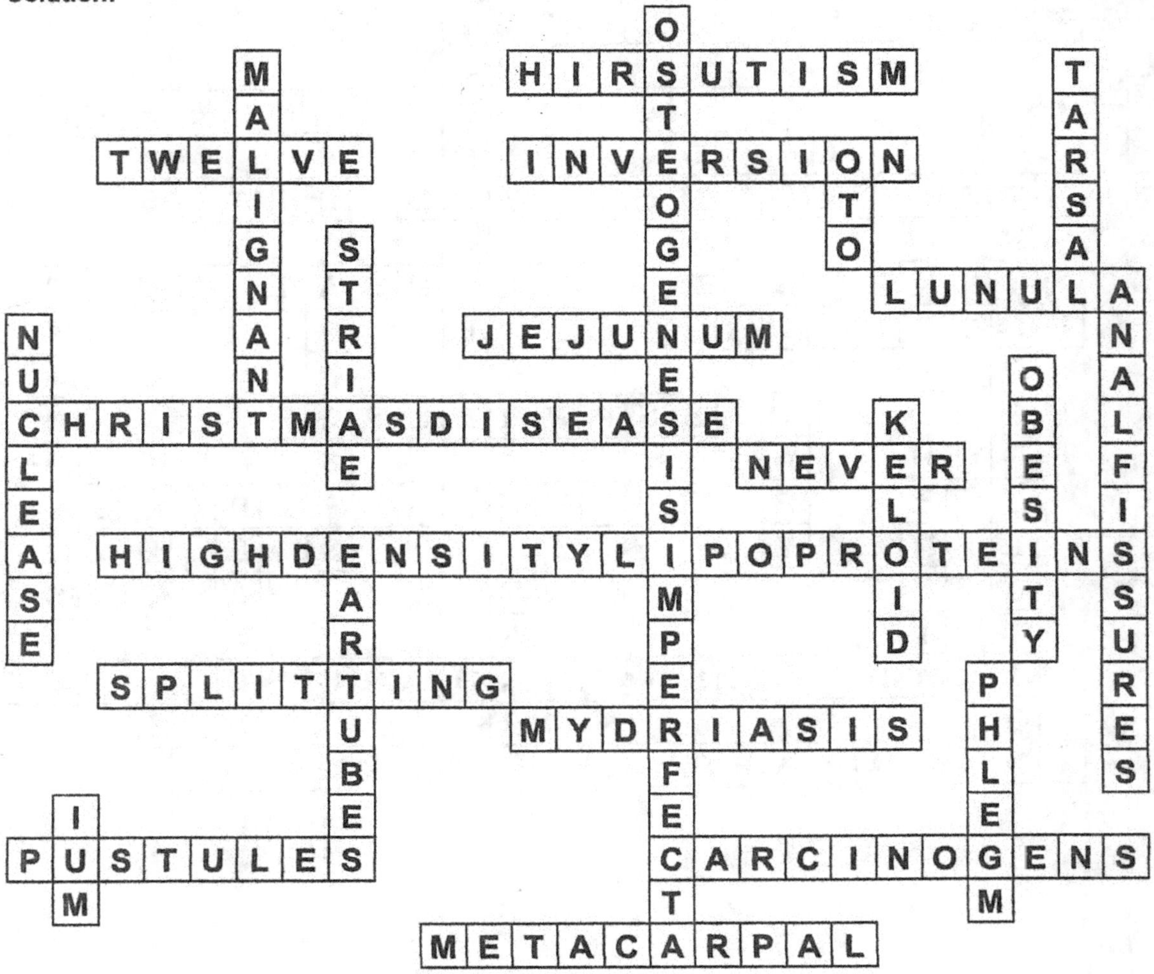

HIRSUTISM

TWELVE

INVERSION

MALIGNANT

STRIAE

OSTEOGENESIS IMPERFECT

TARSAL

ANAL FISSURES

LUNULA

JEJUNUM

NUCLEASE

CHRISTMAS DISEASE

NEVER

KELLOID

OBESITY

HIGH DENSITY LIPOPROTEINS

SPLITTING

ARTUBE

MYDRIASIS

PHLEGM

PUSTULES

IUM

CARCINOGENS

METACARPAL

Solution: # 8

Solution:

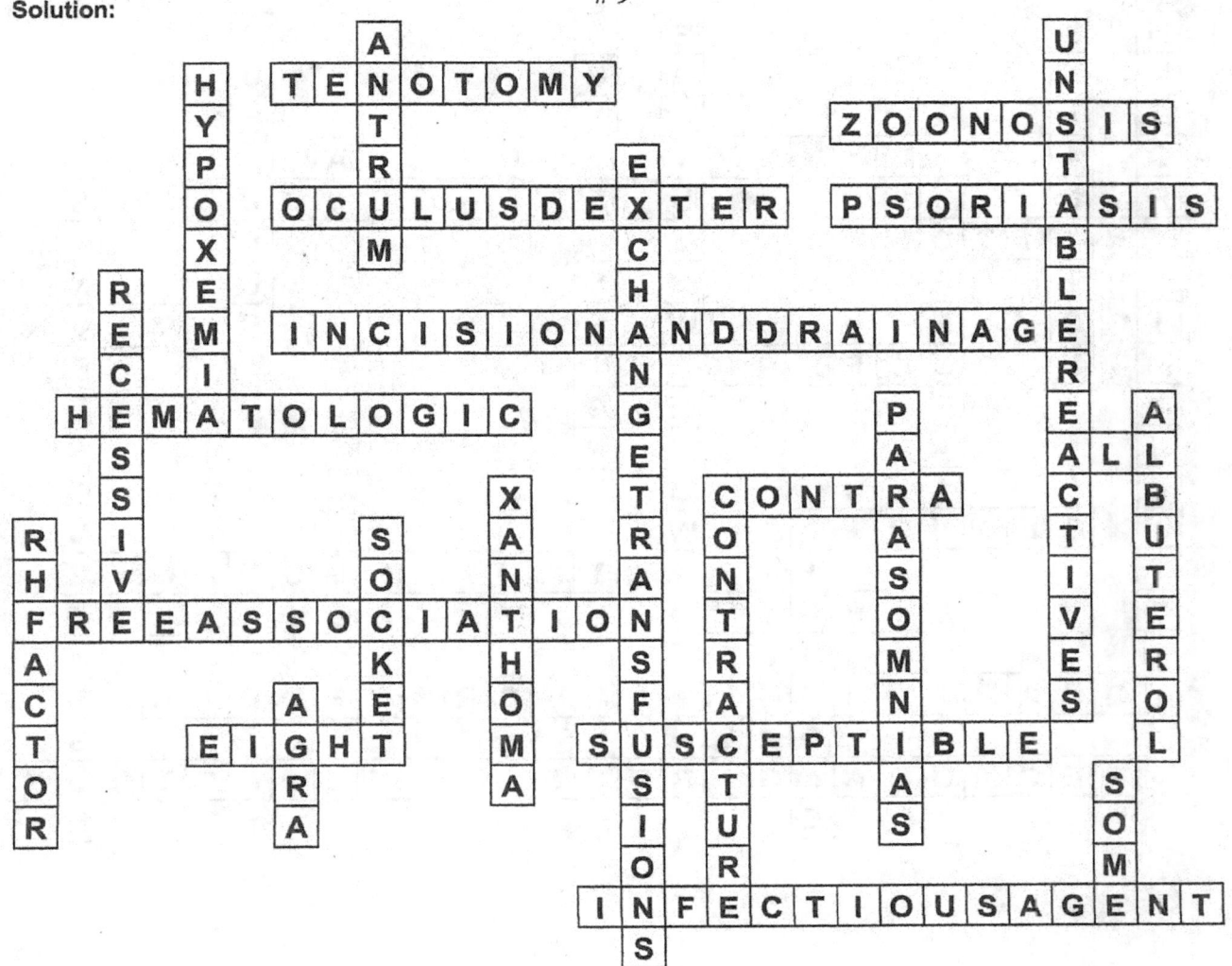

Solution:

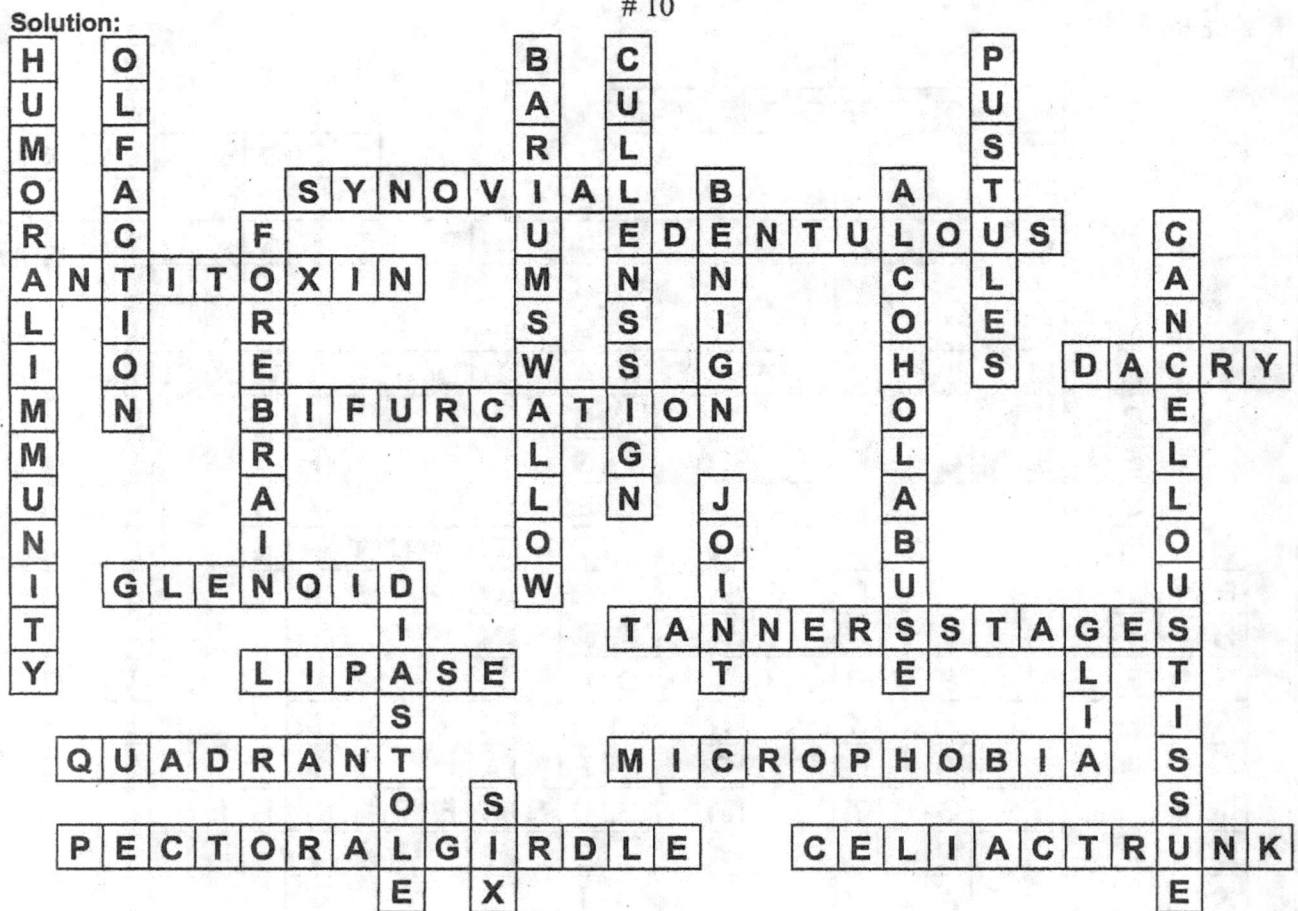

Solution: # 11

A crossword puzzle solution grid containing the following words:

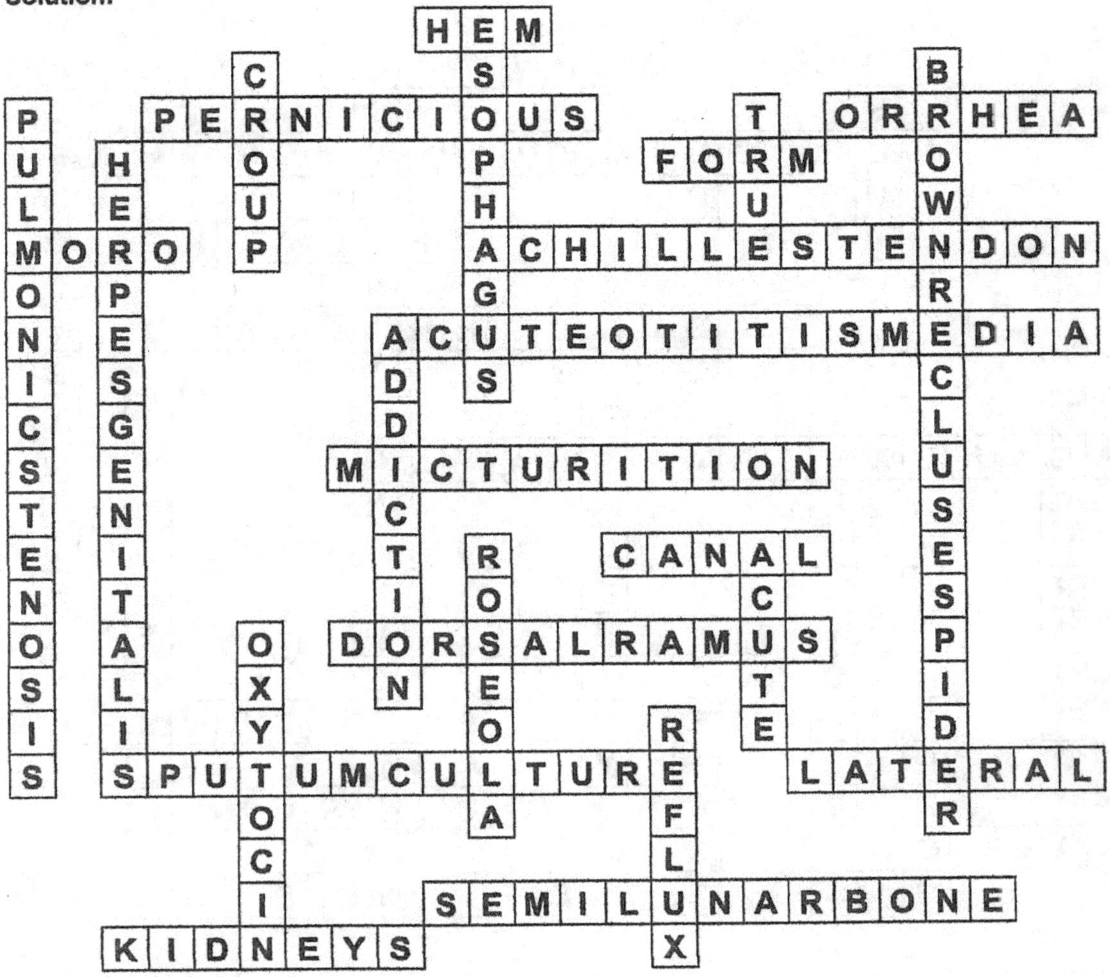

- HEM
- PERNICIOUS
- TORRHEA (ORRHEA)
- CROUP
- FORM
- BROWN
- PULMONICSTENOSIS
- HERPESGENITALIS
- MORO
- ACHILLESTENDON
- TRU
- ACUTEOTITISMEDIA
- ADDICTION
- MICTURITION
- RECLUSESPIDER
- CANAL
- ROSEOLA
- DORSALRAMUS
- ACUTE
- OXYTOCI
- SPUTUMCULTURE
- LATERAL
- REFLUX
- SEMILUNARBONE
- KIDNEYS

Solution:

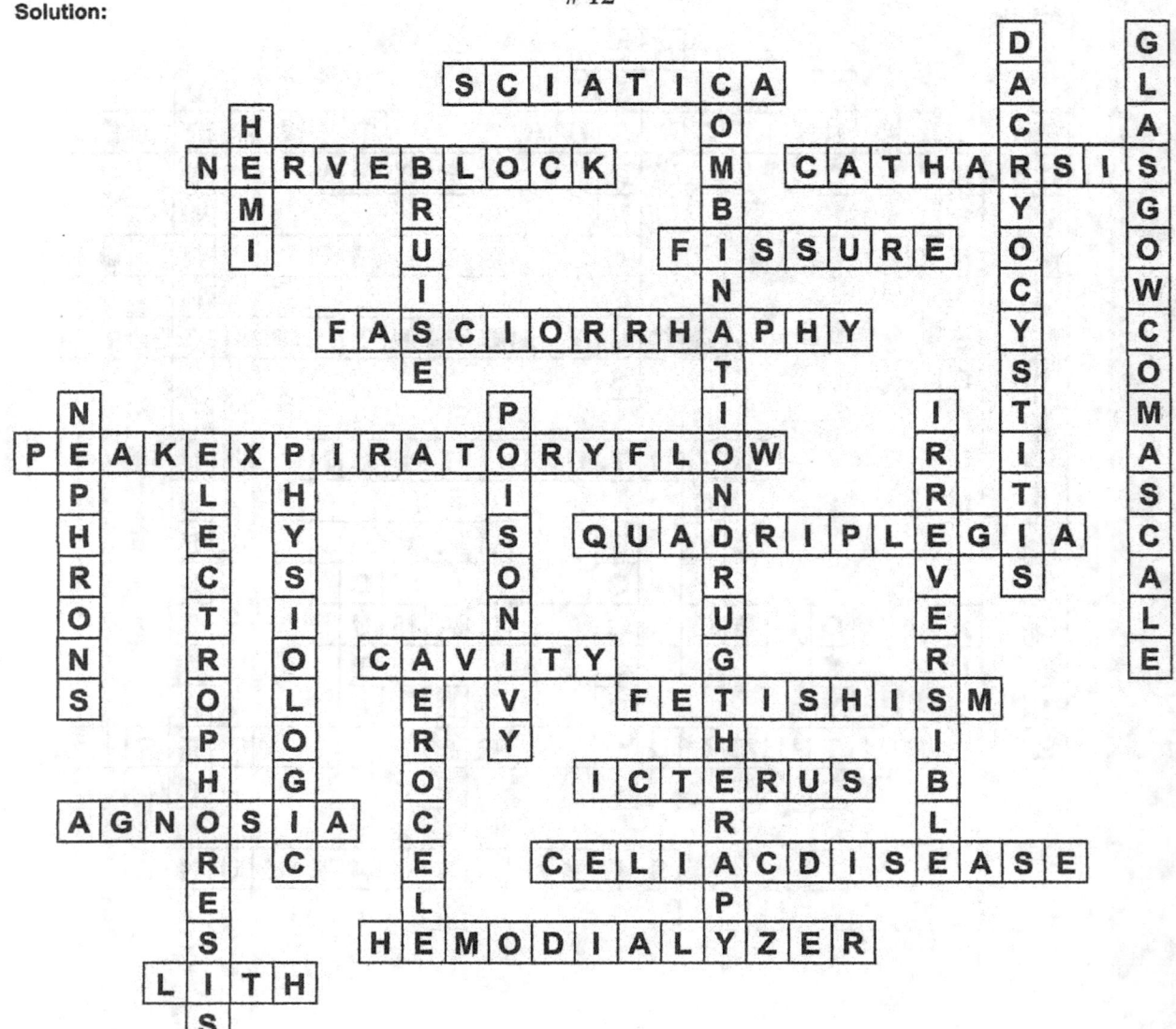

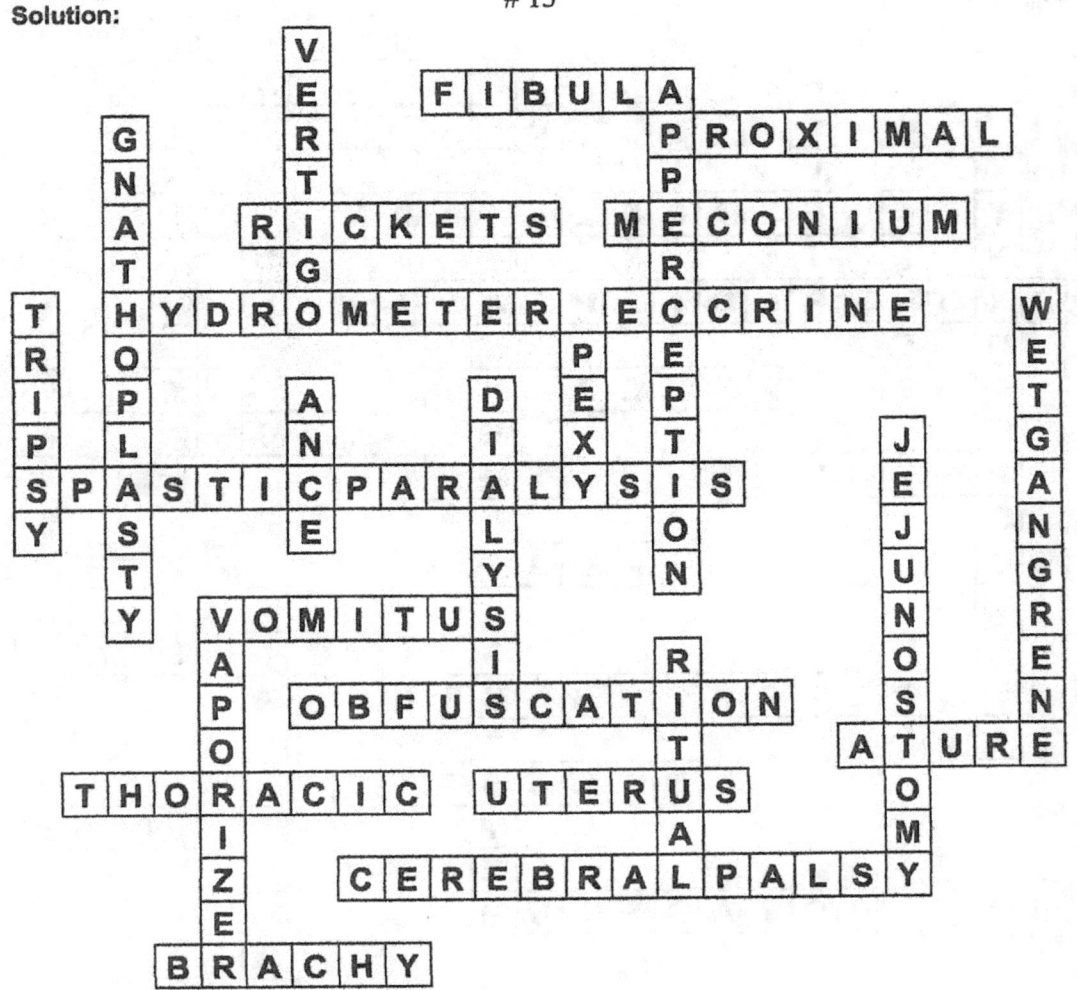

Solution:

A crossword puzzle solution containing the following words:

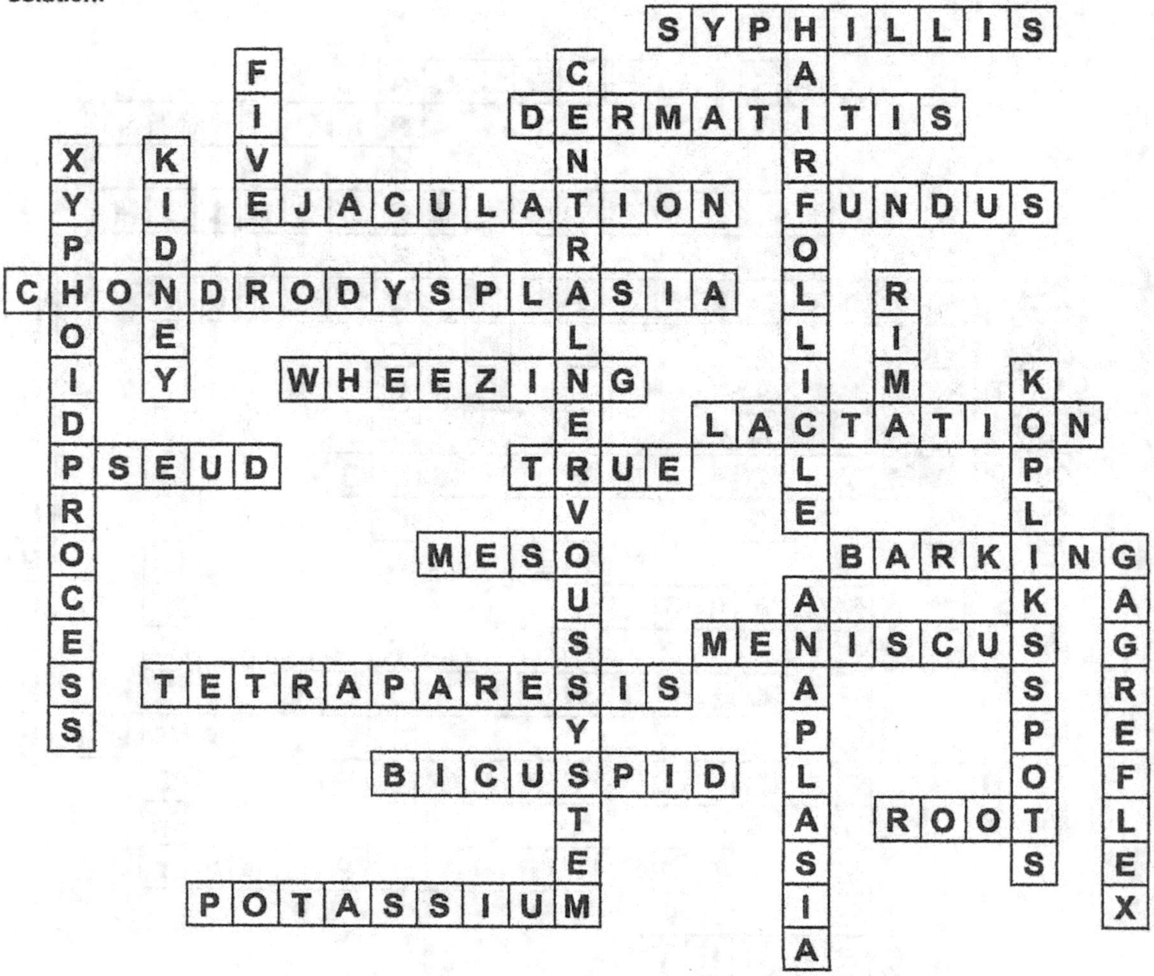

SYPHILLIS

DERMATITIS

FIVE — CENTRAL — AIR

XYPHOID — KIDNEY — EJACULATION — FUNDUS

CHONDRODYSPLASIA — FOLLICLE — RIM

WHEEZING

CHOROID PROCESS — LACTATION — KON PLI

PSEUD — TRUE

MESO — BARKING

TETRAPARESIS — MENISCUS — AGREFLEX

APLASIA — KSS SPOTS

BICUSPID

NERVOUS SYSTEM

ROOTS

POTASSIUM

Solution:

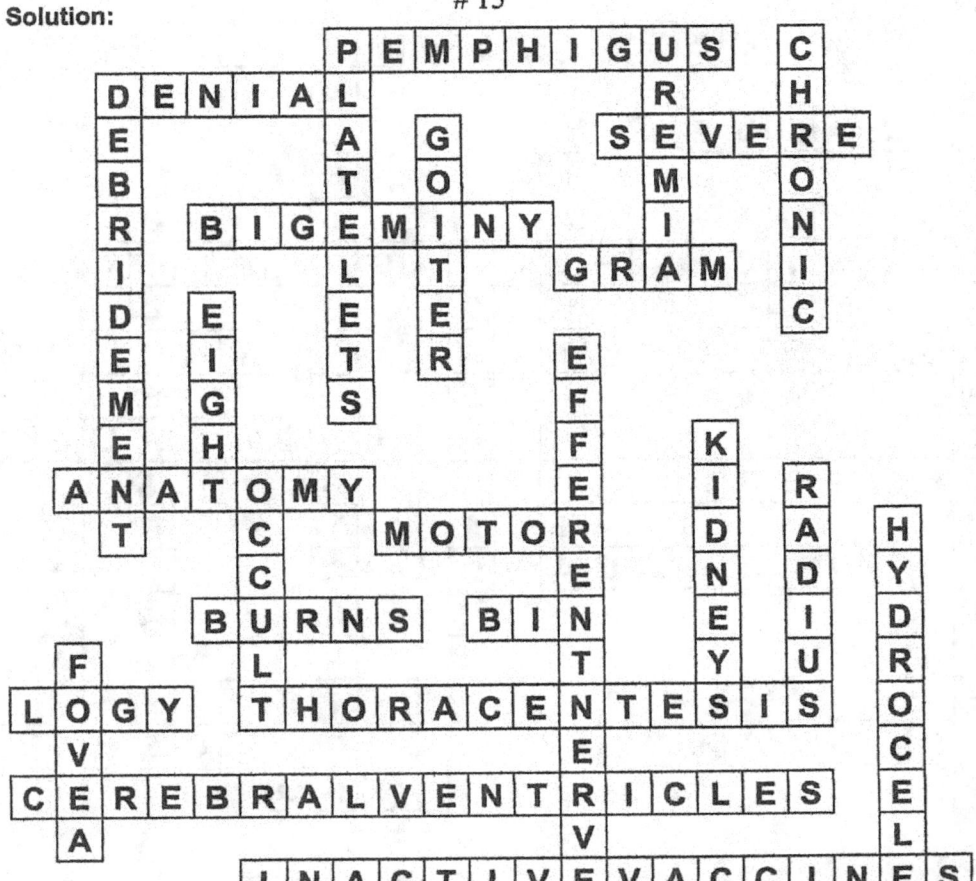

Solution:

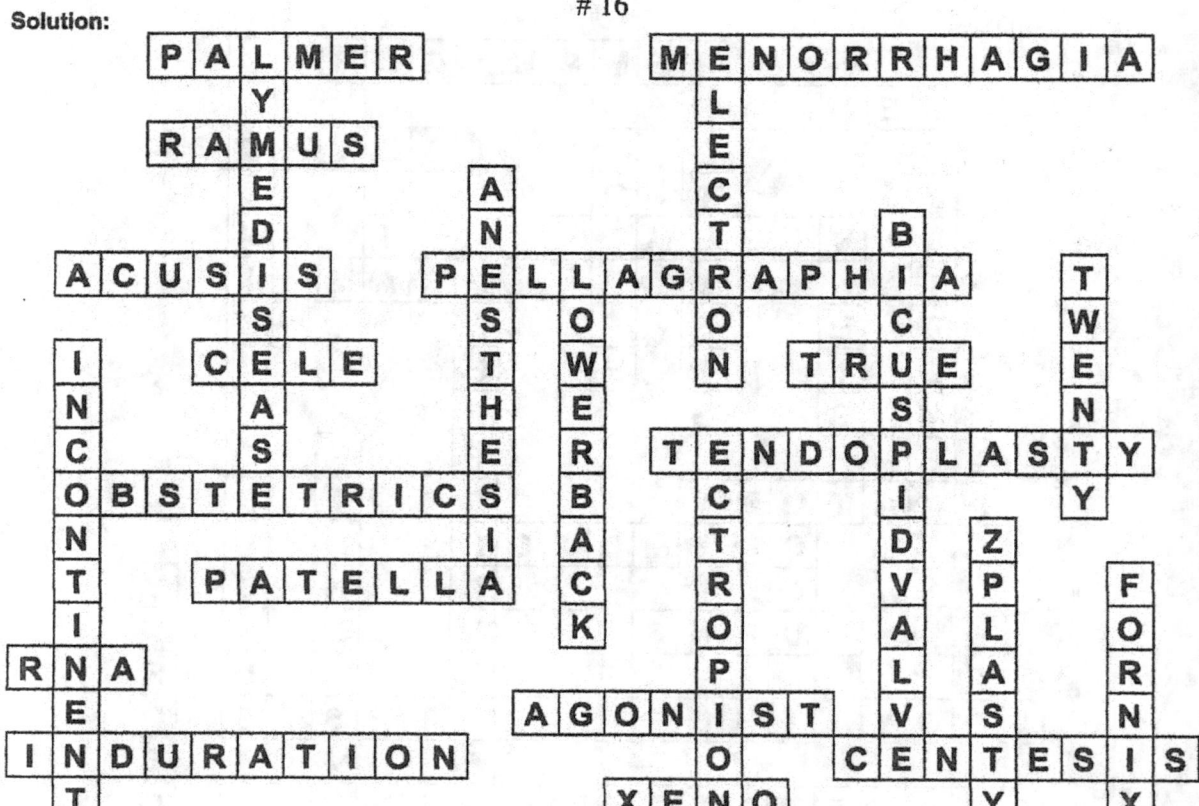

Solution:

17

```
                    A B D O M I N A L
                                  G
                                  G                    C          C
        I N C E N T I V E S P I R O M E T R Y          Y
                                  E          C          S
        P L   M                   G          U          T
        L     E   P E C T U S E X C A V A T U M          I
        A     N               G          E              T
        S     O   Z Y G O M A T I C B O N E S            I
        M     R           N       B      S              S
              R           A       L
        A I R E M B O L I S M     B I L A T E R A L      V
    P         H           A       Q                      I
    H         E   P I N W O R M S Q                      B
    O         A           C       U                      I
    B             R U B E O L A   X E N O G R A F T      C
    I                     L   V   F                      E
G A L L B L A D D E R D I S E A S E   T E N E S M U S
                          I   S   I              C
    N E P H R O T O X I C A   S   U              Z
                          A   U                  E
                          L Y M E D I S E A S E  M
```

Solution:

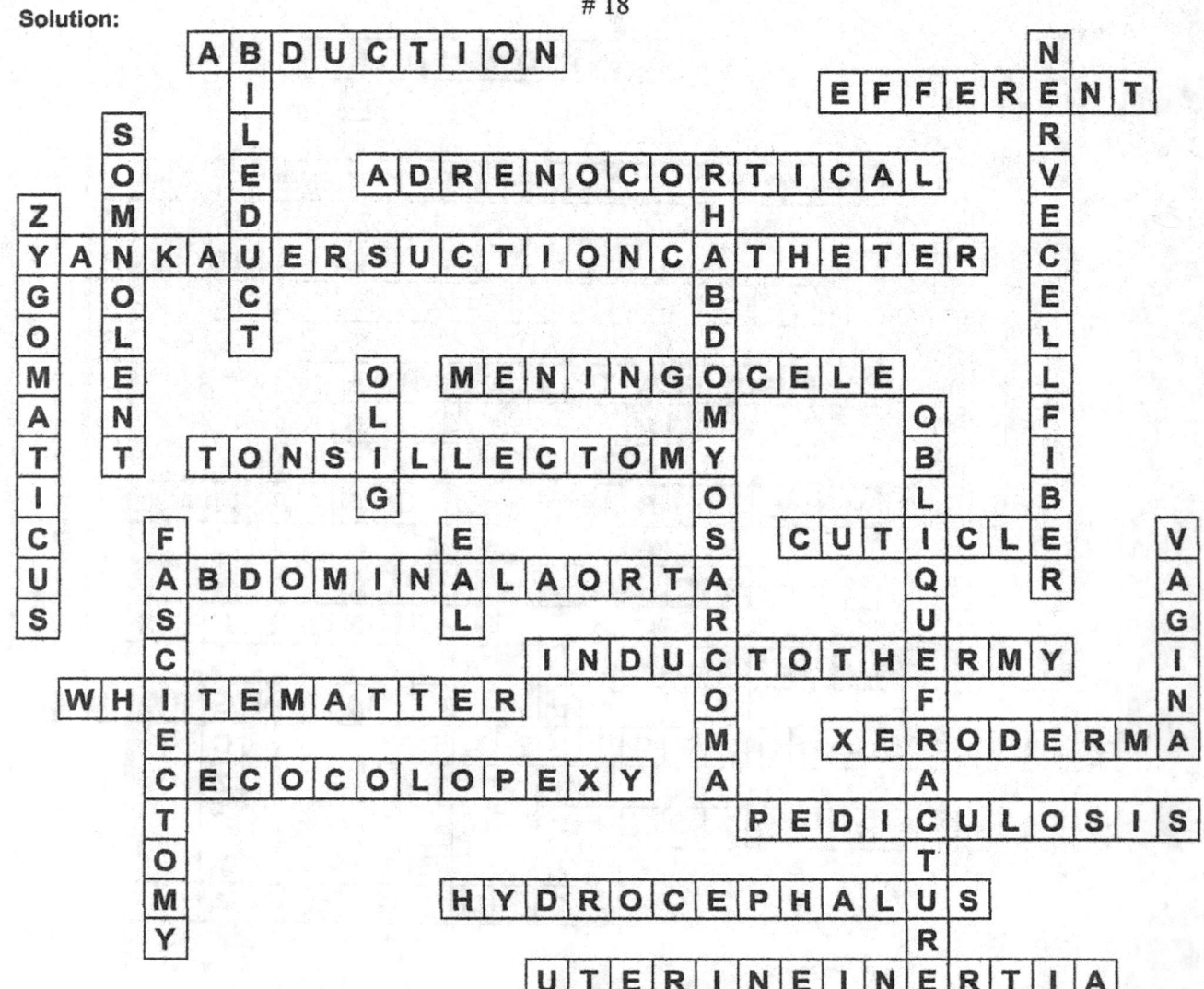

Solution:

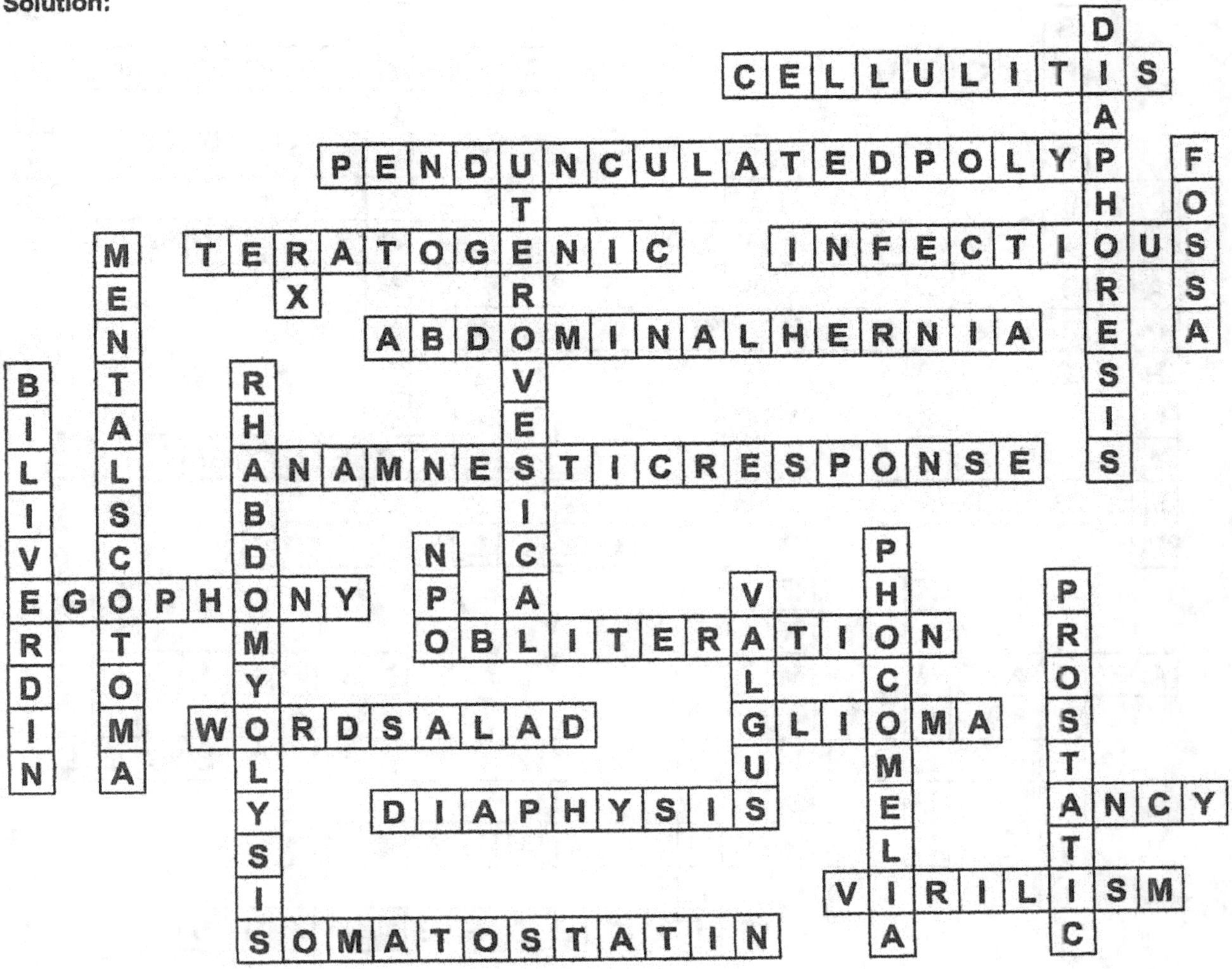

CELLULITIS
DIAPHORESIS
PENDUNCULATEDPOLYP
FOSSA
TERATOGENIC
INFECTIOUS
MENTALSCOTOMA
RX
UTEROVESICAL
ABDOMINALHERNIA
BILIVERDIN
RHABDOMYOLYSIS
ANAMNESTICRESPONSE
NPO
PHOCOMELIA
EGOPHONY
VALGUS
PROSTATIC
OBLITERATION
WORDSALAD
GLIOMA
DIAPHYSIS
ANCY
VIRILISM
SOMATOSTATIN

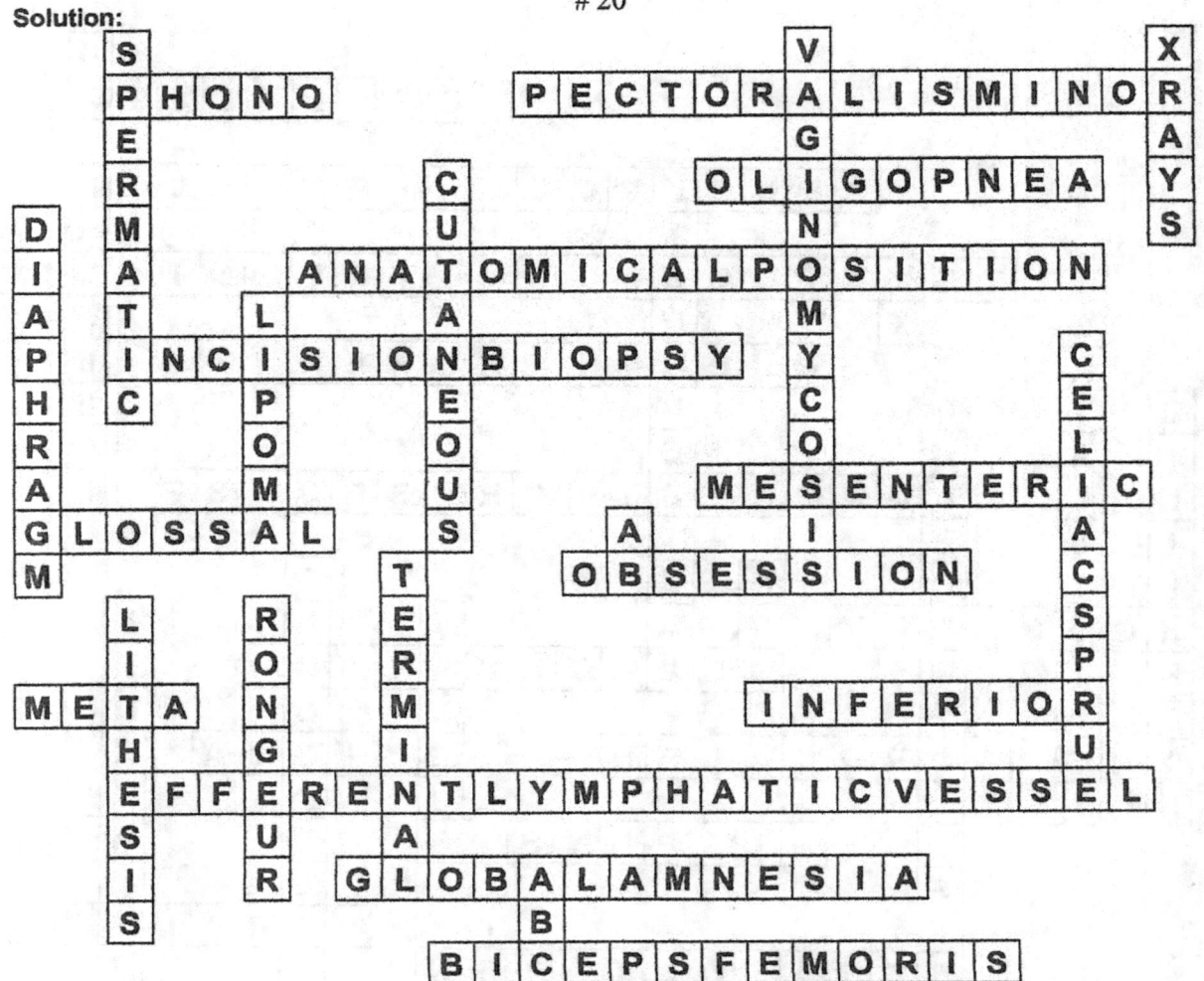

Solution:

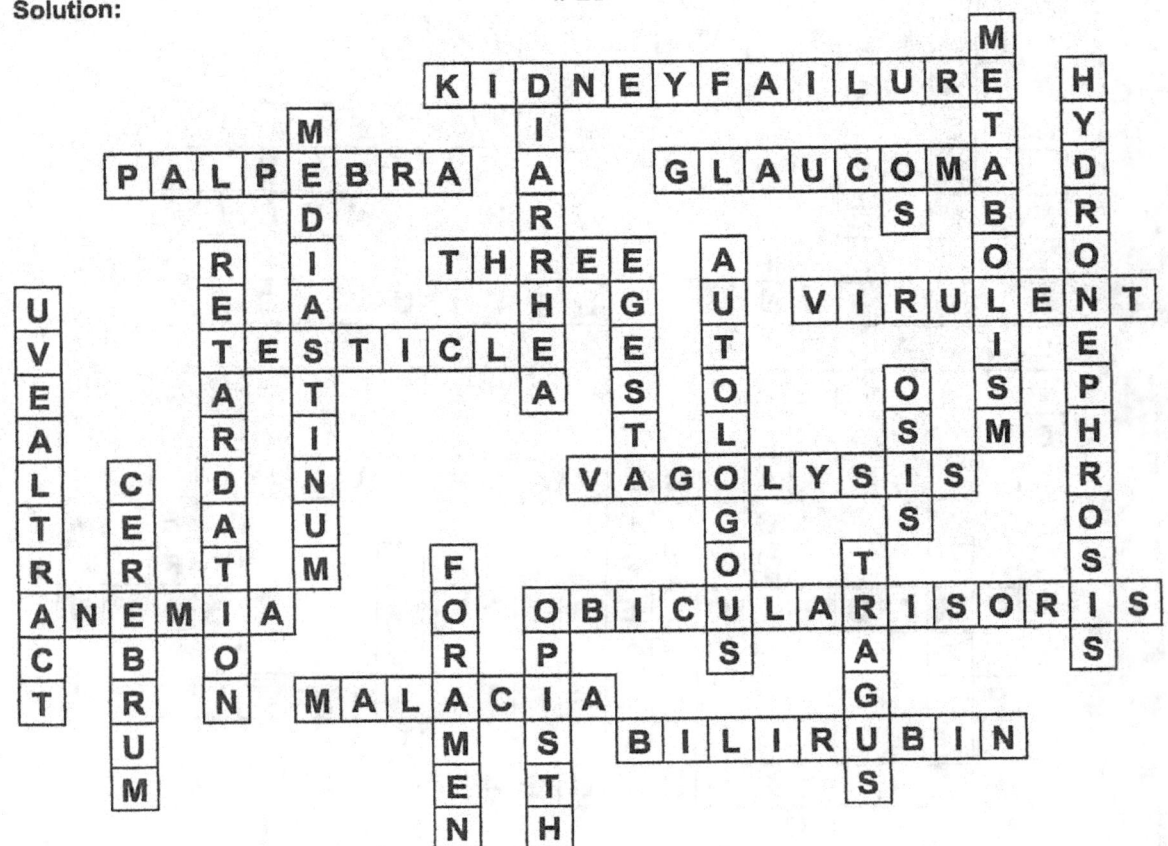

Solution:

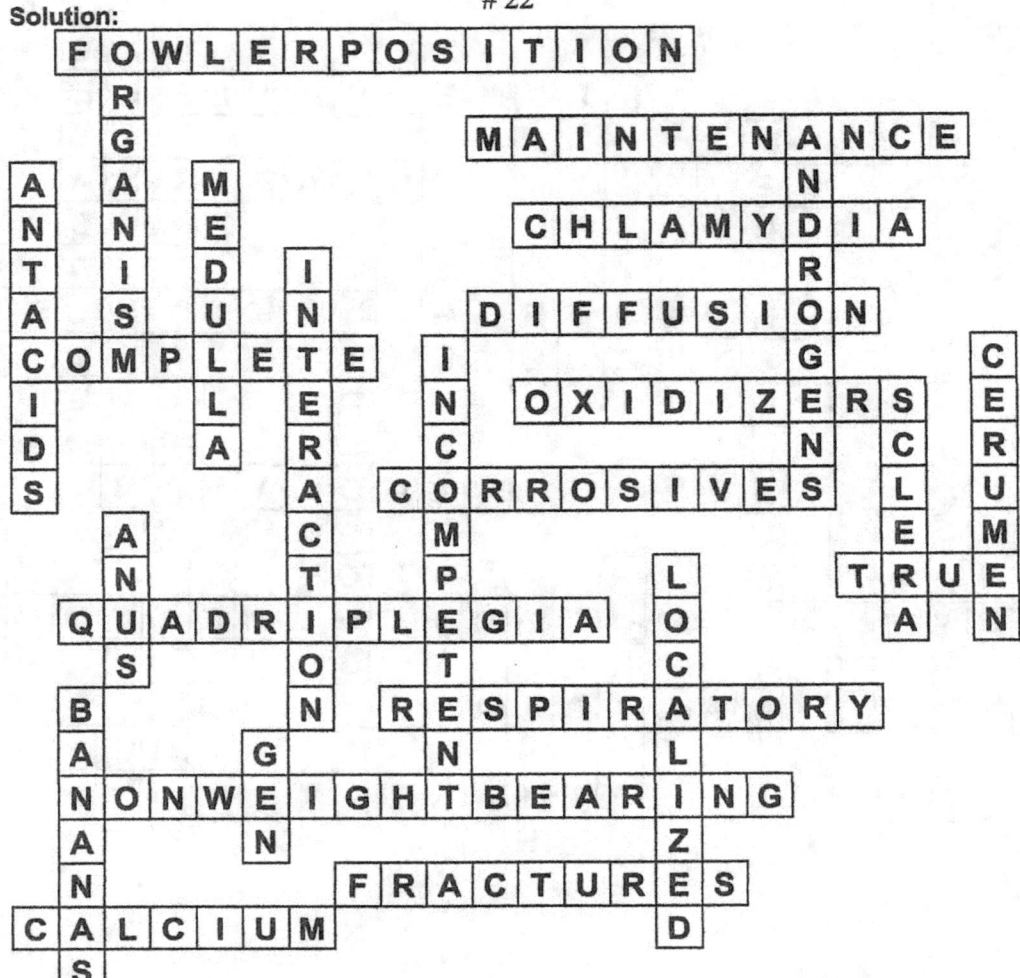

Solution:

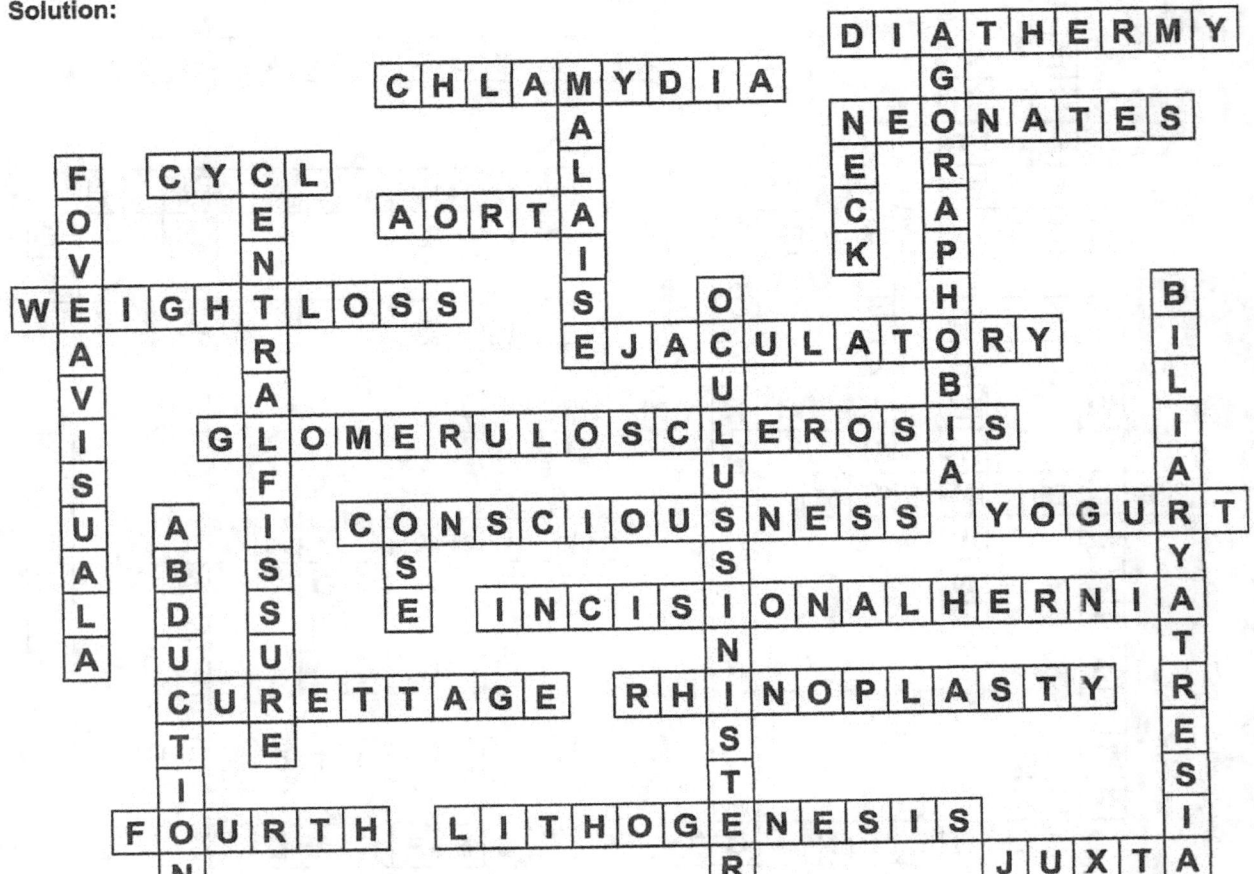

Solution:

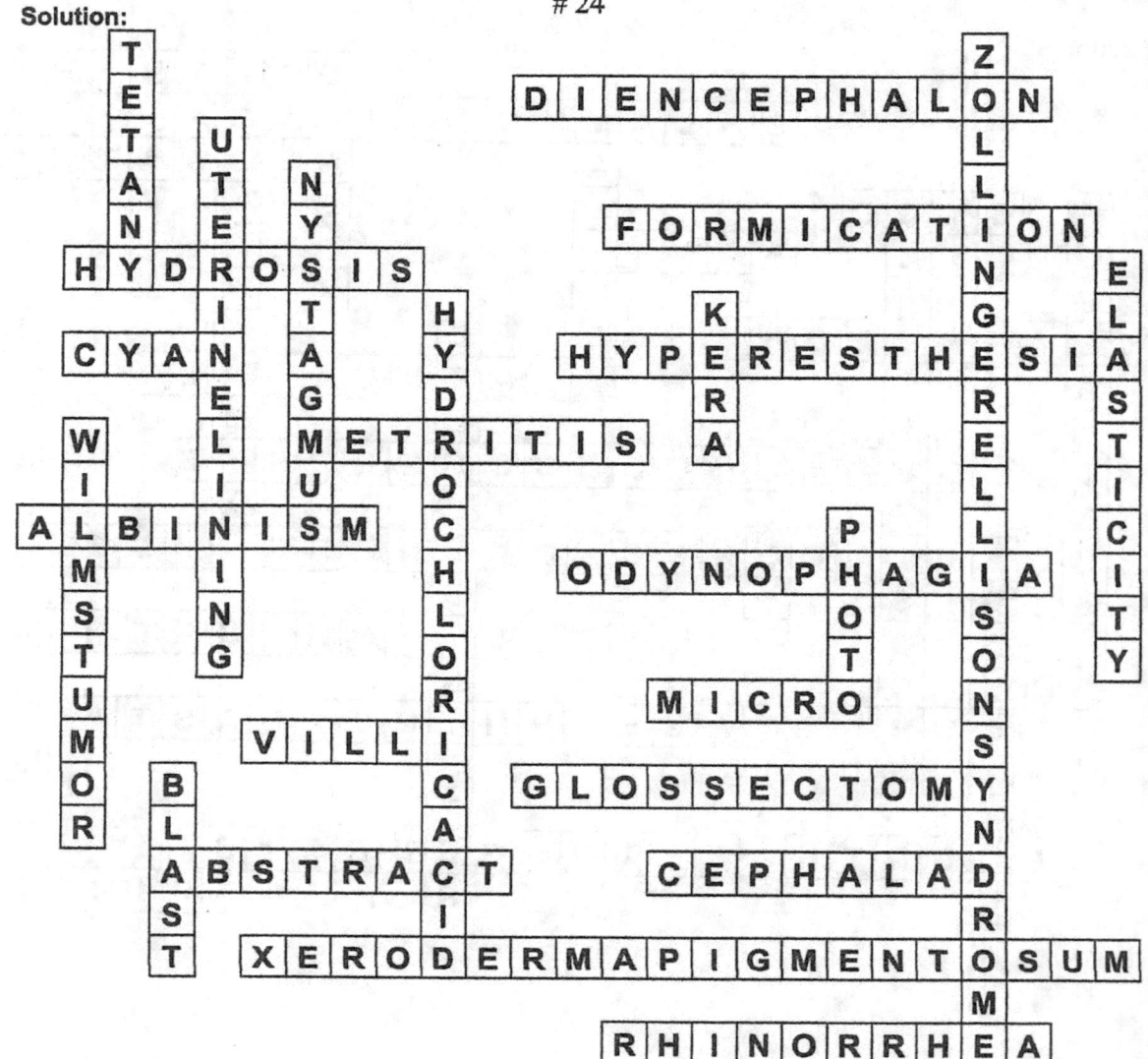

Solution:

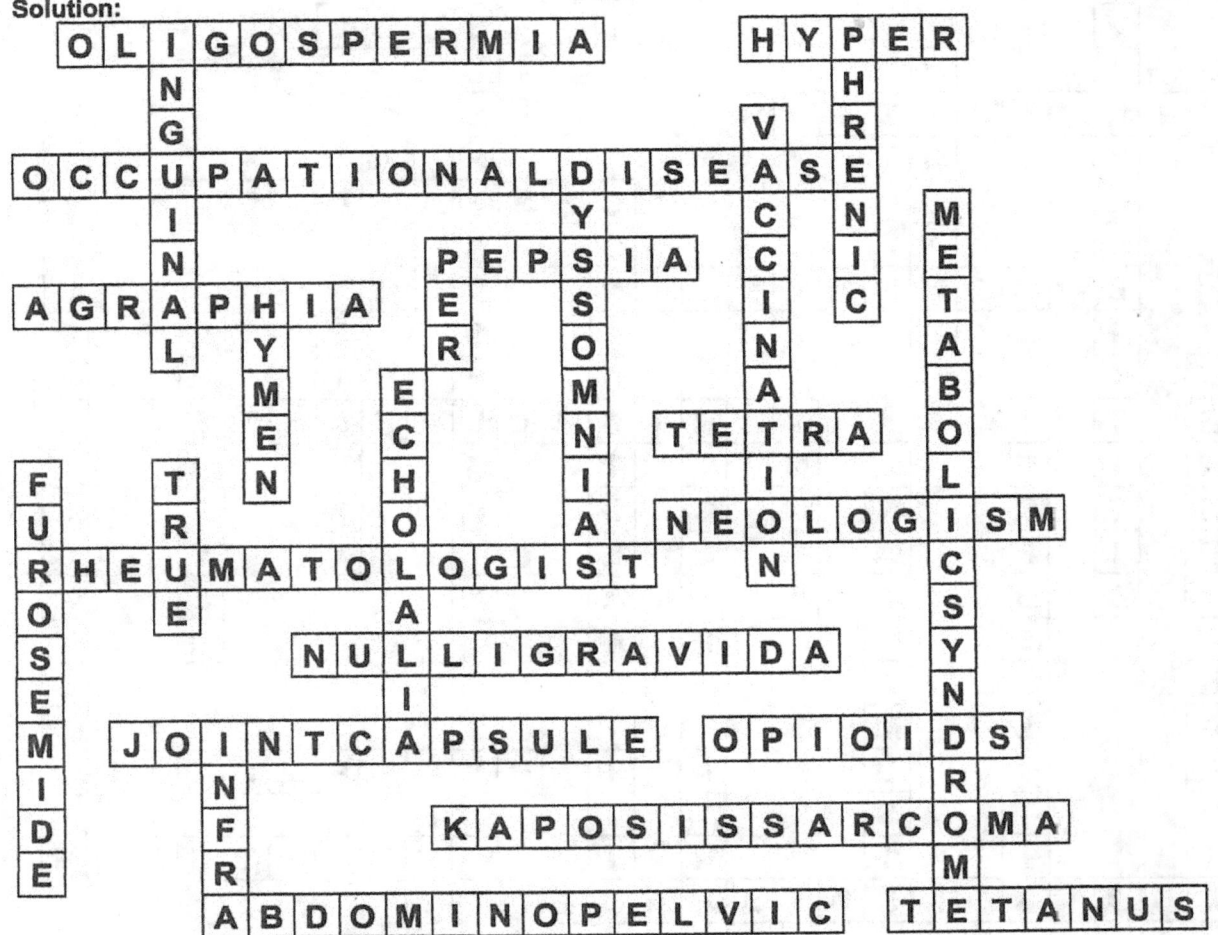

Solution:

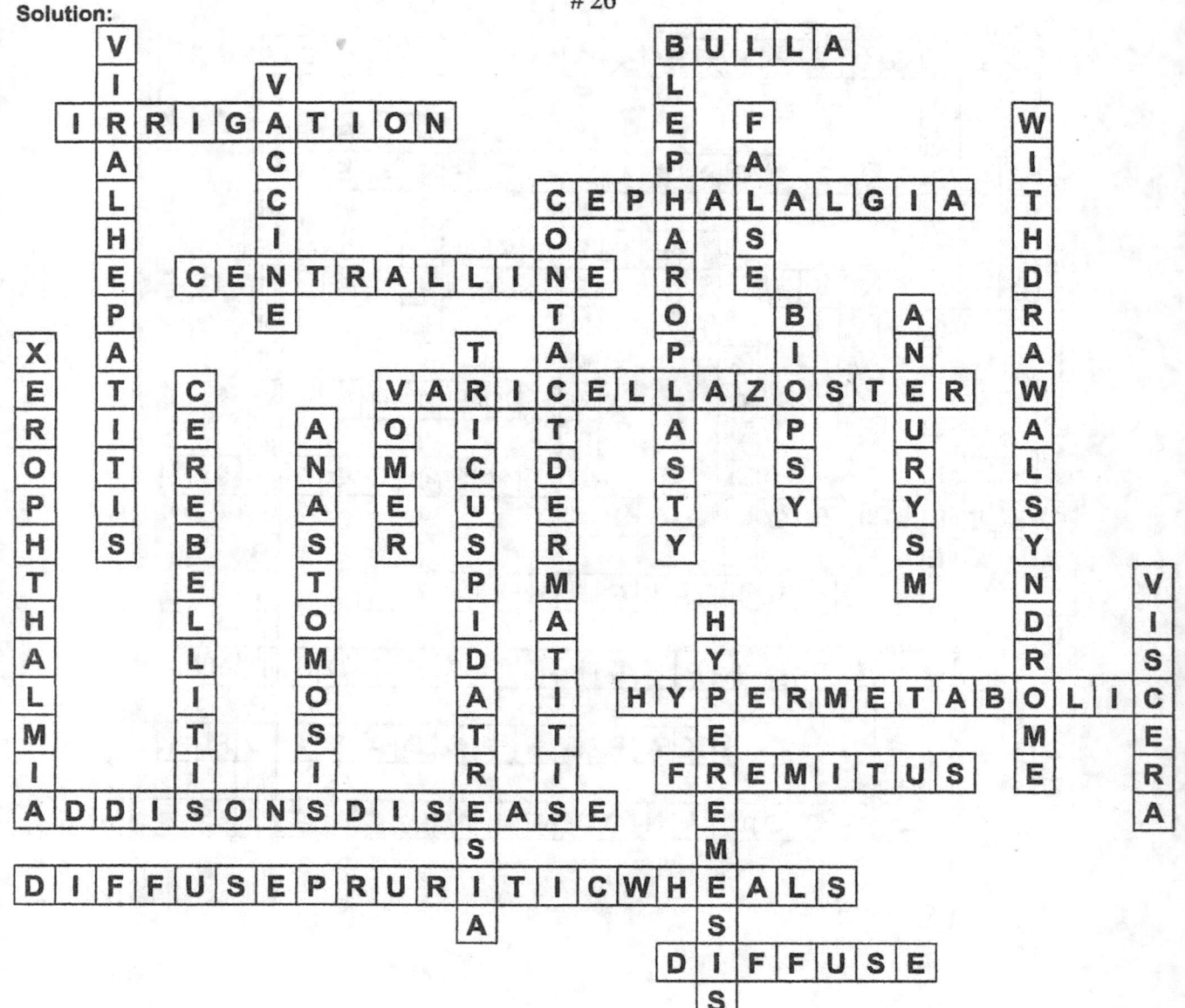

27

Solution:

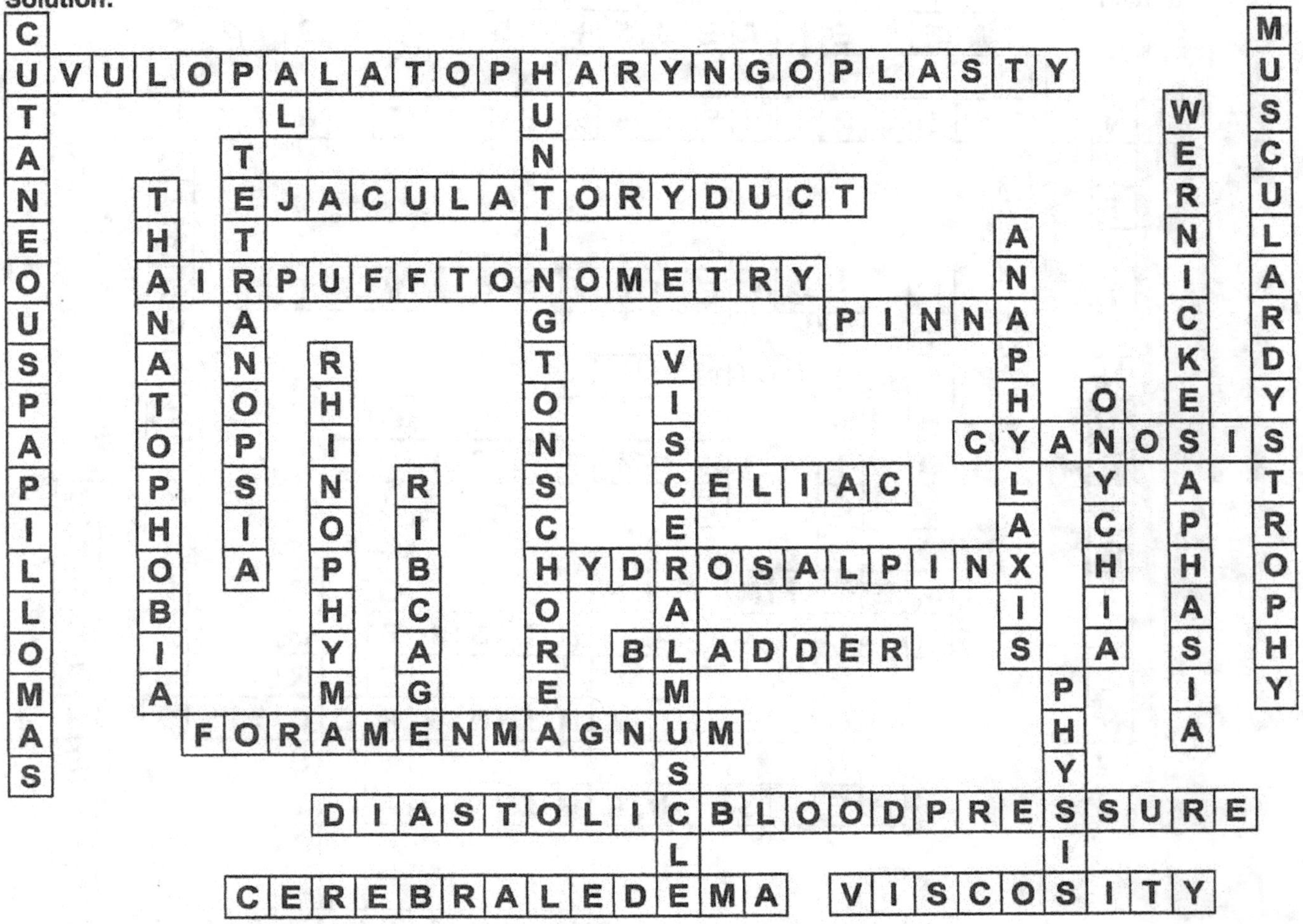
CUTANEOUSPAPILLOMAS
UVULOPALATOPHARYNGOPLASTY
AL
HUNTINGTONSCHOREA
TETRANOPSIA
EJACULATORYDUCT
THANATOPHOBIA
AIRPUFFTONOMETRY
PINNA
ANAPHYLAXIS
WERNICKESAPHASIA
MUSCULARDYSTROPHY
RHINOPHYMA
VISCERALMUSCLE
ONYCHIA
CYANOSIS
CELIAC
RIBCAGE
HYDROSALPINX
BLADDER
PHYSIS
FORAMENMAGNUM
DIASTOLICBLOODPRESSURE
CEREBRALEDEMA
VISCOSITY

Solution:

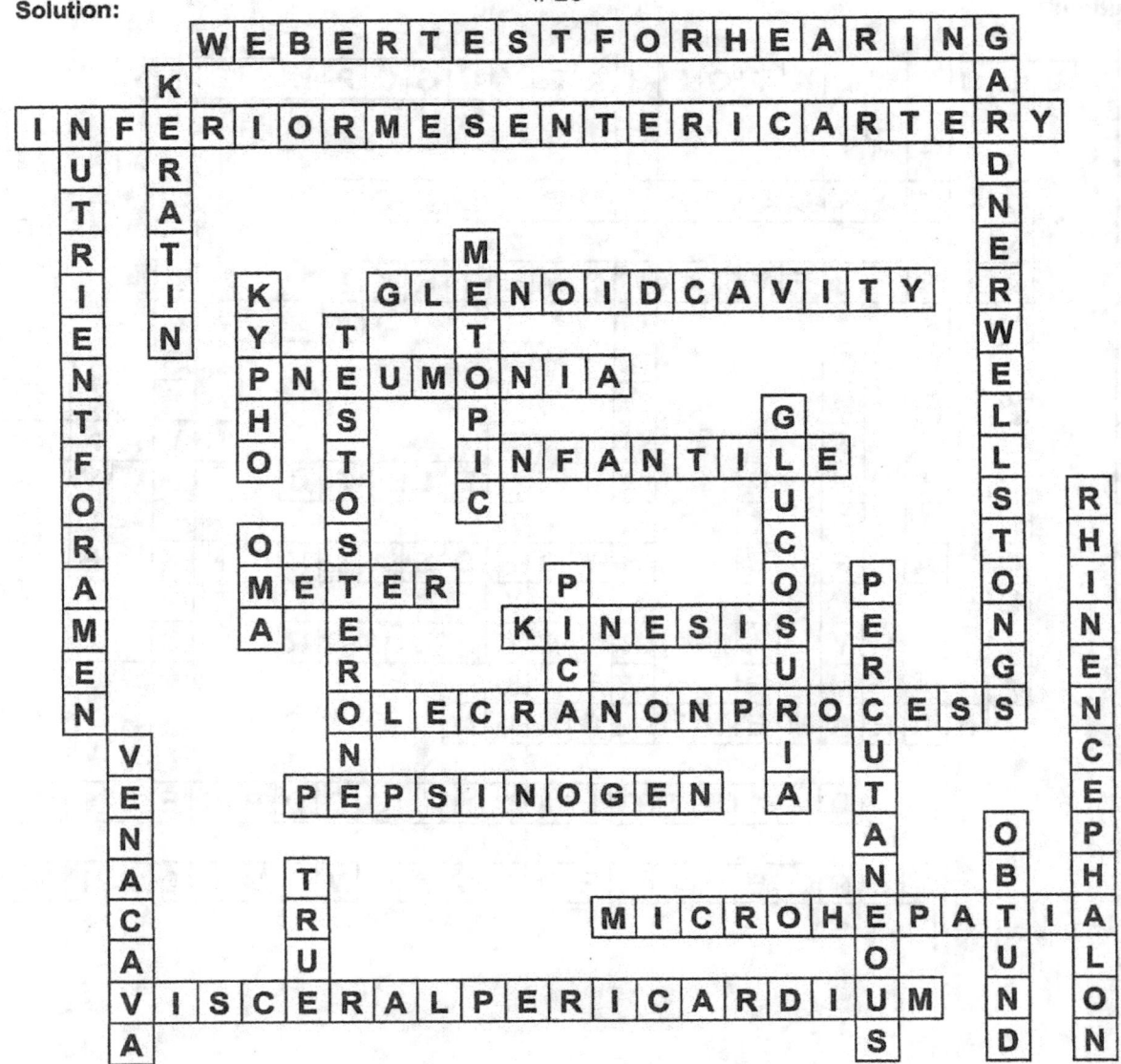

Solution:

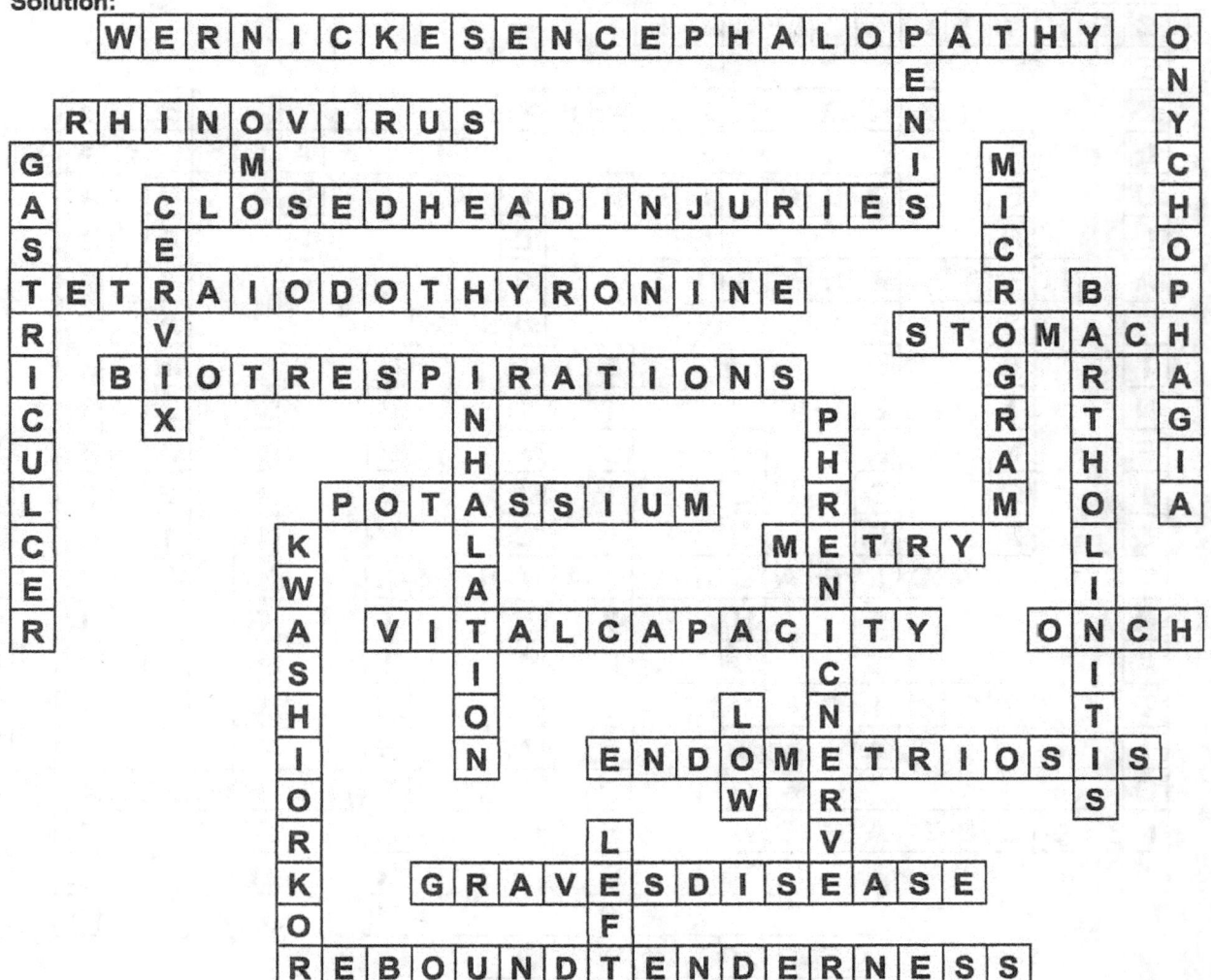

Solution:

Crossword solution grid #30

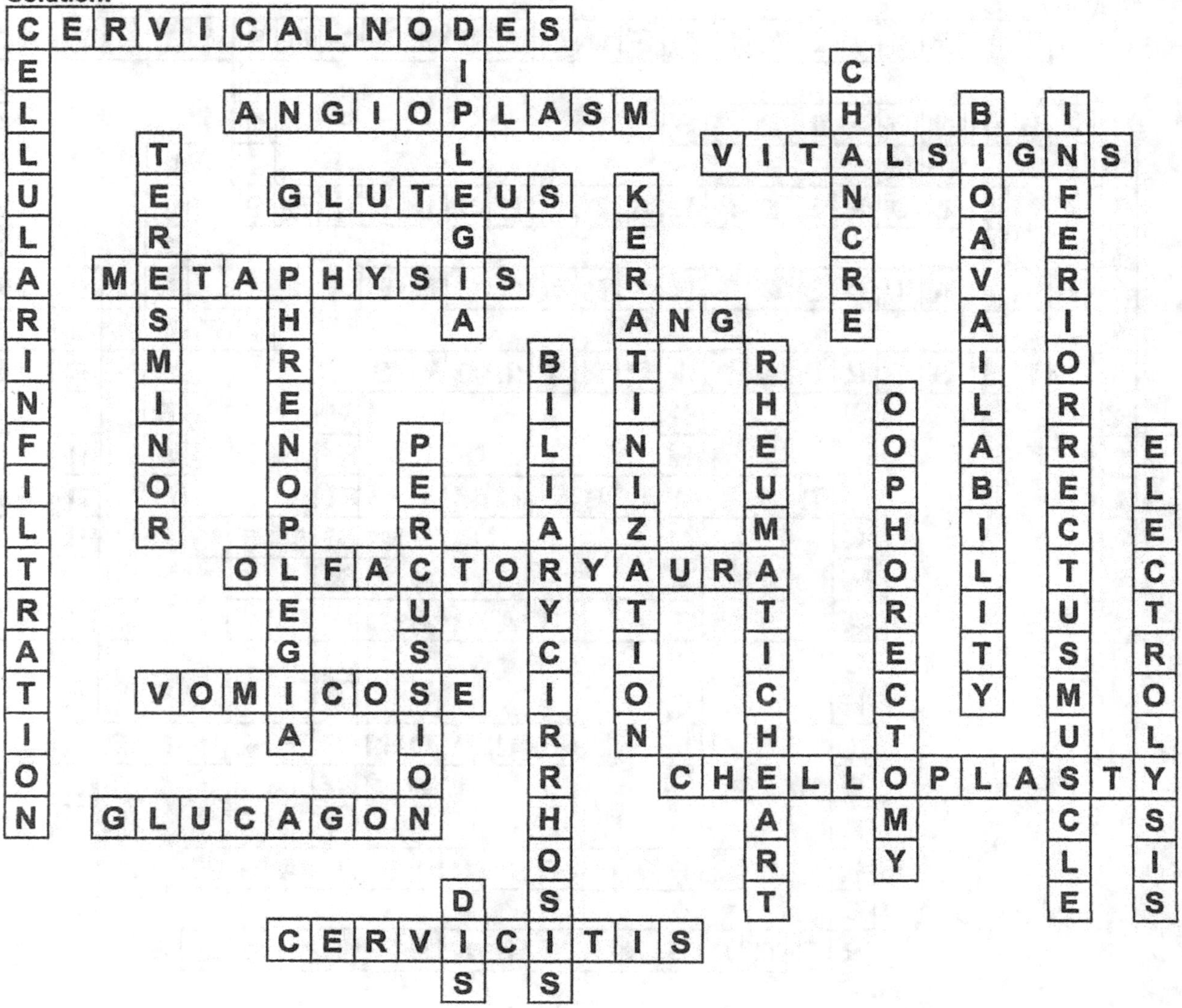

Across:
- CERVICALNODES
- ANGIOPLASM
- VITALSIGNS
- GLUTEUS
- METAPHYSIS
- OLFACTORY
- AURA
- VOMICOSE
- CHELLOPLASTY
- GLUCAGON
- CERVICITIS

Down:
- CELLULARINFILTRATION
- TERMSMINOR
- PHRENOPLEG
- ILIGIA
- KERATINIZATION
- CHANCRE
- BIOAVAILABILITY
- INFERIORRECTUSMUSCLE
- ELECTROLYSIS
- PERCUSSION
- BILIARYCIRRHOSIS
- RHEUMATICHEART
- OOPHORECTOMY
- DISS

Solution:

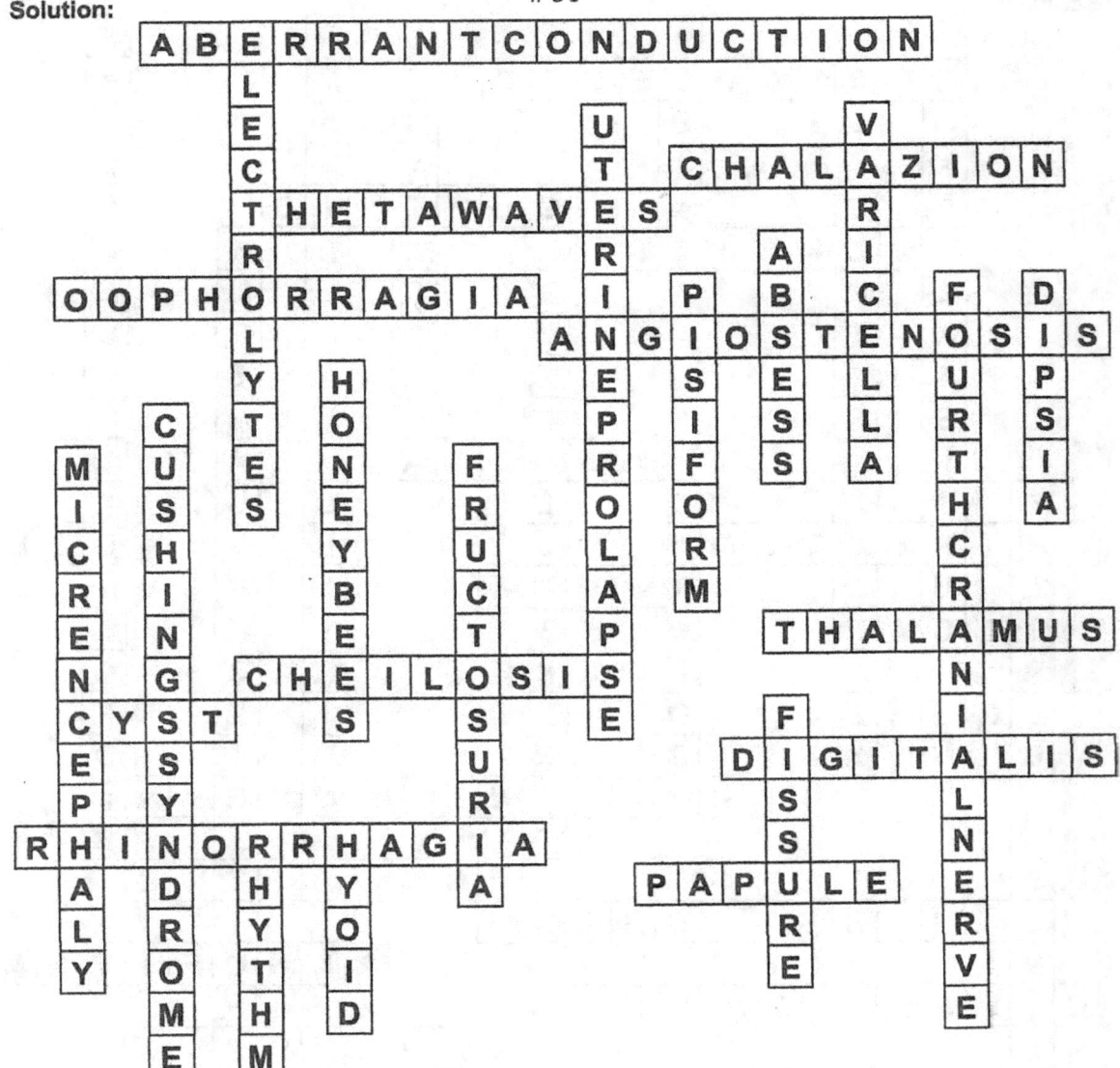

Solution:

Crossword puzzle grid (# 32) with the following answers:

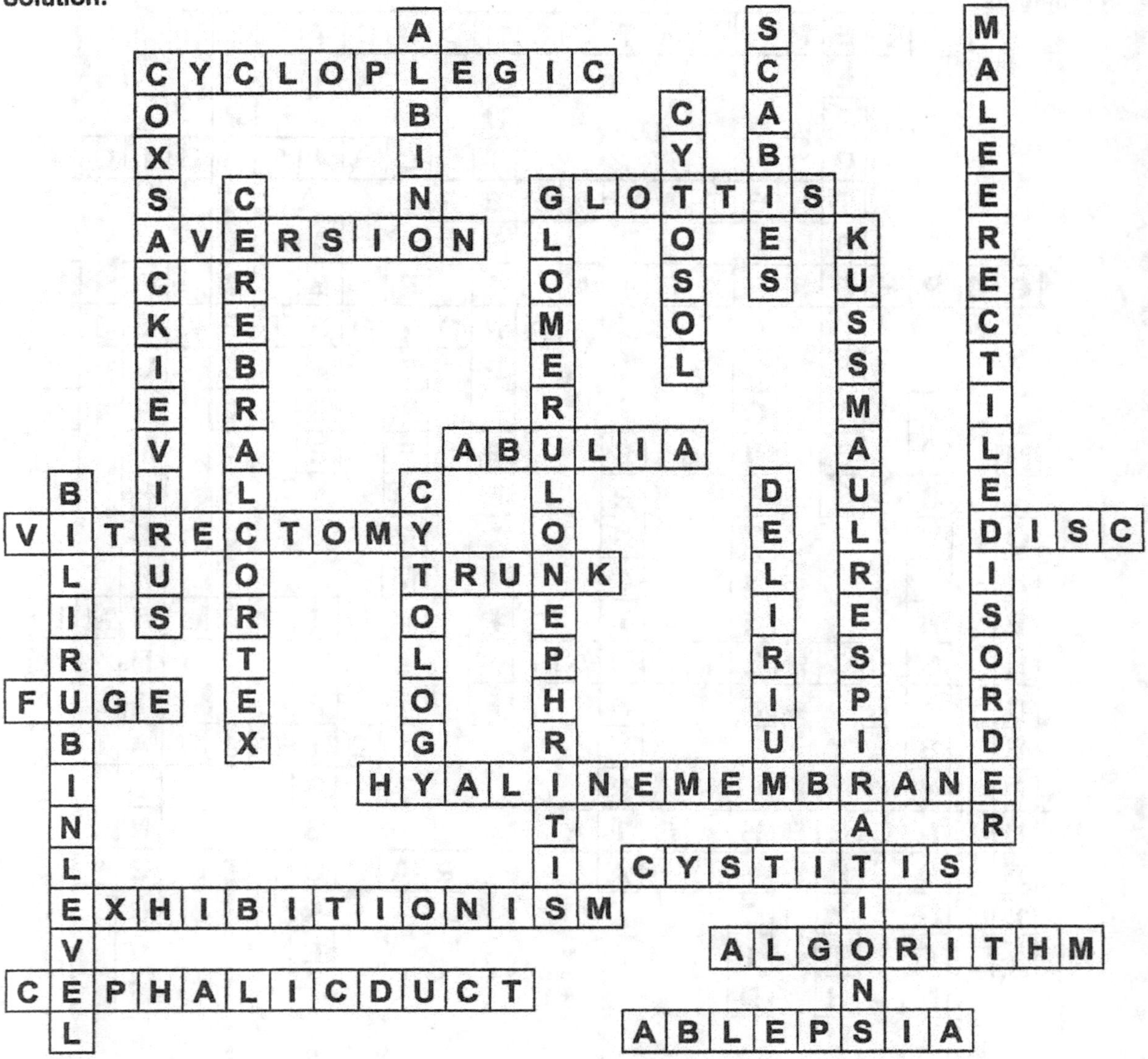

- CYCLOPLEGIC
- ALBININ (ALBIN)
- COXSACKIEVIRUS
- AVERSION
- CEREBRAL CORTEX
- GLOTTIS
- GLOMERULONEPHRITIS
- CYTOSOL
- SCABIES
- KUSSMAULRESPIRATION
- MALE ERECTILE DISORDER
- ABULIA
- VITRECTOMY
- CYTOLOGY
- DELIRIUM
- DISC
- BILIRUBIN FUGE (BILIRUBIN LEVEL)
- FUGE
- TRUNK
- HYALINE MEMBRANE
- CYSTITIS
- EXHIBITIONISM
- ALGORITHM
- CEPHALIC DUCT
- ABLEPSIA

Solution:

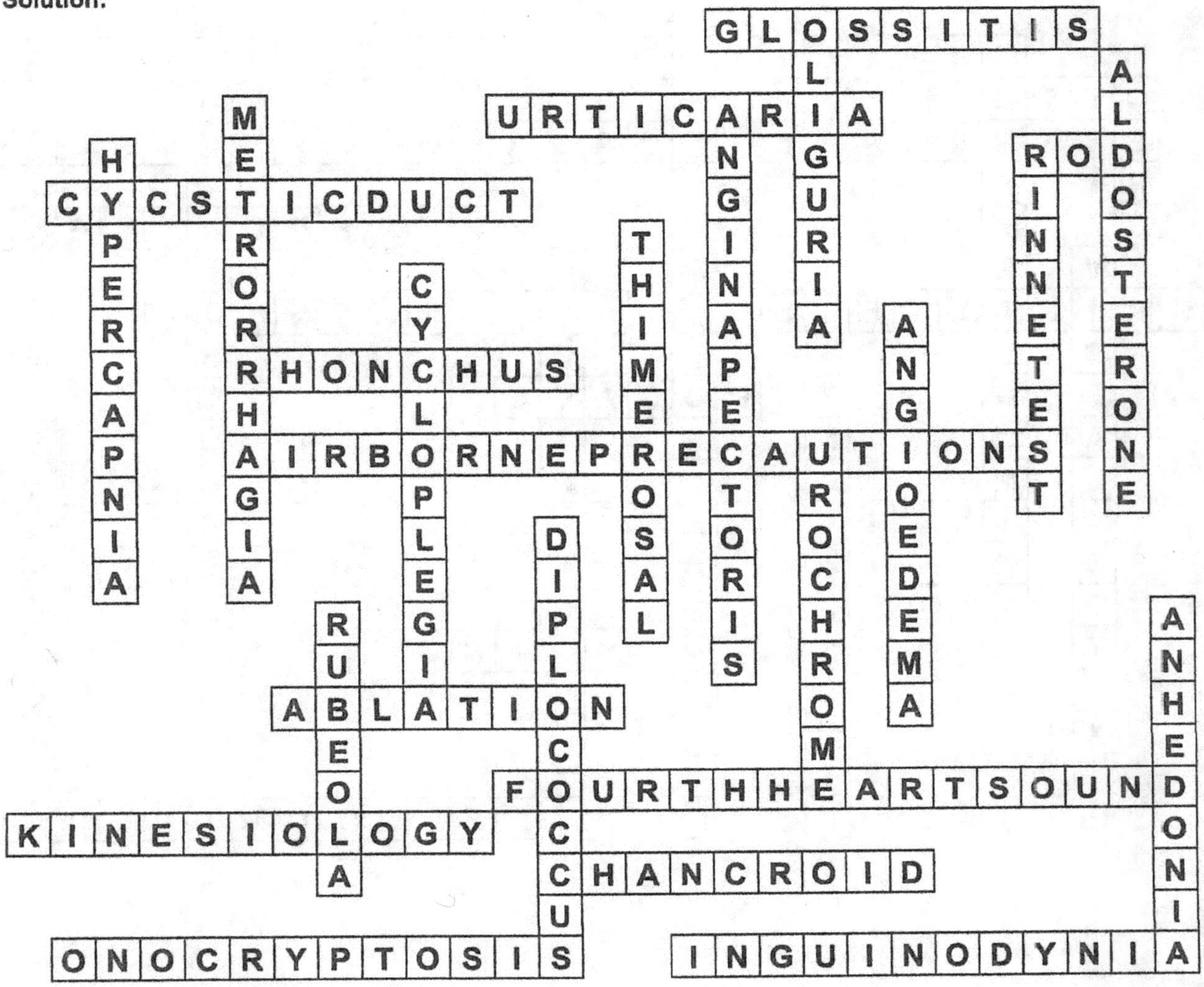

A crossword puzzle solution grid containing the following words:

GLOSSITIS

URTICARIA

METRORRHAGIA

CYCSTICDUCT

HYPERCAPNIA

RHONCHUS

AIRBORNEPRECAUTIONS

ABLATION

KINESIOLOGY

ONOCRYPTOSIS

FOURTHHEARTSOUND

CHANCROID

INGUINODYNIA

LIGURIA

ANGINAPECTORIS

THIMEROSAL

ANGIOEDEMA

RINNETEST

ALDOSTERONE

ANHEDONIA

RUBEOLA

CYLPLEGI

DIPLOCOCCUS

UROCHROM

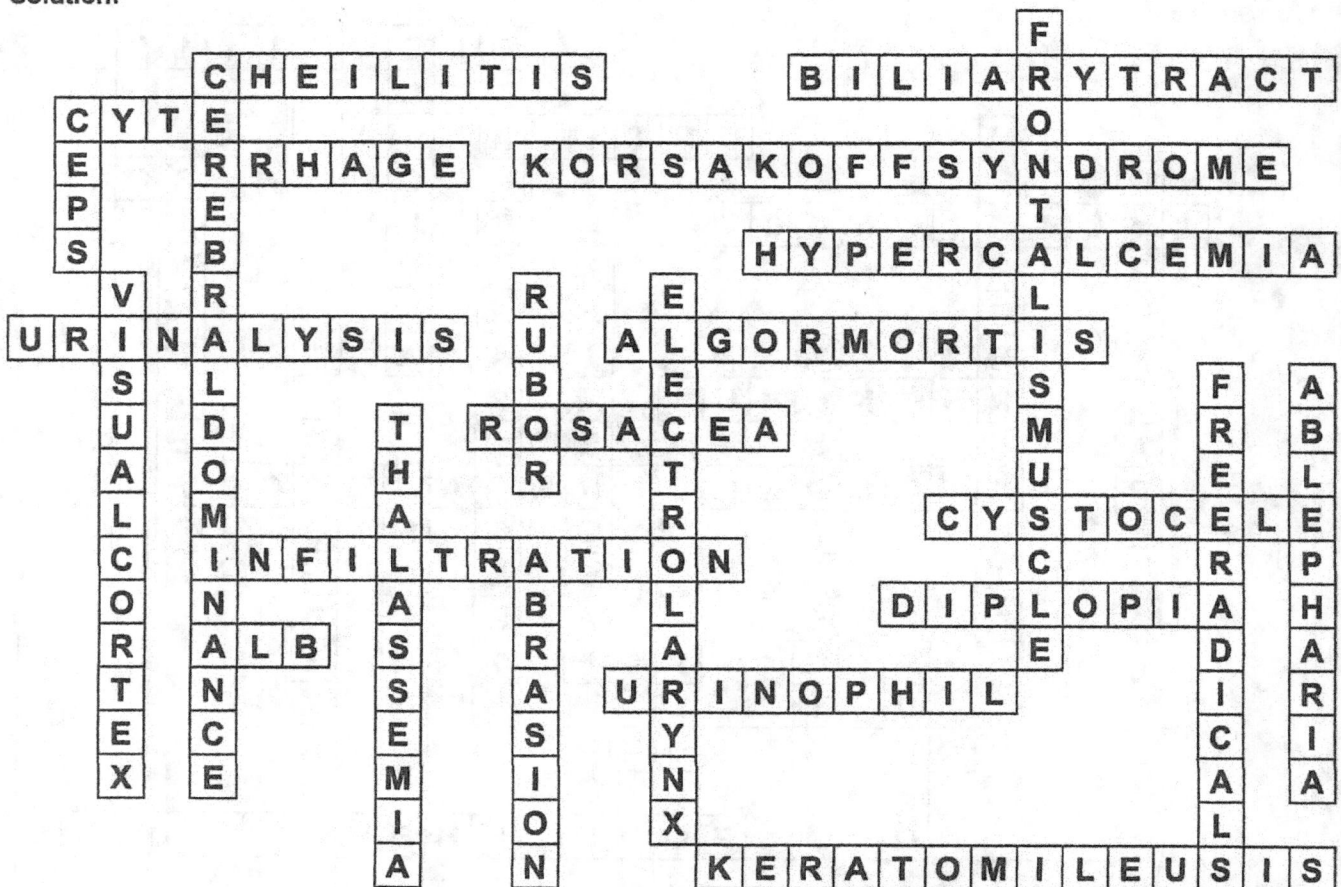

Solution:

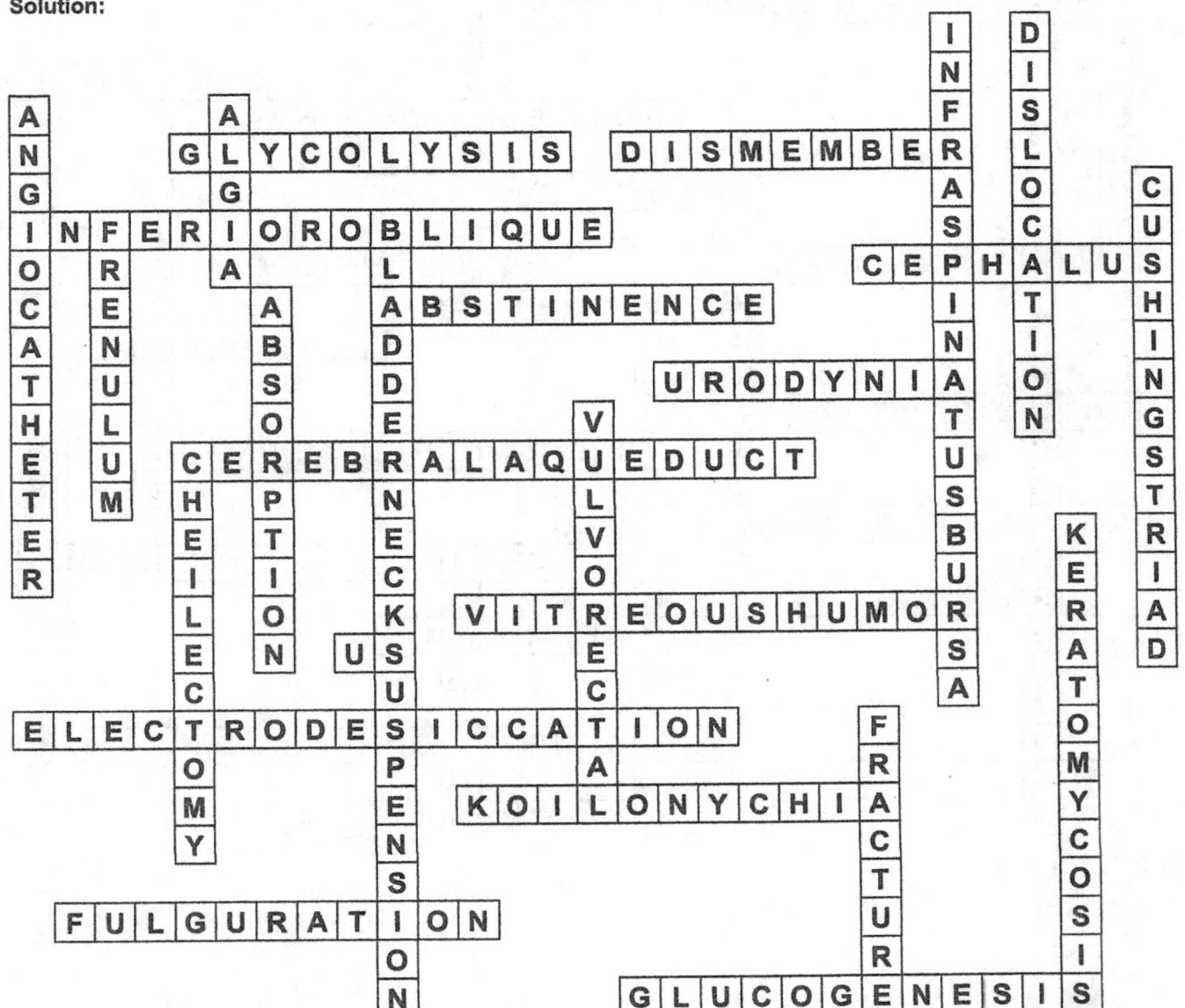

Solution:

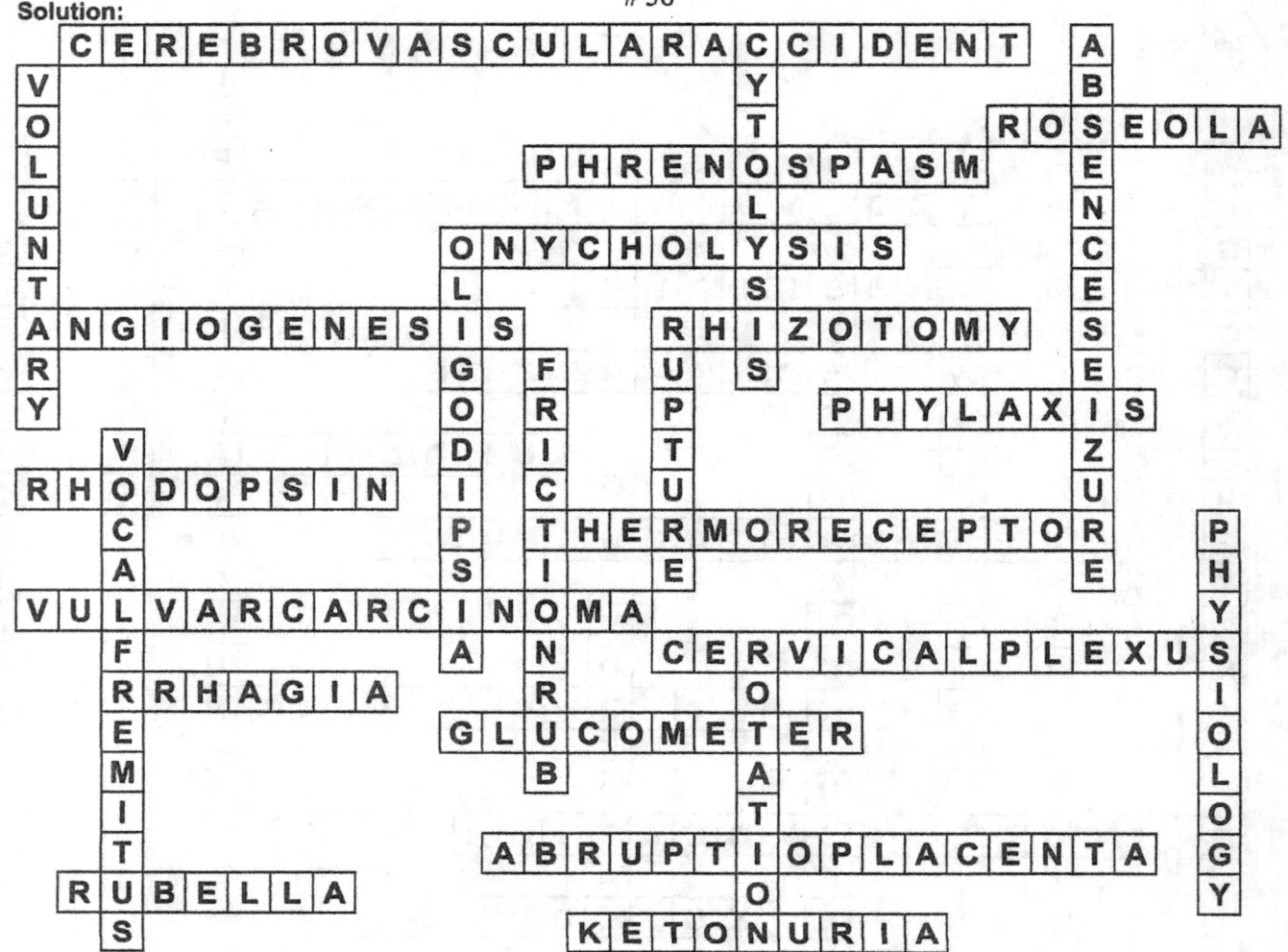

Solution:

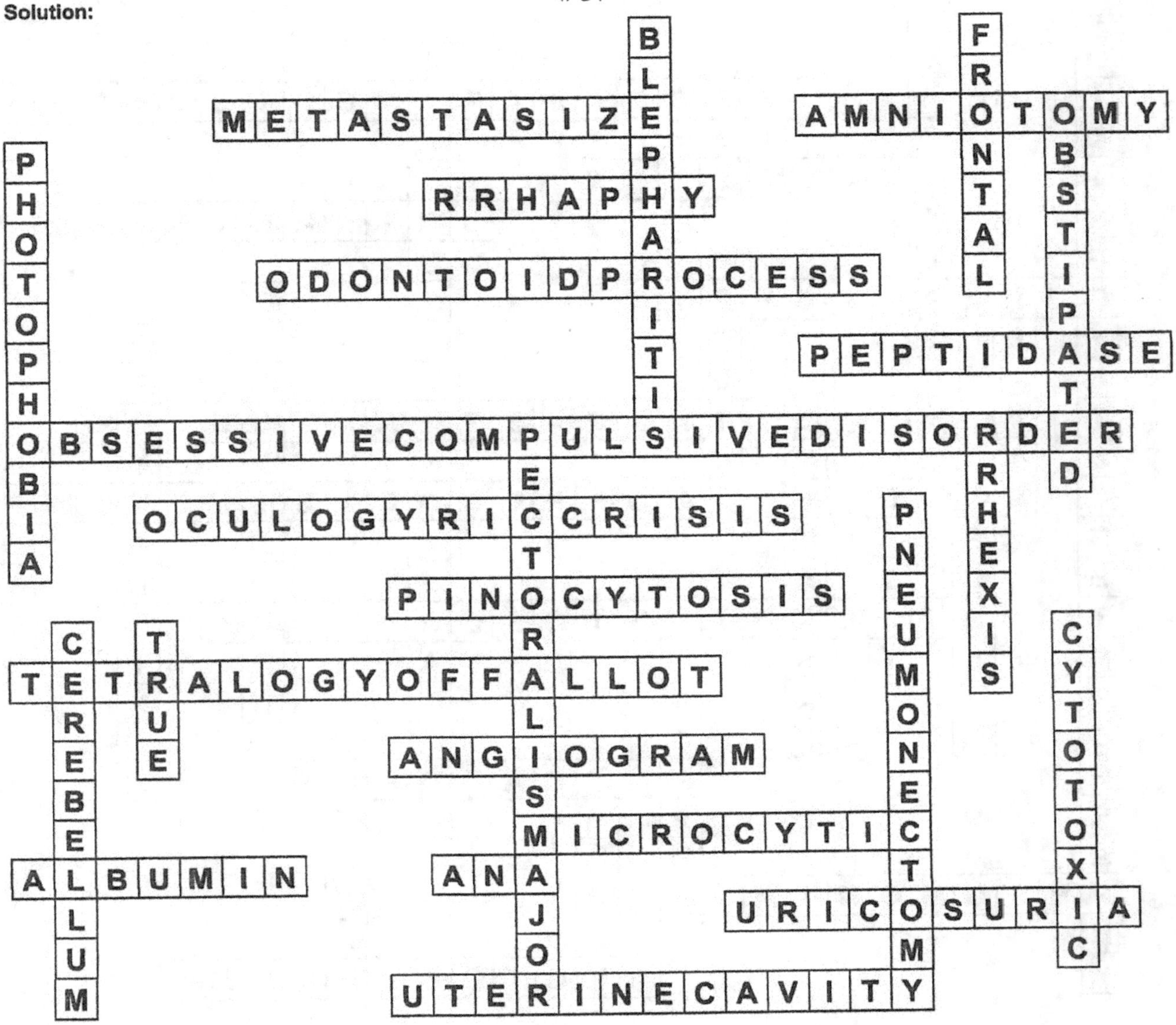

METASTASIZE

BLEPHARITIS (vertical)

RRHAPHY

ODONTOIDPROCESS

FRONTAL (vertical)

AMNIOTOMY

OBSTIPATED (vertical)

PEPTIDASE

PHOTOPHOBIA (vertical)

OBSESSIVECOMPULSIVEDISORDER

OCULOGYRICCRISIS

PECTORALISMAJOR (vertical)

RRHEXIS (vertical)

PINOCYTOSIS

PNEUMONECTOMY (vertical)

TETRALOGYOFFALLOT

CEREBELLUM (vertical)

TRUE (vertical)

ANGIOGRAM

CYTOTOXIC (vertical)

MICROCYTIC

ALBUMIN

ANA

URICOSURIA

UTERINECAVITY

Solution:

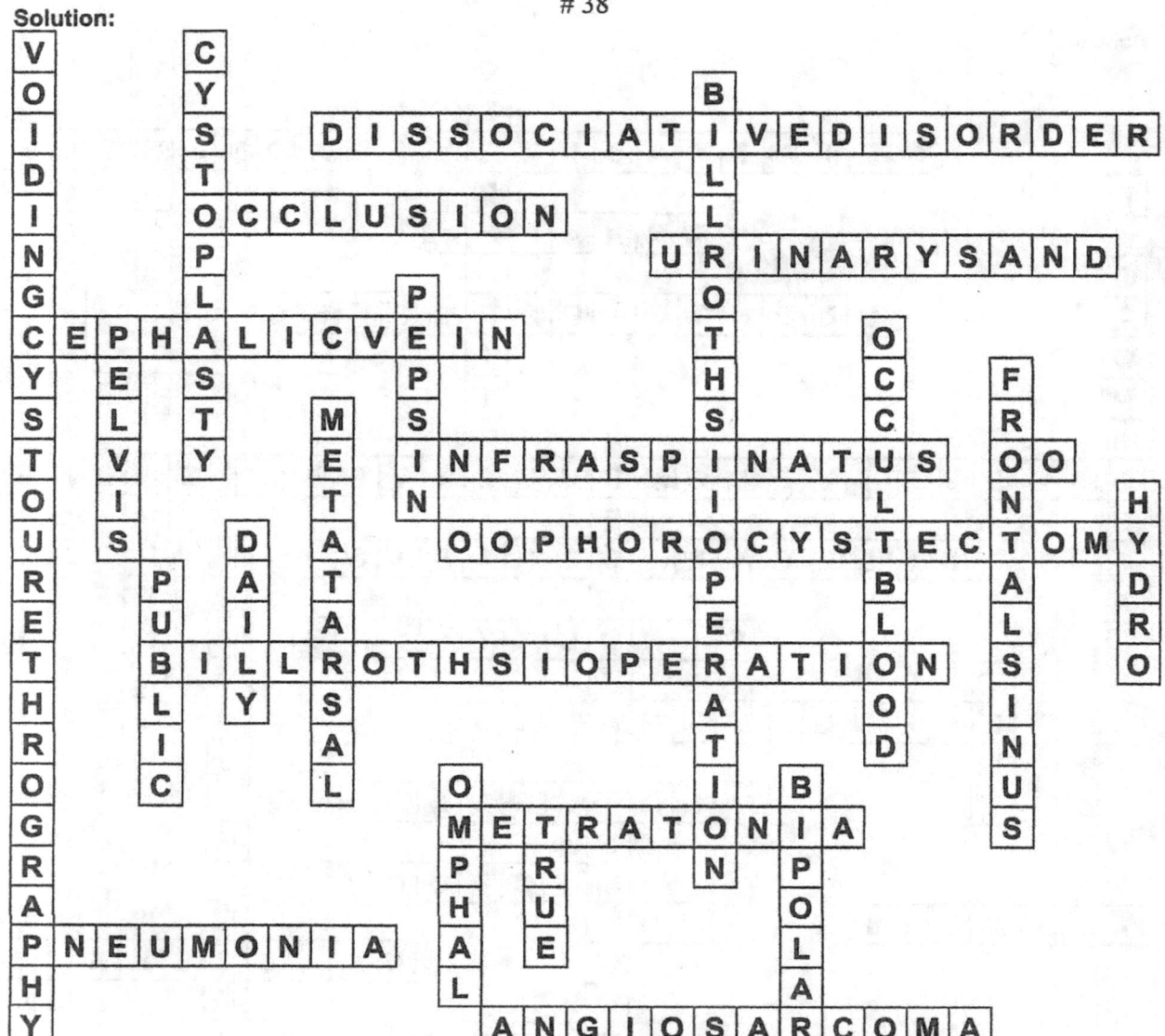

Solution:

A crossword puzzle solution grid containing the following words:

- PIAMATER
- RIGHTLUNG
- ENCE (ENCEPTICULCER / ENCEPHAL...)
- ALBUMINURIA
- PINEALGLAND
- OBSTRUCTIVESHOCK
- ROTATORCUFF
- RHEUMATOIDARTHRITIS
- AMB
- RUGA
- FRAGILEXSYNDROME
- OCULOMOTOR
- EJECTIONFRACTION
- FRONTALLOBE
- ANGIOPLASTY
- CYSTOTOMY
- AMNION
- UROSTOMY
- ANACUSIS
- EMESIS
- AMYL
- DIGITALSUBTRACTIONANGIOGRAPHY
- RHE / RRHE
- OCCIPITALIS

Solution:

40

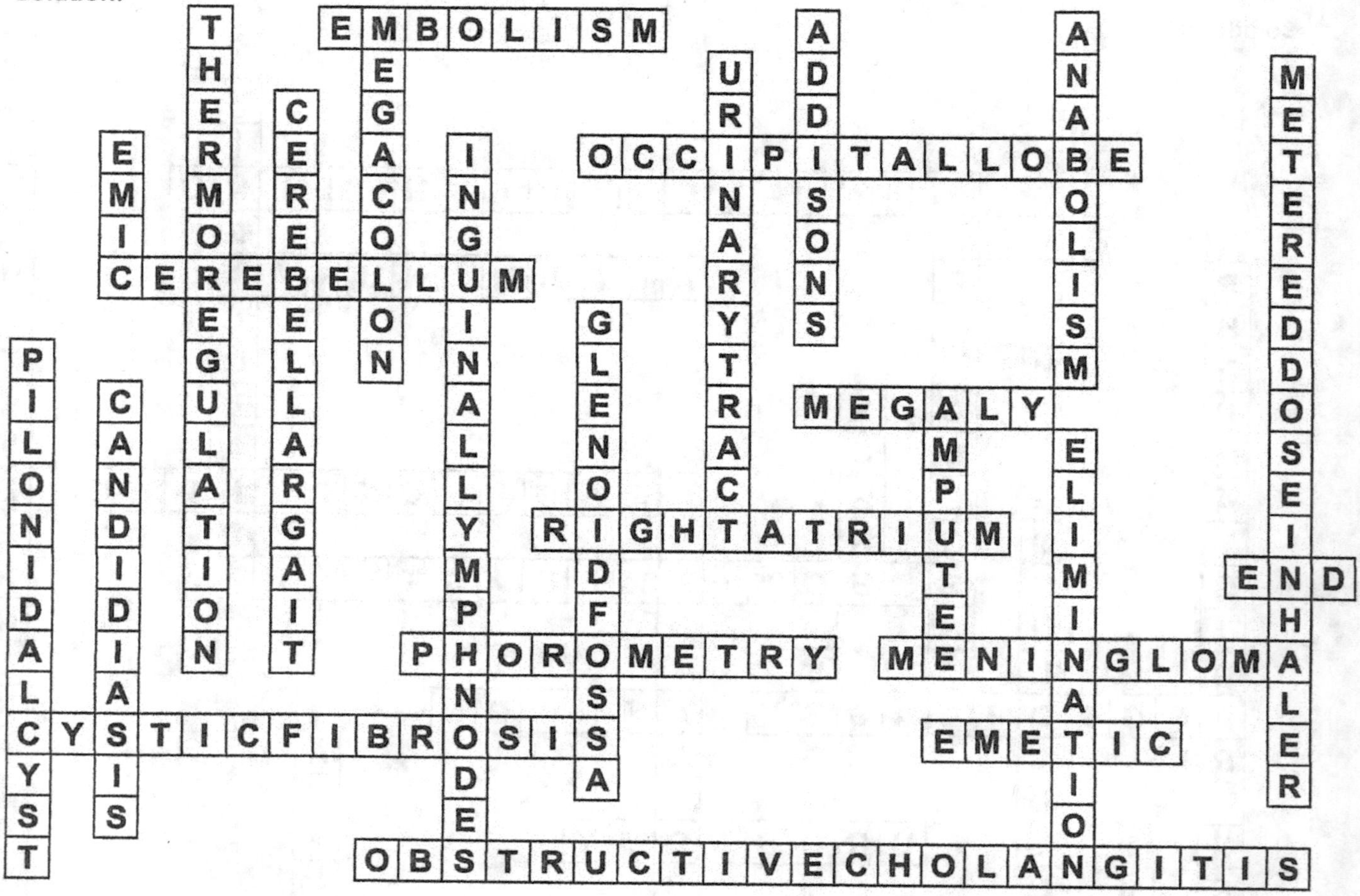
EMBOLISM
THERMOREGULATION
MEGACOLON
URINARYTRACT
ADDISONS
ANABOLISM
METEREDDOSEINHALER
CEREBELLARGAIT
INGUINALLYMPHNODE
OCCIPITALLOBE
EMIC
CEREBELLUM
GLENOIDFOSSA
PILONIDALCYST
CANDIDIASIS
MEGALY
AMPUTEE
ELIMINATION
RIGHTATRIUM
END
PHOROMETRY
MENINGLOMA
EMETIC
CYSTICFIBROSIS
OBSTRUCTIVECHOLANGITIS

Solution:

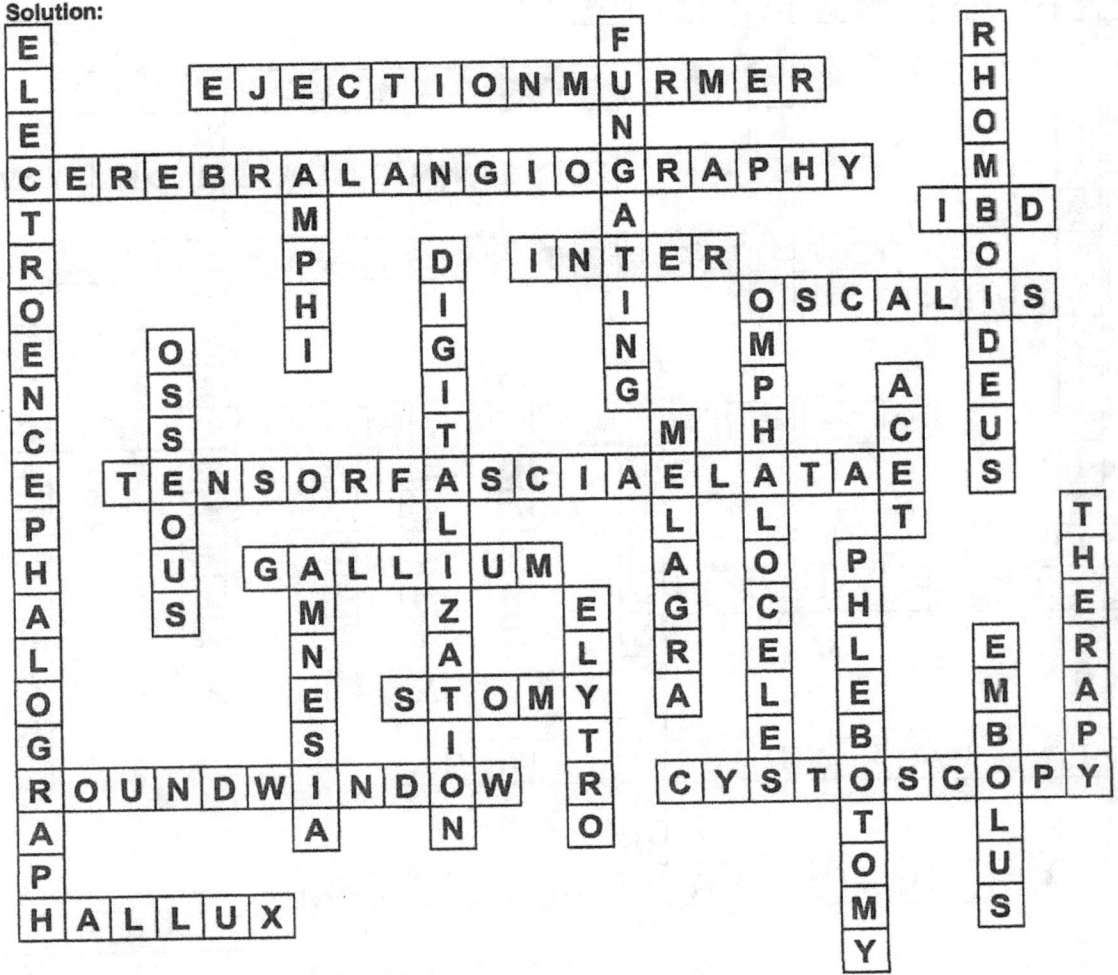

Solution:

A crossword puzzle solution grid containing the following words:

Across / Down words:

- PHOTOABLATION
- RORSCHACHTEST
- URINETURBIDITY
- OBSTRUCTIVEJAUNDICE
- ANALGESIA
- TRUE
- PEG
- PELVICINFLAMMATORYDISEASE
- OCCIPITALBONE
- INFERIORVENACAVA
- CEPHALICPRESENTATION
- GLOMERULARFILTRATION
- ONYCHOMYCOSIS
- RIGHTVENTRICLE
- ALGOPHOBIA
- RIGHTCORONARY
- ELECTROENCEPHALOGRAM
- THIRDDEGREEBURN
- DILATEDFUNDUSCOPY
- OLOGIST
- SELENIC
- ANALYTE
- ROSACEIFORM
- CYSTOSTOMY
- ORIF

Solution:

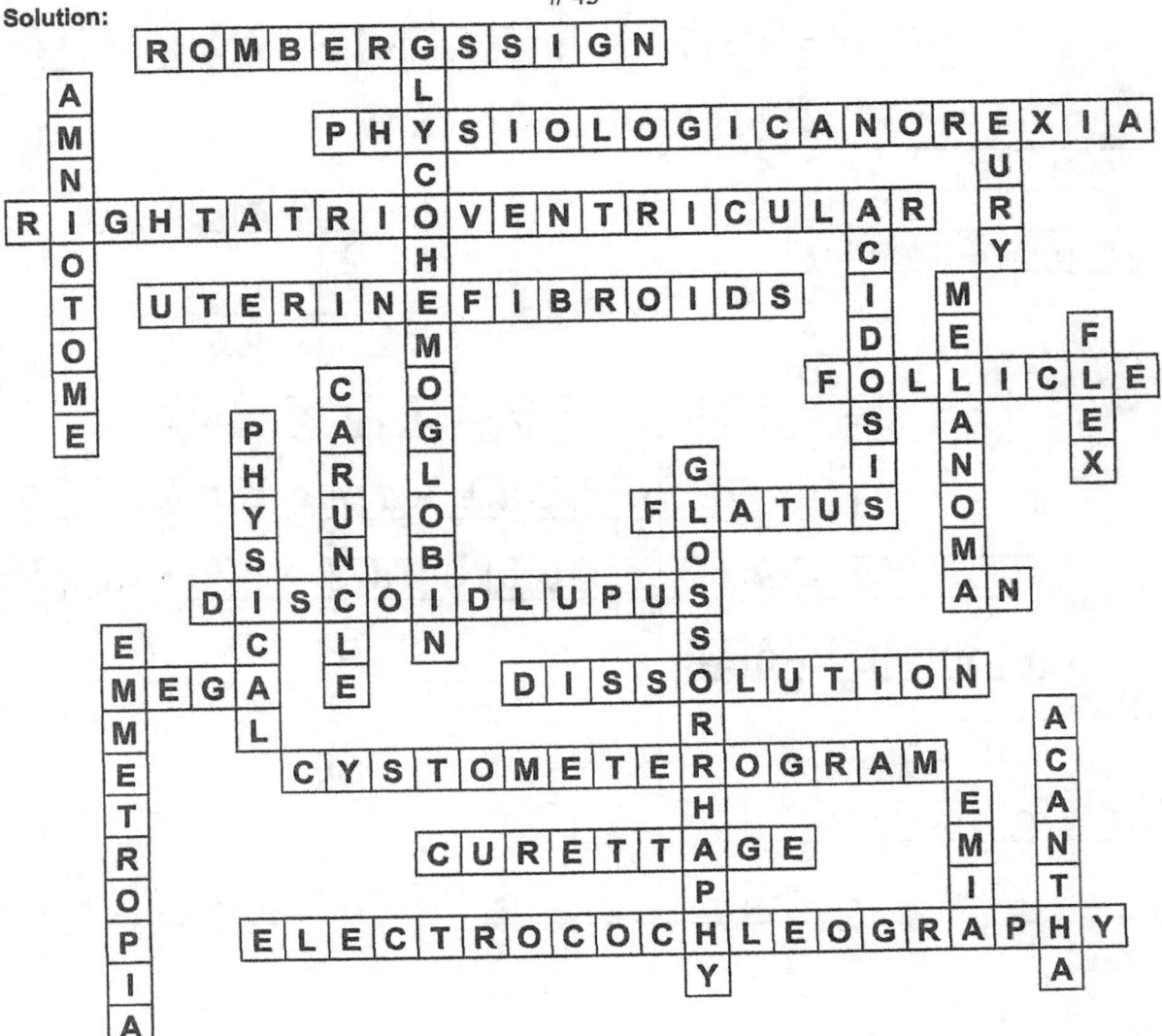

Solution:

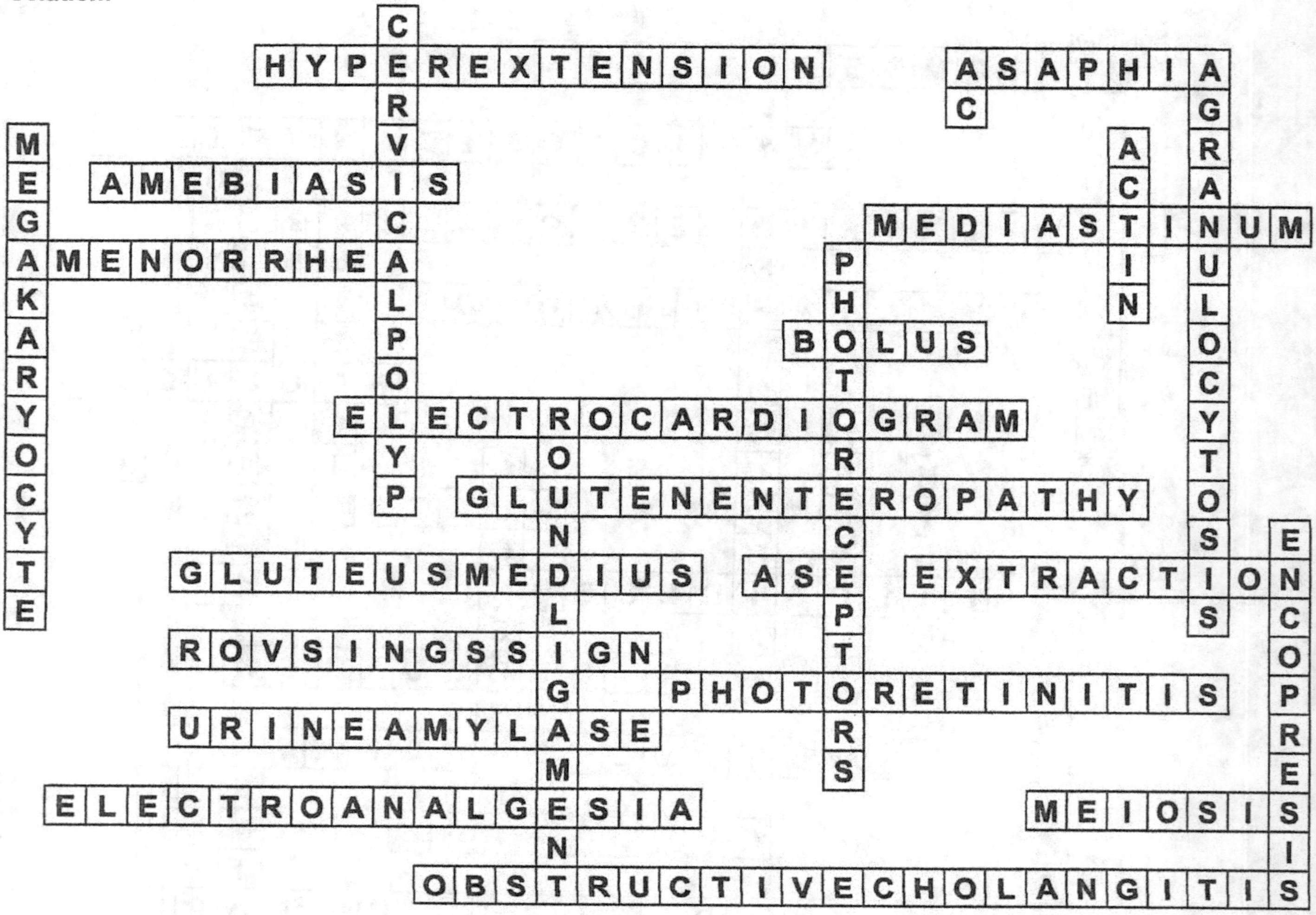
CERVICALPOLYP
HYPEREXTENSION
ASAPHIA
AC
AGRANULOCYTOSIS
ACTIN
MEGAKARYOCYTE
AMEBIASIS
MEDIASTINUM
AMENORRHEA
PHOTORECEPTORS
BOLUS
ELECTROCARDIOGRAM
ROUNDLIGAMENT
GLUTENENTEROPATHY
GLUTEUSMEDIUS
ASE
EXTRACTION
ENCOPRESIS
ROVSINGSSIGN
PHOTORETINITIS
URINEAMYLASE
ELECTROANALGESIA
MEIOSIS
OBSTRUCTIVECHOLANGITIS

Solution:

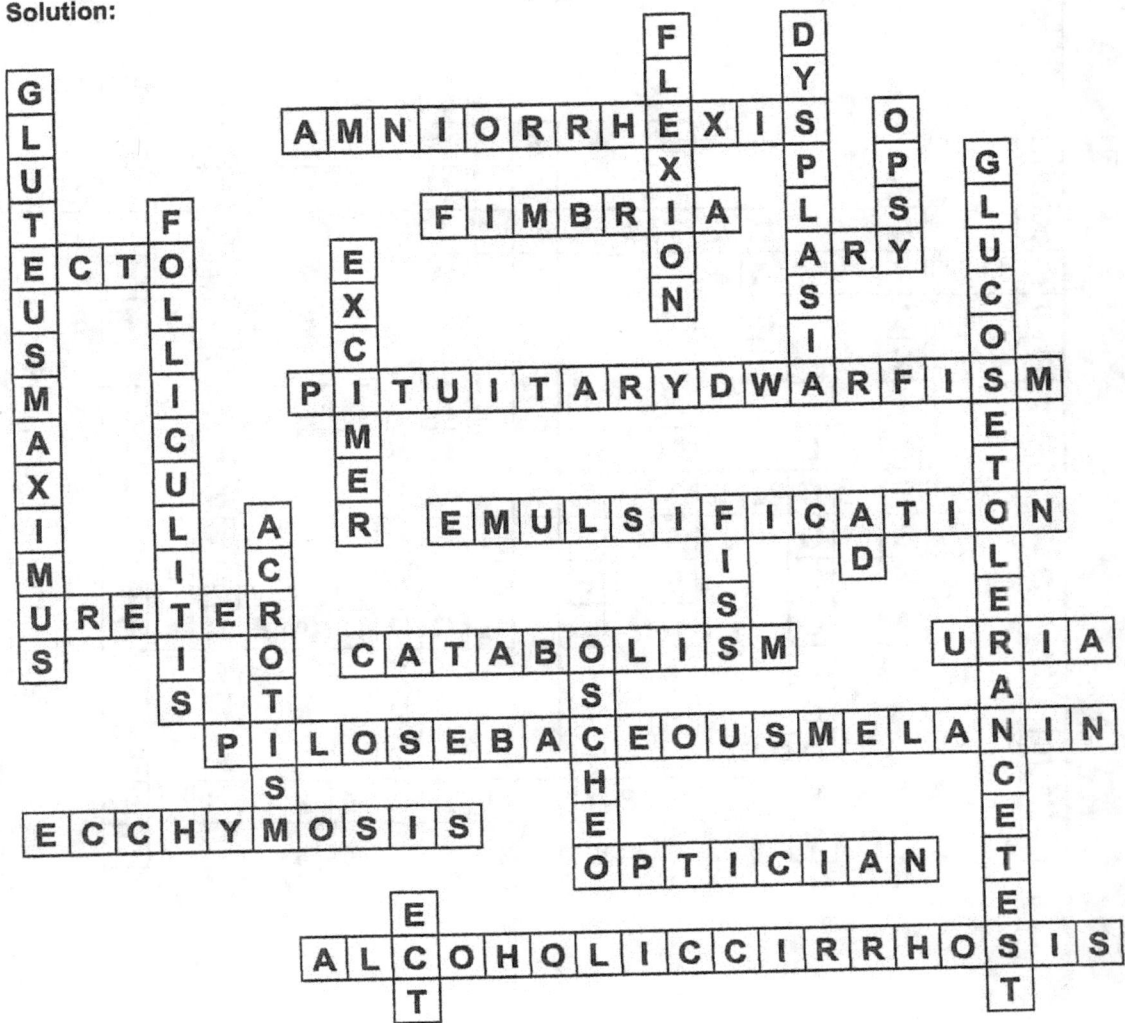

Solution:

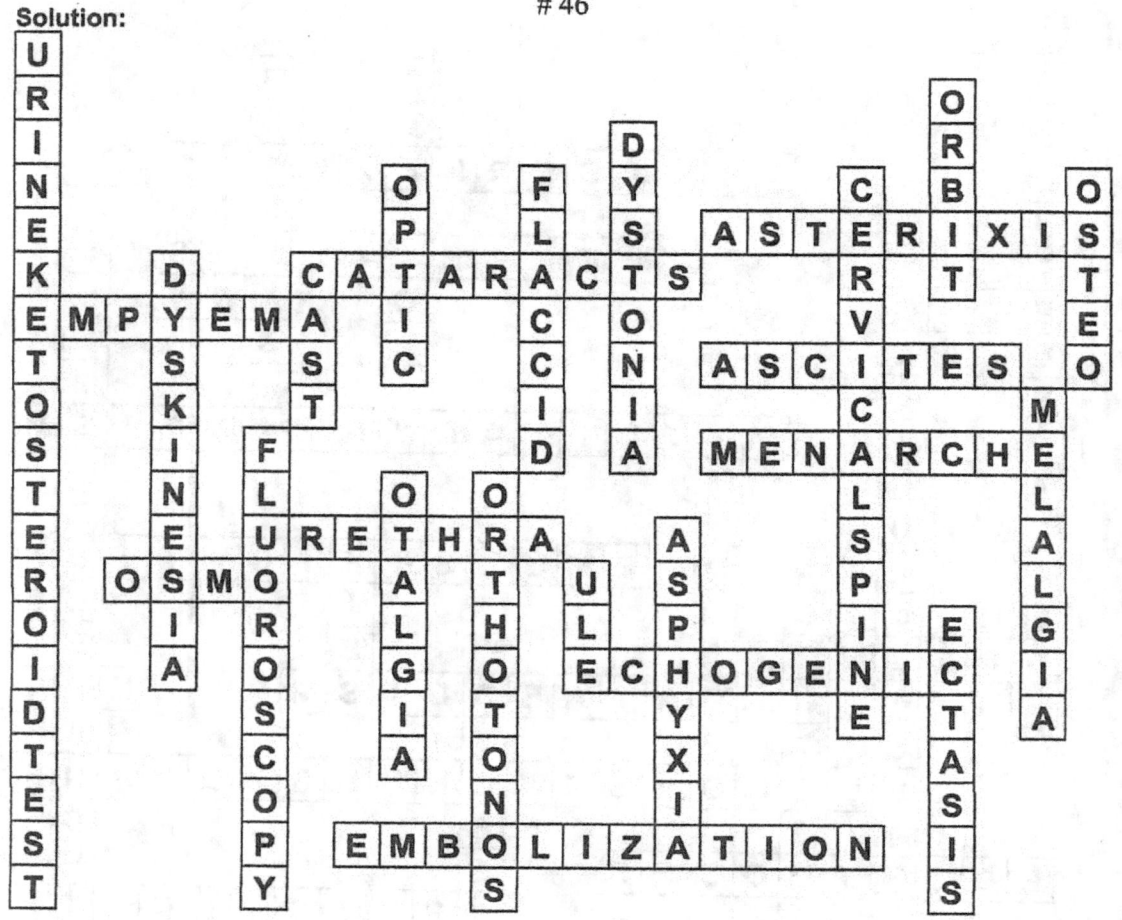

Solution:

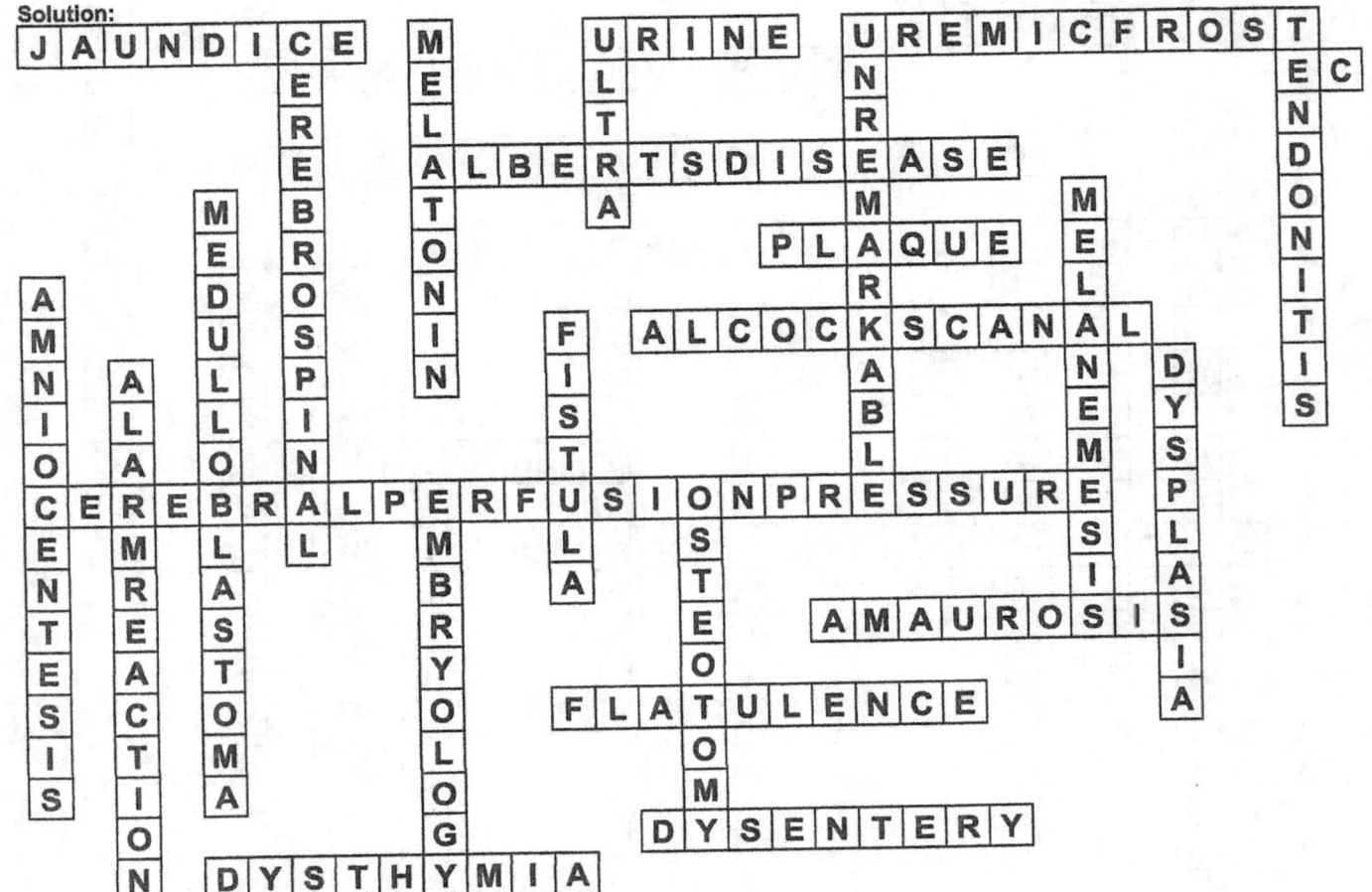

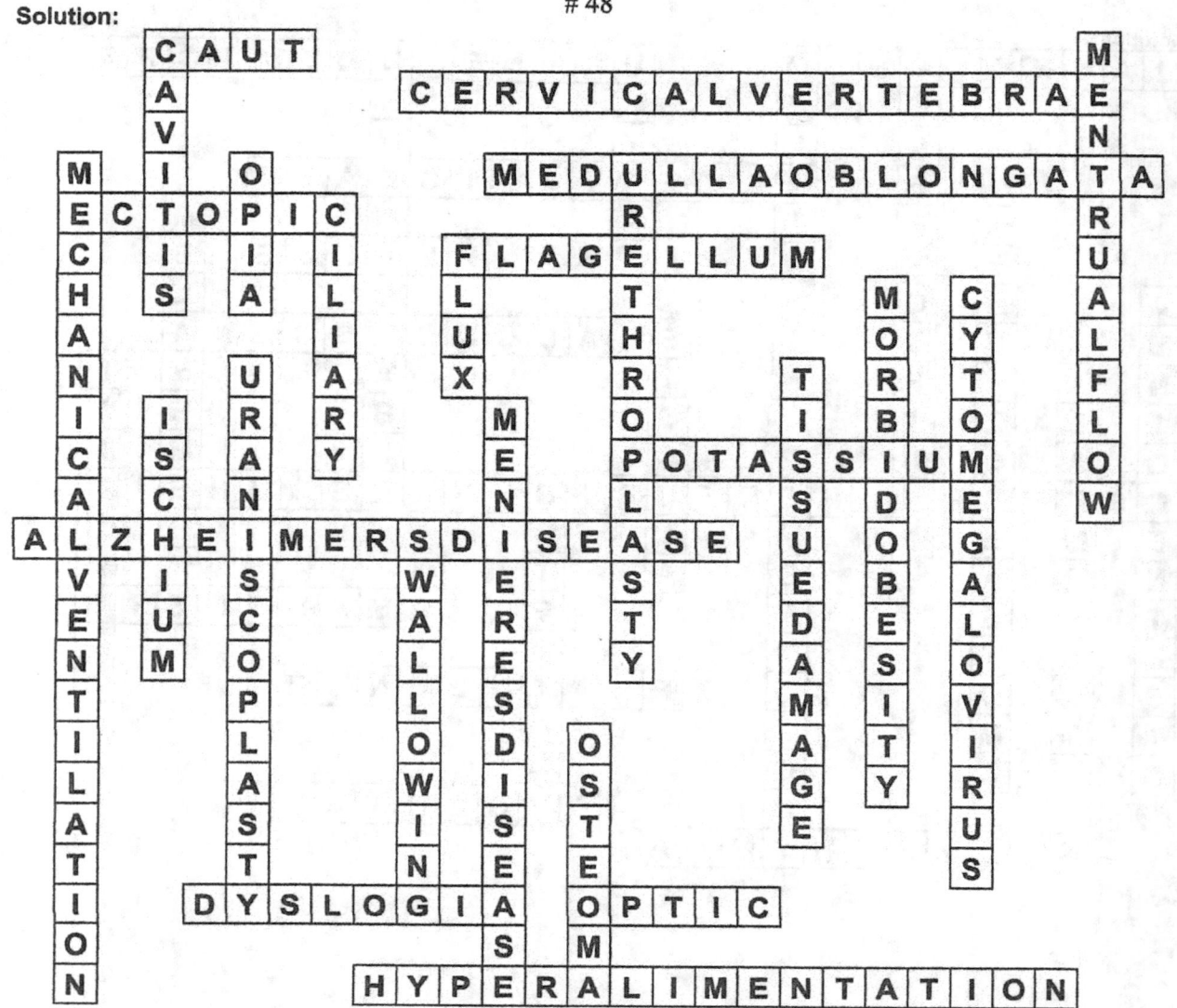

Solution:

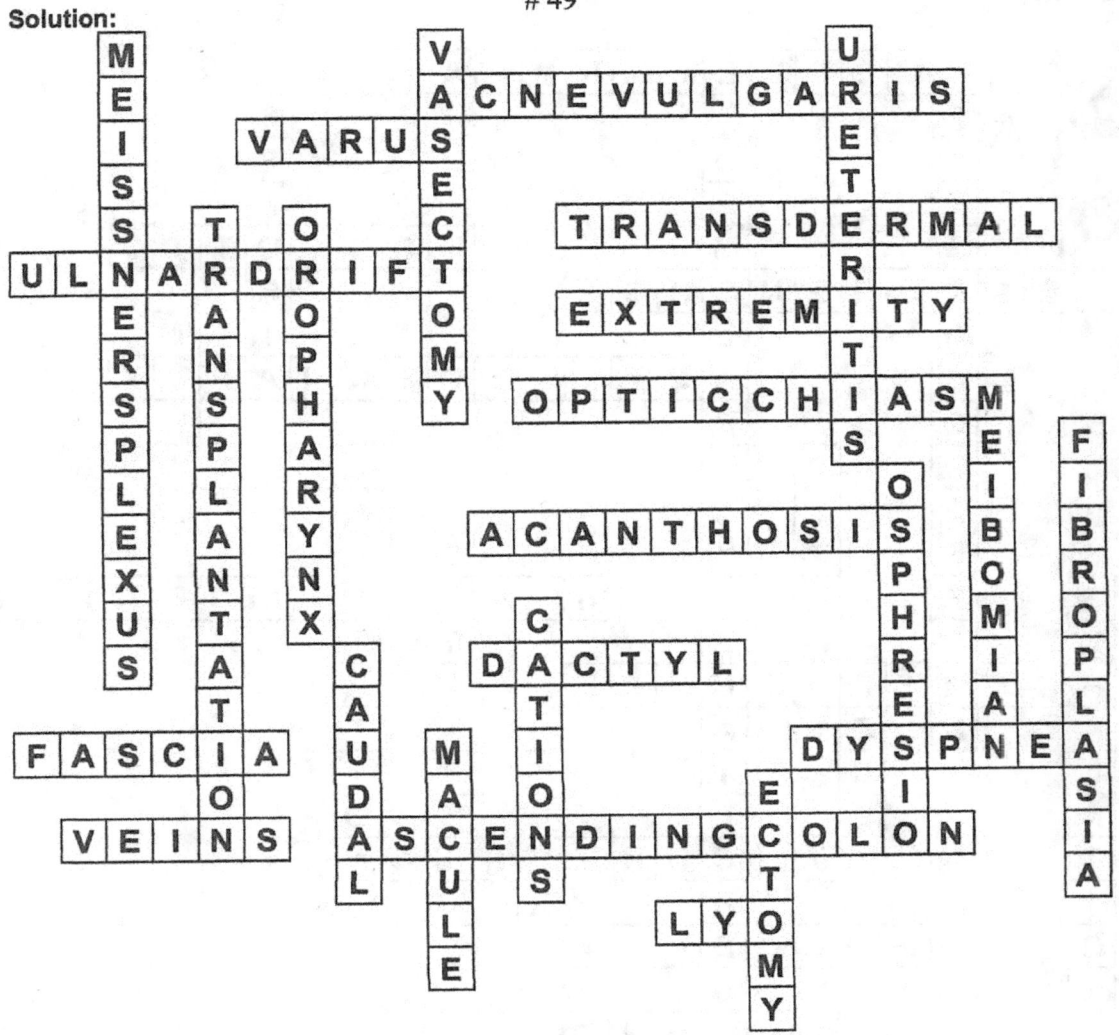

Solution:

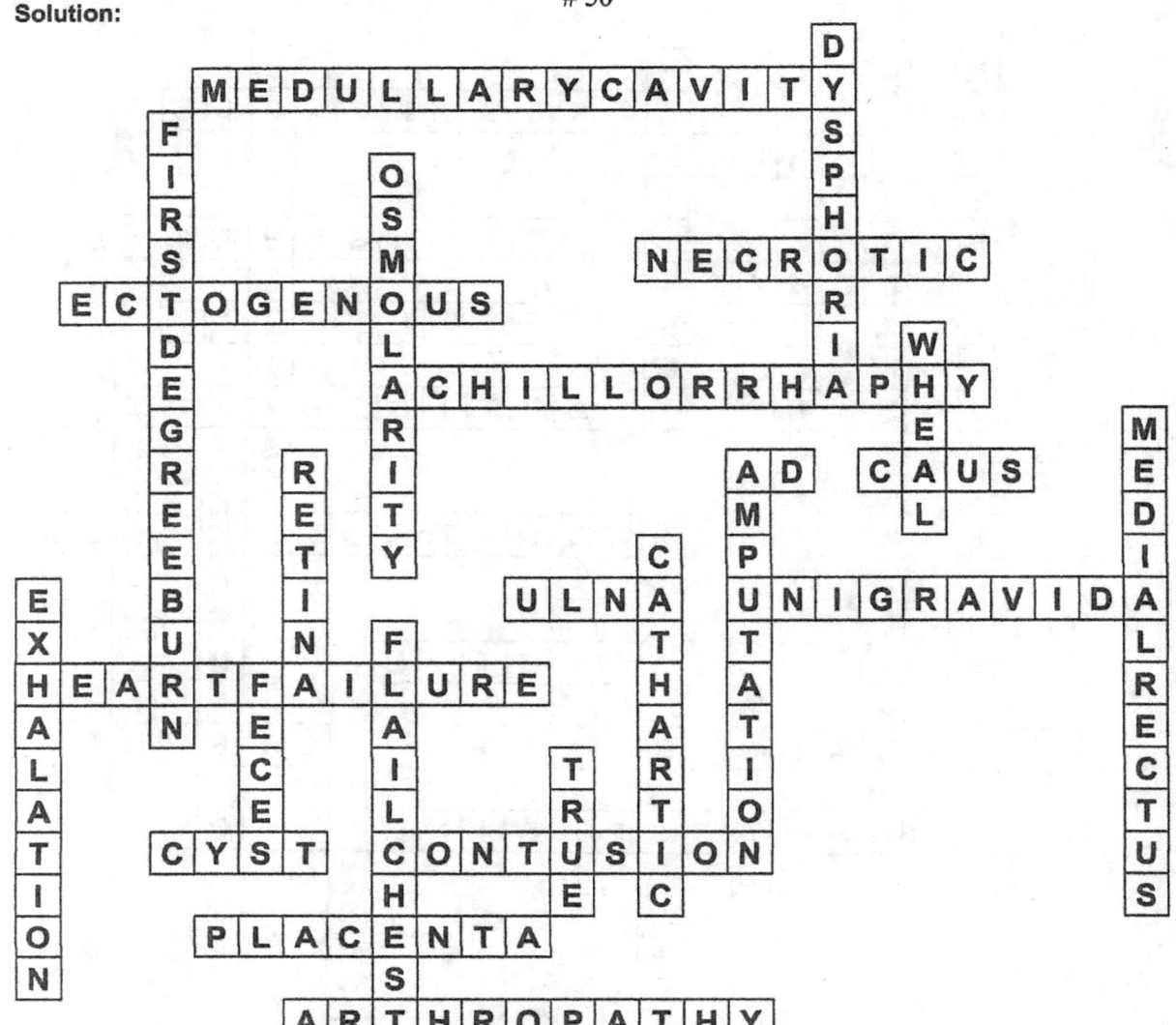

Solution:

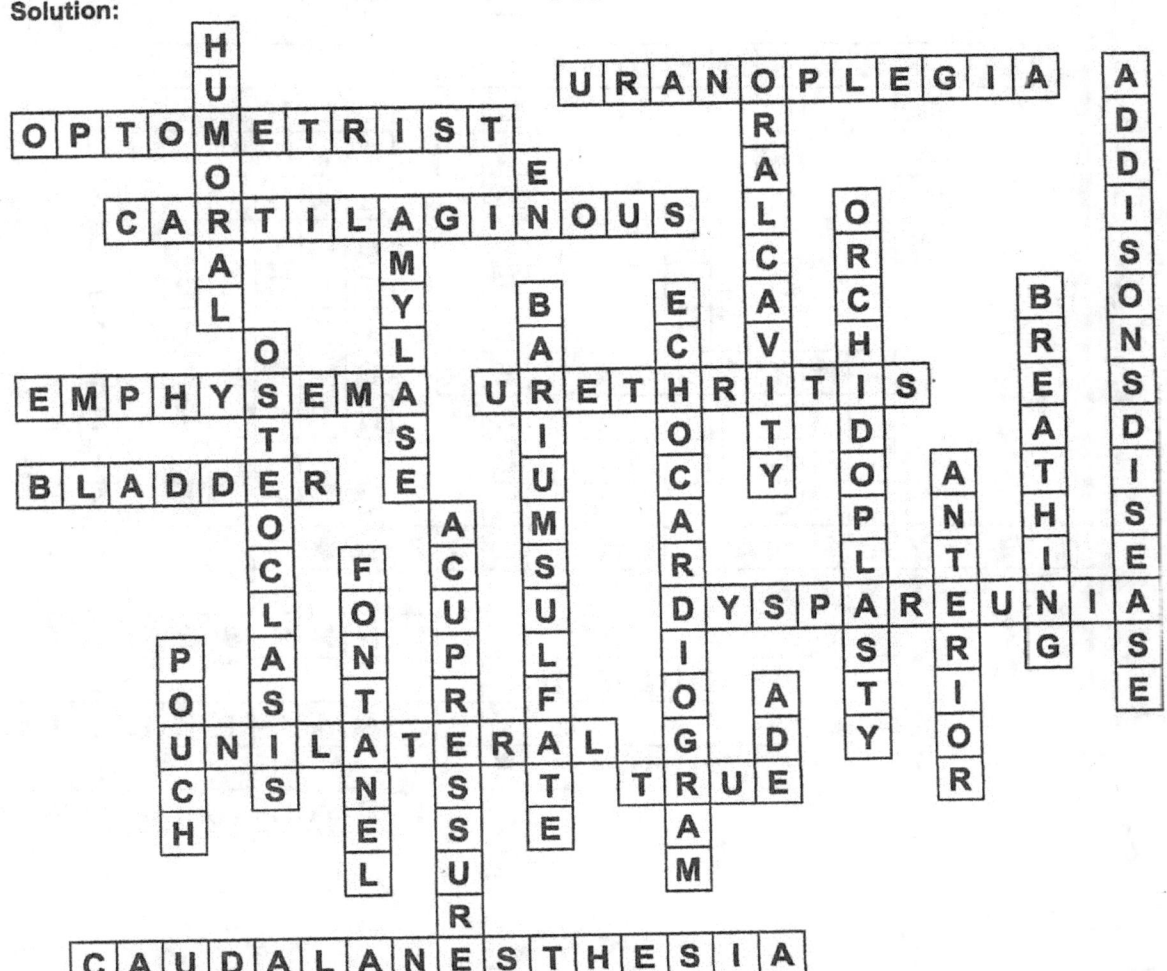

Solution:

52

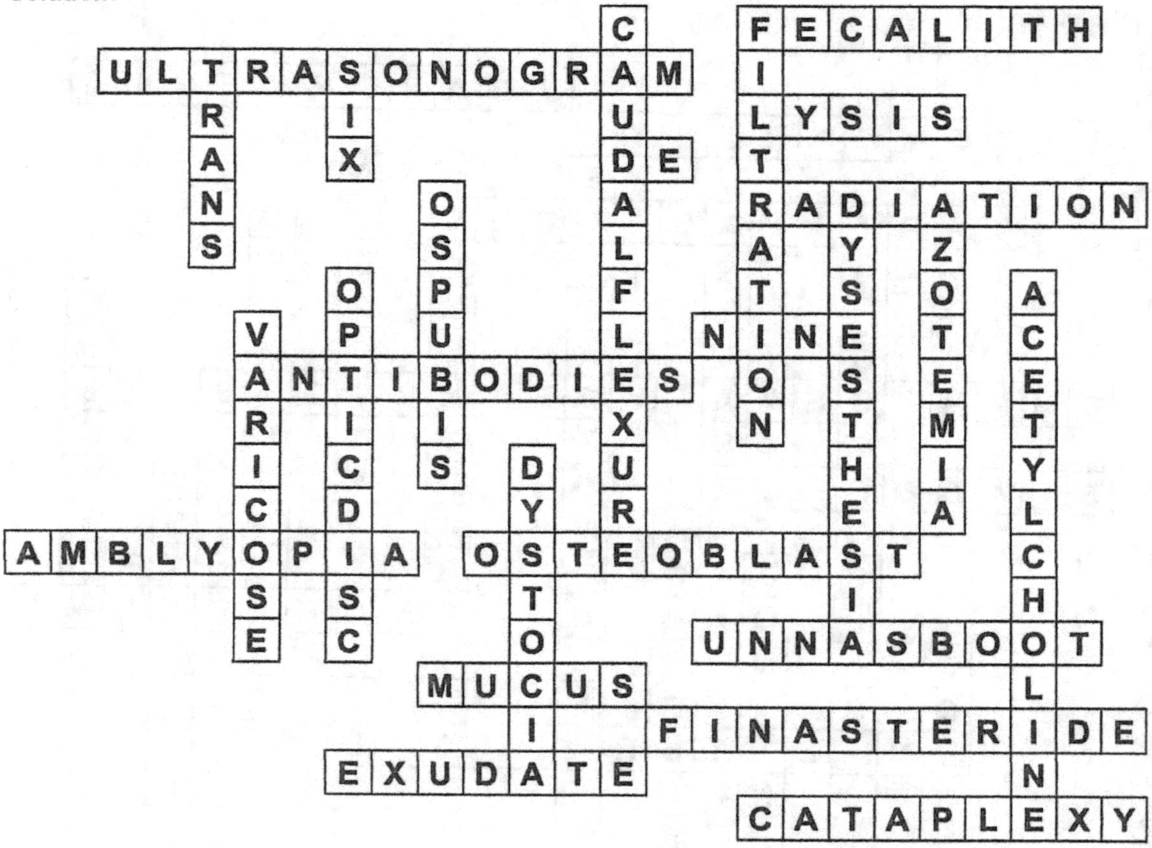

A crossword puzzle solution grid containing the following words:

Across:
- ULTRASONOGRAM
- FECALITH
- LYSIS
- RADIATION
- ANTIBODIES
- NINE
- AMBLYOPIA
- OSTEOBLAST
- UNNASBOOT
- MUCUS
- FINASTERIDE
- EXUDATE
- CATAPLEXY

Down:
- CAUDAL FLEXURE
- FILTRATION
- SIX
- TRANS
- OPTIC DISC
- OPUS
- VARICOSE
- DYSTOCIA
- ANESTHESIA
- AZOTEMIA
- ACETYLCHOLIN

Solution:

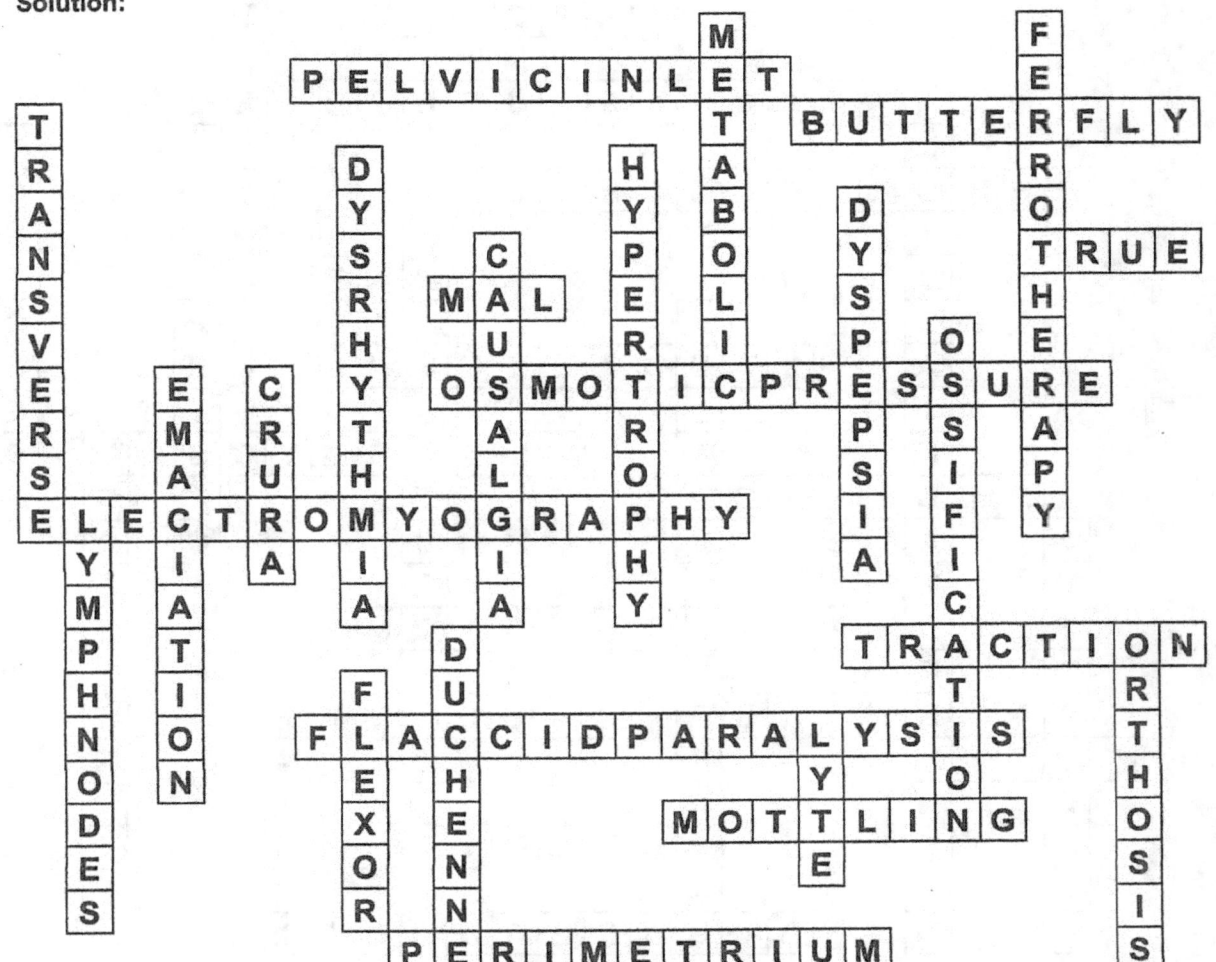

Solution:

Solution:

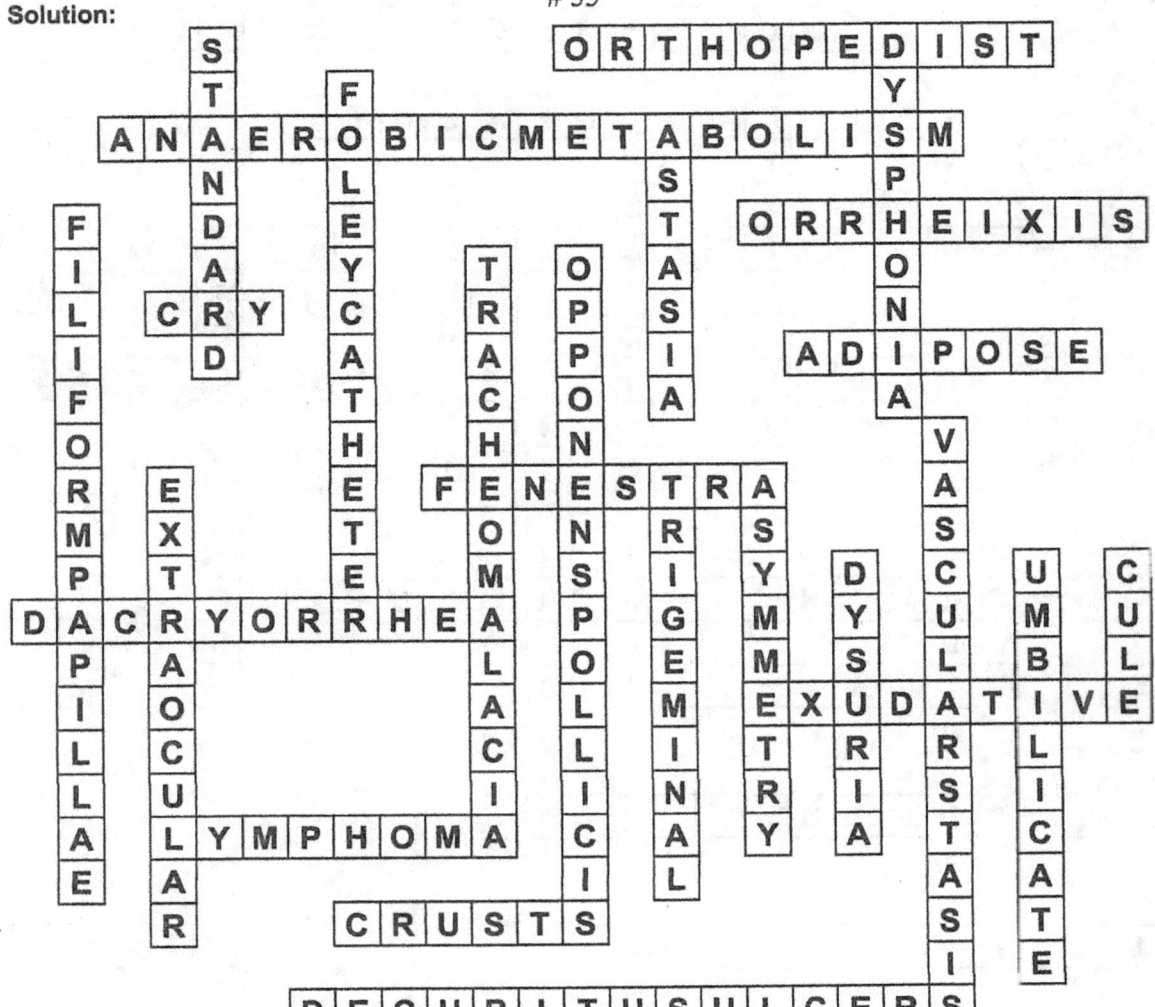

Solution:

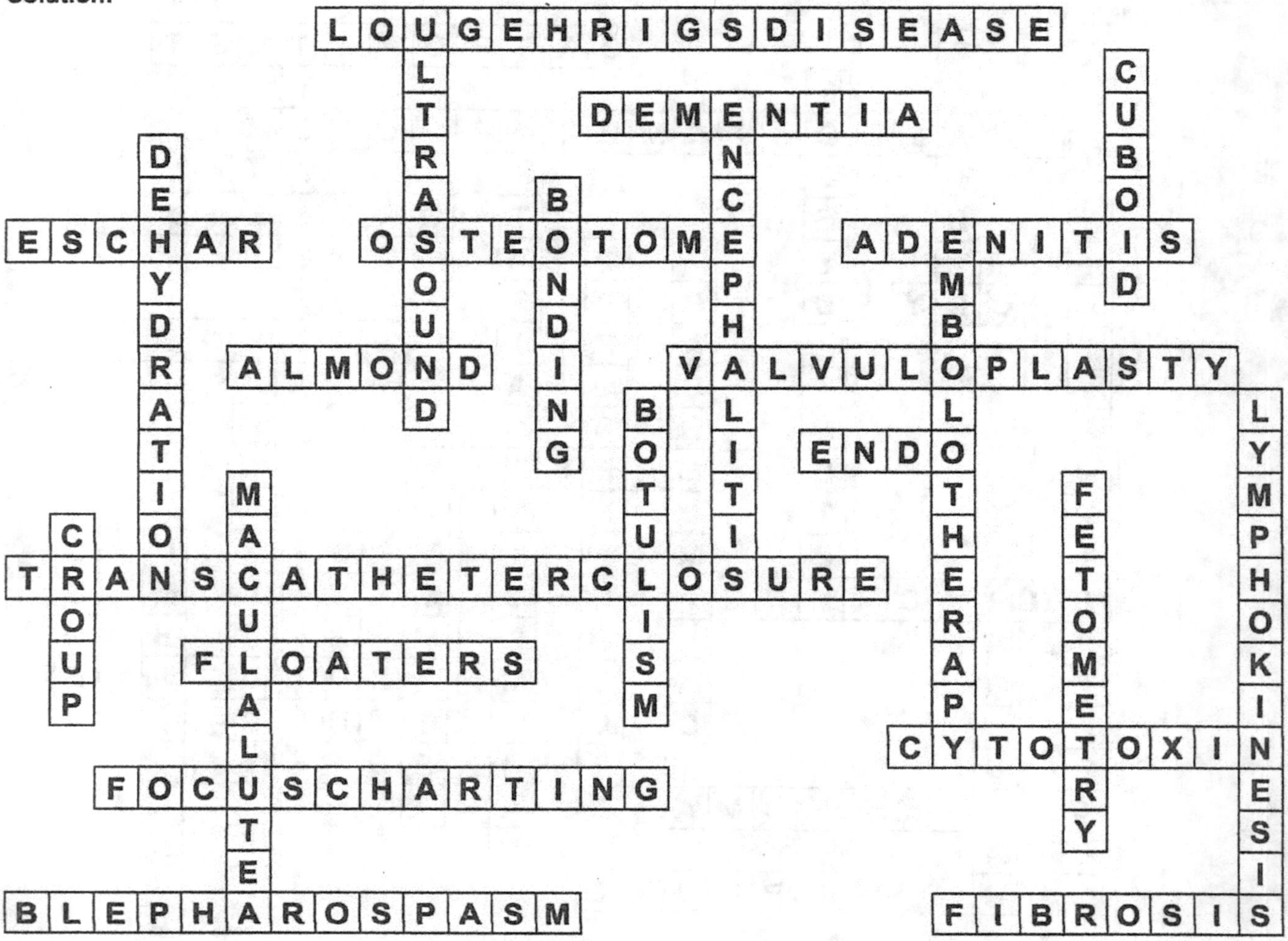

56

A crossword puzzle solution grid containing the following words:

Across:
- LOUGEHRIGSDISEASE
- DEMENTIA
- ESCHAR
- OSTEOTOME
- ADENITIS
- ALMOND
- VALVULOPLASTY
- ENDO
- TRANSCATHETERCLOSURE
- FLOATERS
- CYTOTOXIN
- FOCUSCHARTING
- BLEPHAROSPASM
- FIBROSIS

Down:
- ULTRASOUND
- ENCEPHALITIS
- CUBOID
- DEHYDRATION
- BONDING
- EMBOLOTHERAPY
- BOTULISM
- MACULAACUTE (MACULA ACUTE)
- COUP
- FETOMETRY
- LYMPHOKINESIS

Solution:

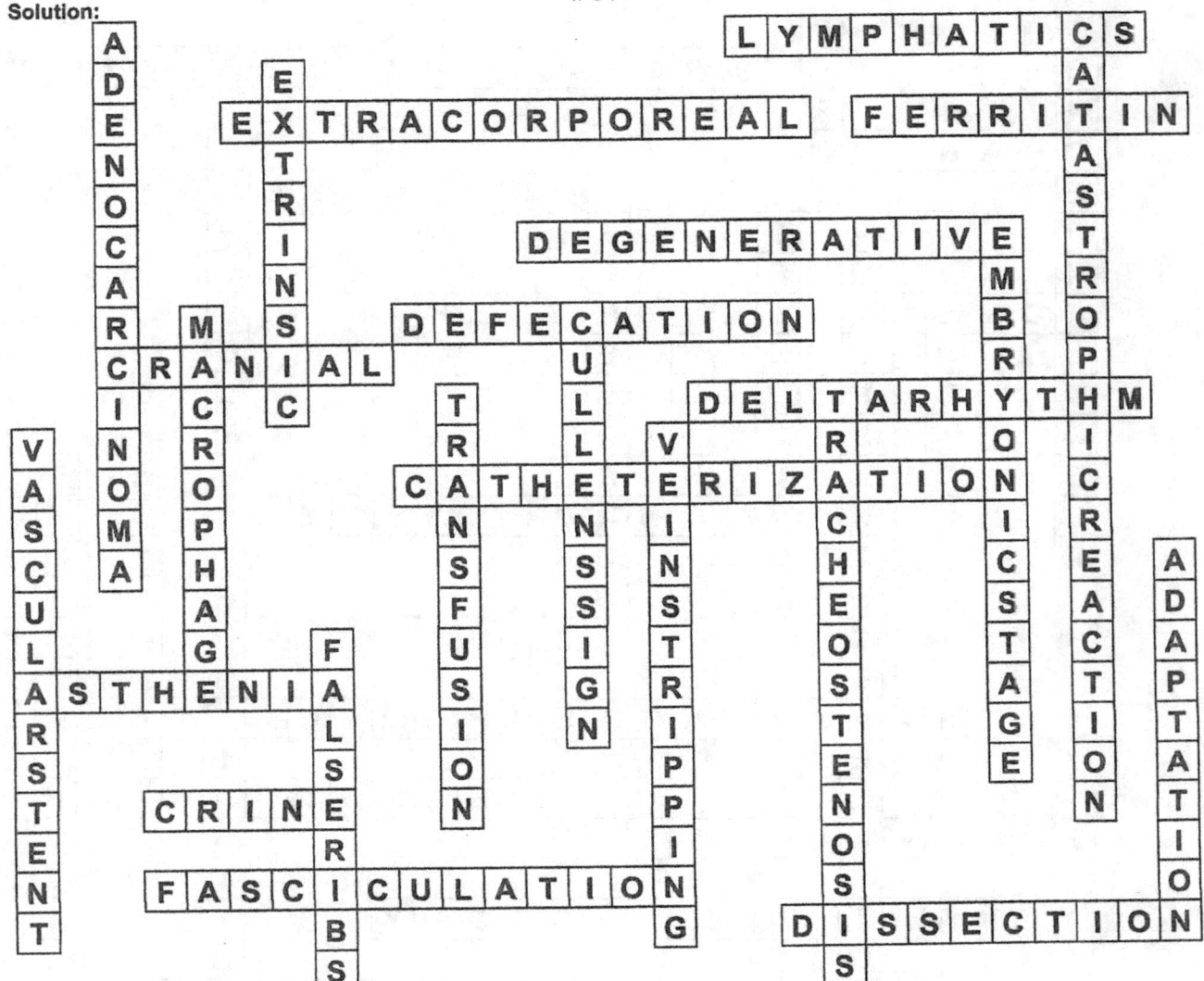

Solution:

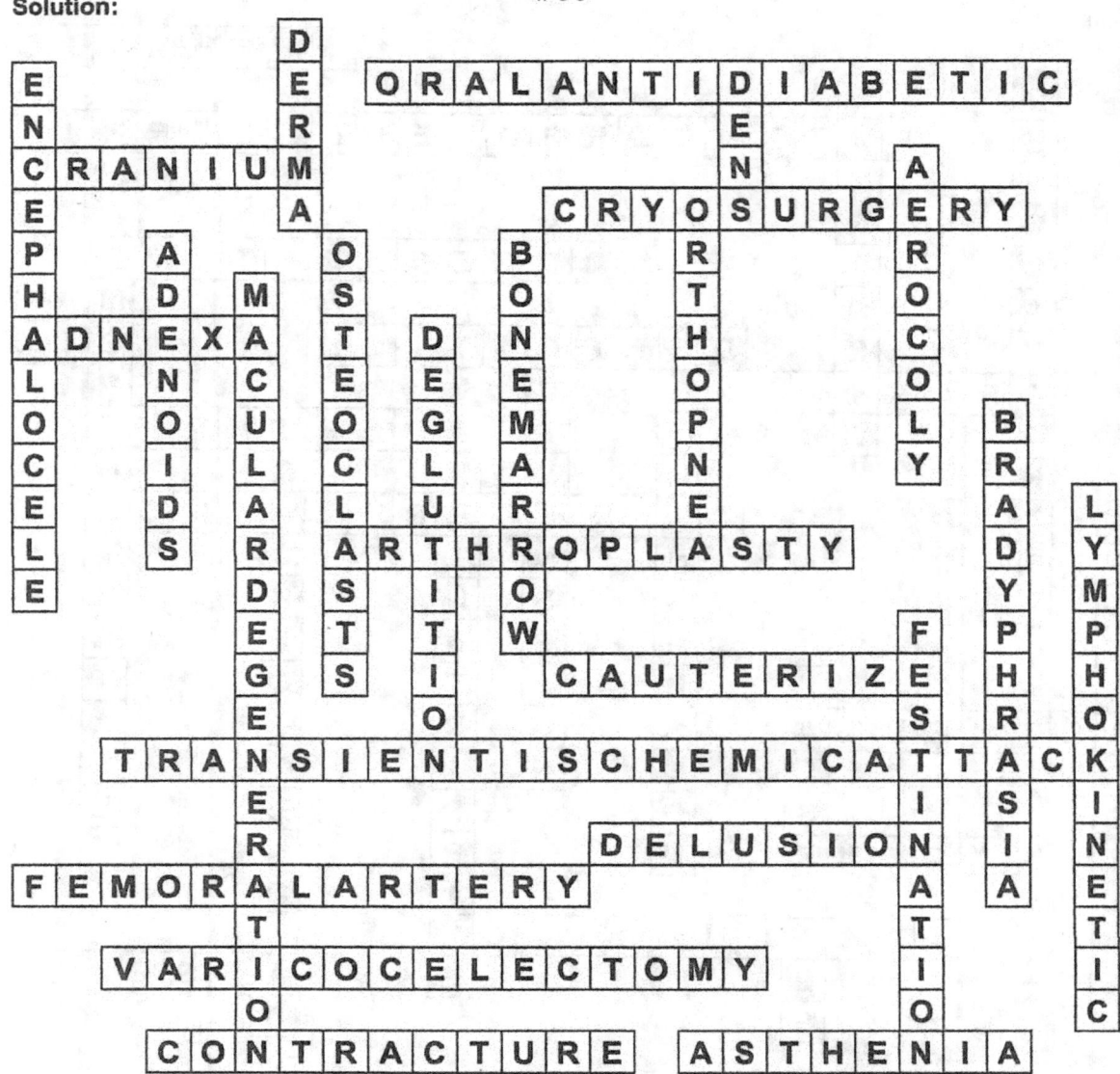

Solution:

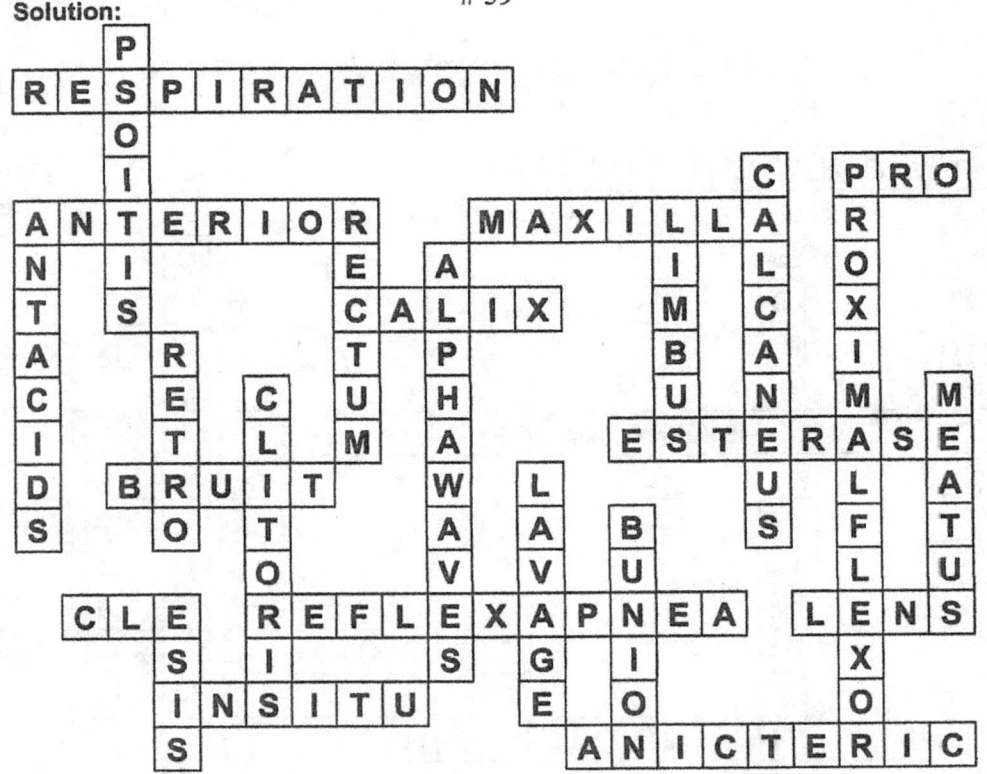

Across / Down entries (crossword solution grid):

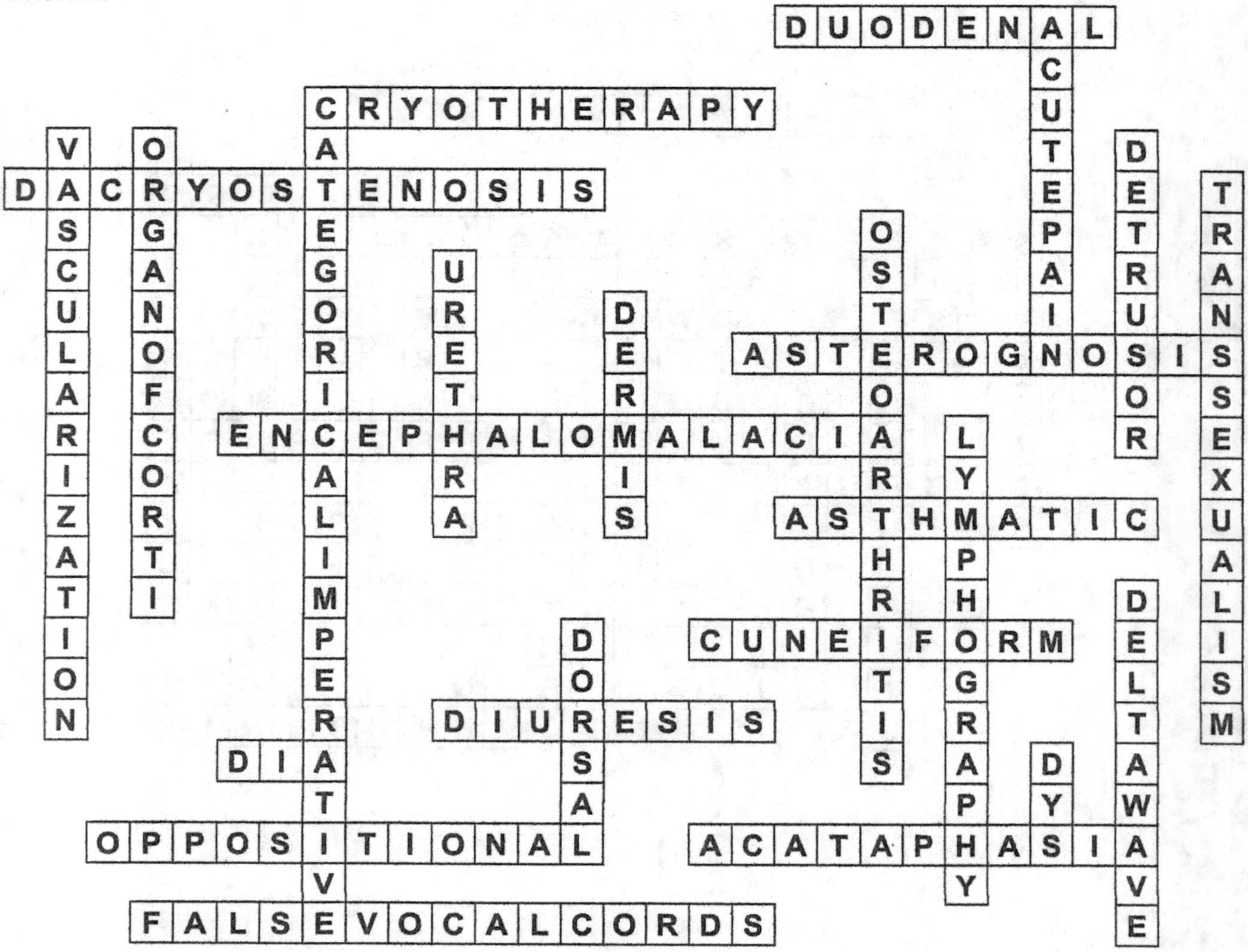

DUODENAL

CRYOTHERAPY

DACRYOSTENOSIS

ASTEROGNOSIS

ENCEPHALOMALACIA

ASTHMATIC

CUNEIFORM

DIURESIS

DIA

OPPOSITIONAL

ACATAPHASIA

FALSEVOCALCORDS

VASCULARIZATION

ORGANOFCORTI

CATEGORIAL

ALIMPERATIVE

URETHRA

DERMIS

OSTEOARTHRITIS

ACUTEPAIN

DETRUSOR

TRANSSEXUALISM

LYMPHPHGRAPHY

DELTAWAVE

DORSA

DY

61

Solution:

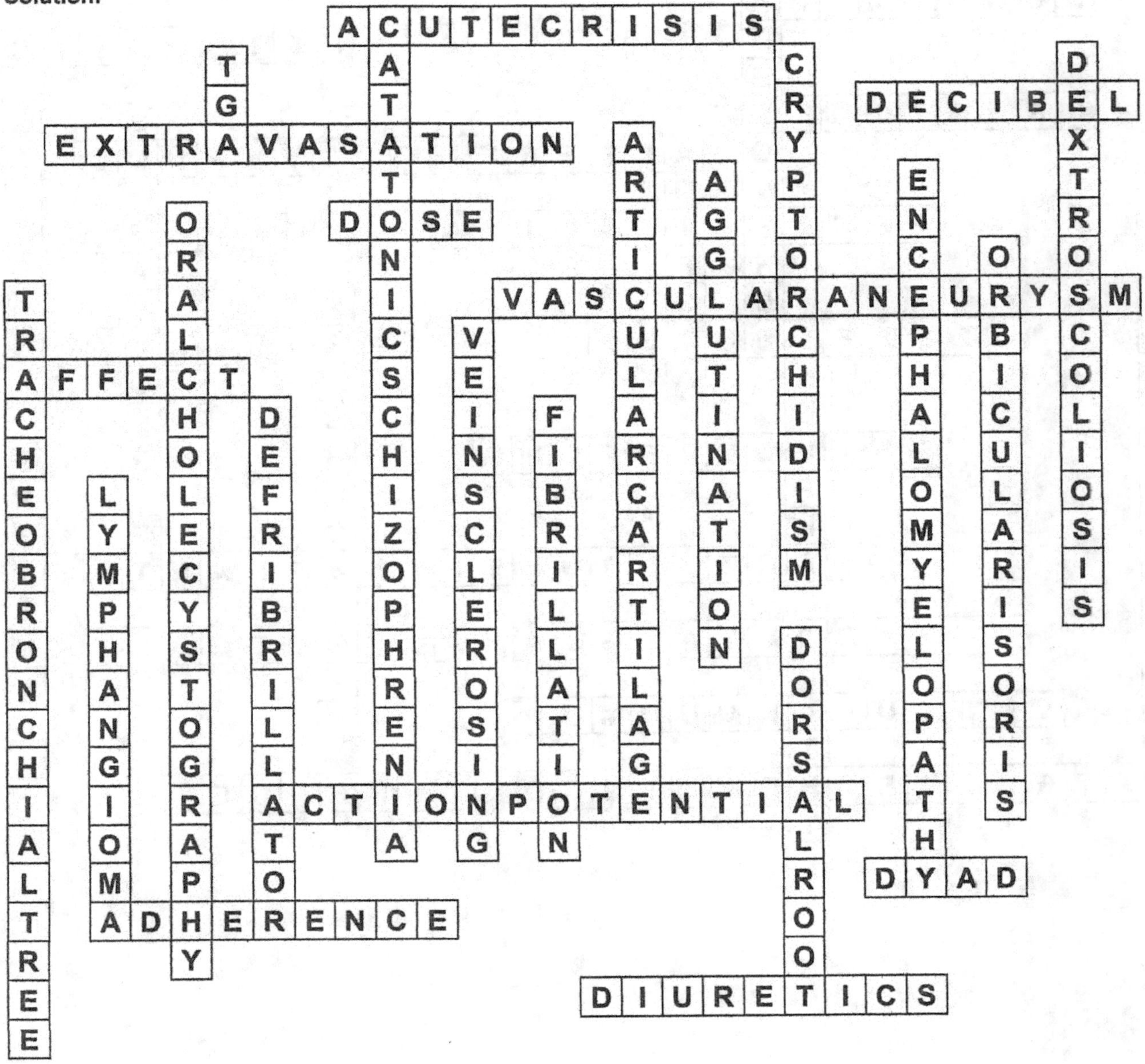
ACUTECRISIS
CATATONICSCHIZOPHRENIA
TGA
EXTRAVASATION
DOSE
DECIBEL
DEXTROSCOLIOSIS
CRYPTORCHIDISM
ARTICULARCARTILAGE
AGGLUTINATION
ENCEPHALOMYELOPATHY
ORBICULARISORIS
VASCULARANEURYSM
ORALCHOLECYSTOGRAPHY
TRACHEOBRONCHIALTREE
AFFECT
VEINSCLEROSING
FIBRILLATION
DEFIBRILLATOR
LYMPHANGIOMA
ACTIONPOTENTIAL
DORSALROOT
DYAD
ADHERENCE
DIURETICS

Solution:

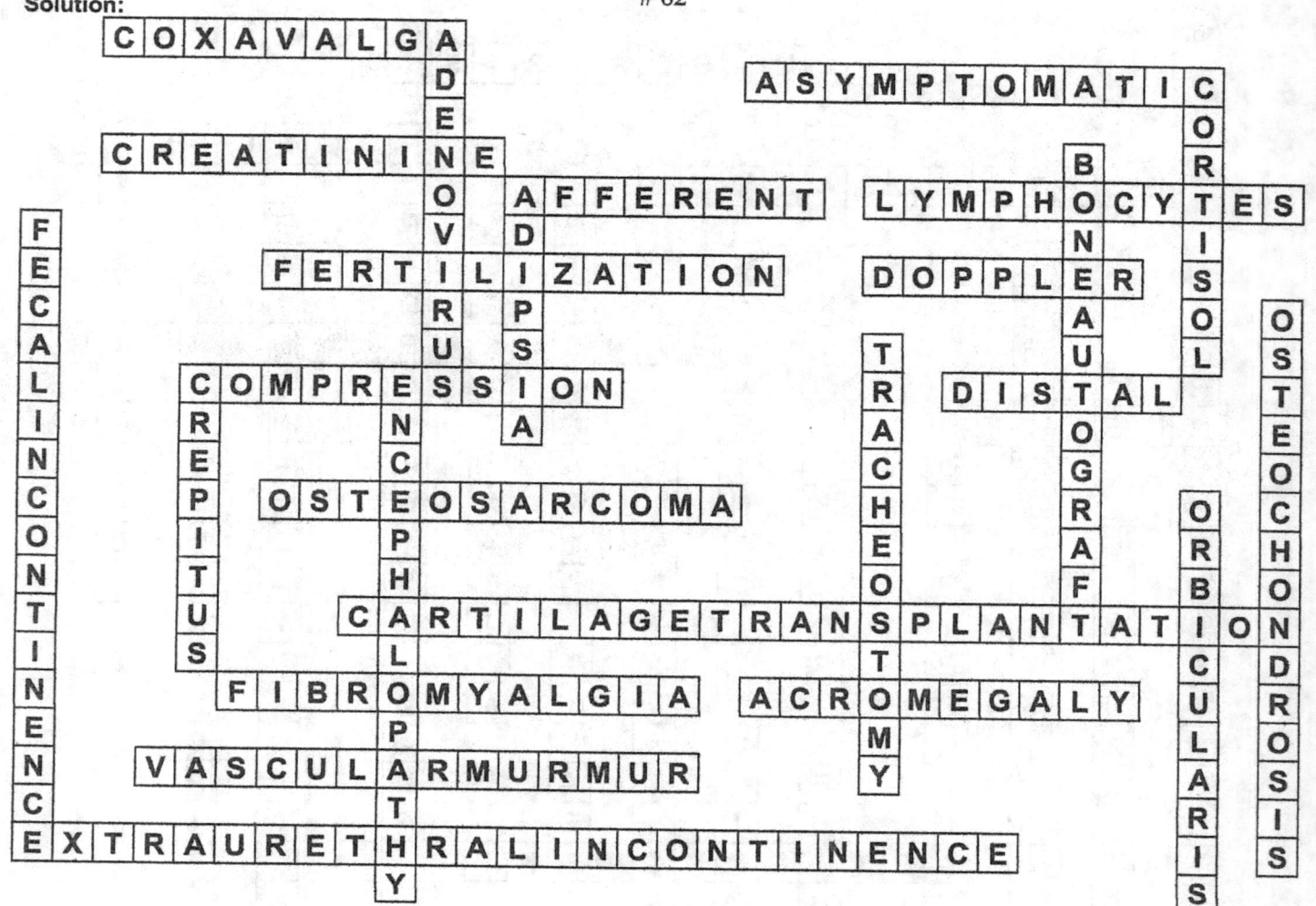

Solution:

Crossword puzzle solution grid containing the following words:

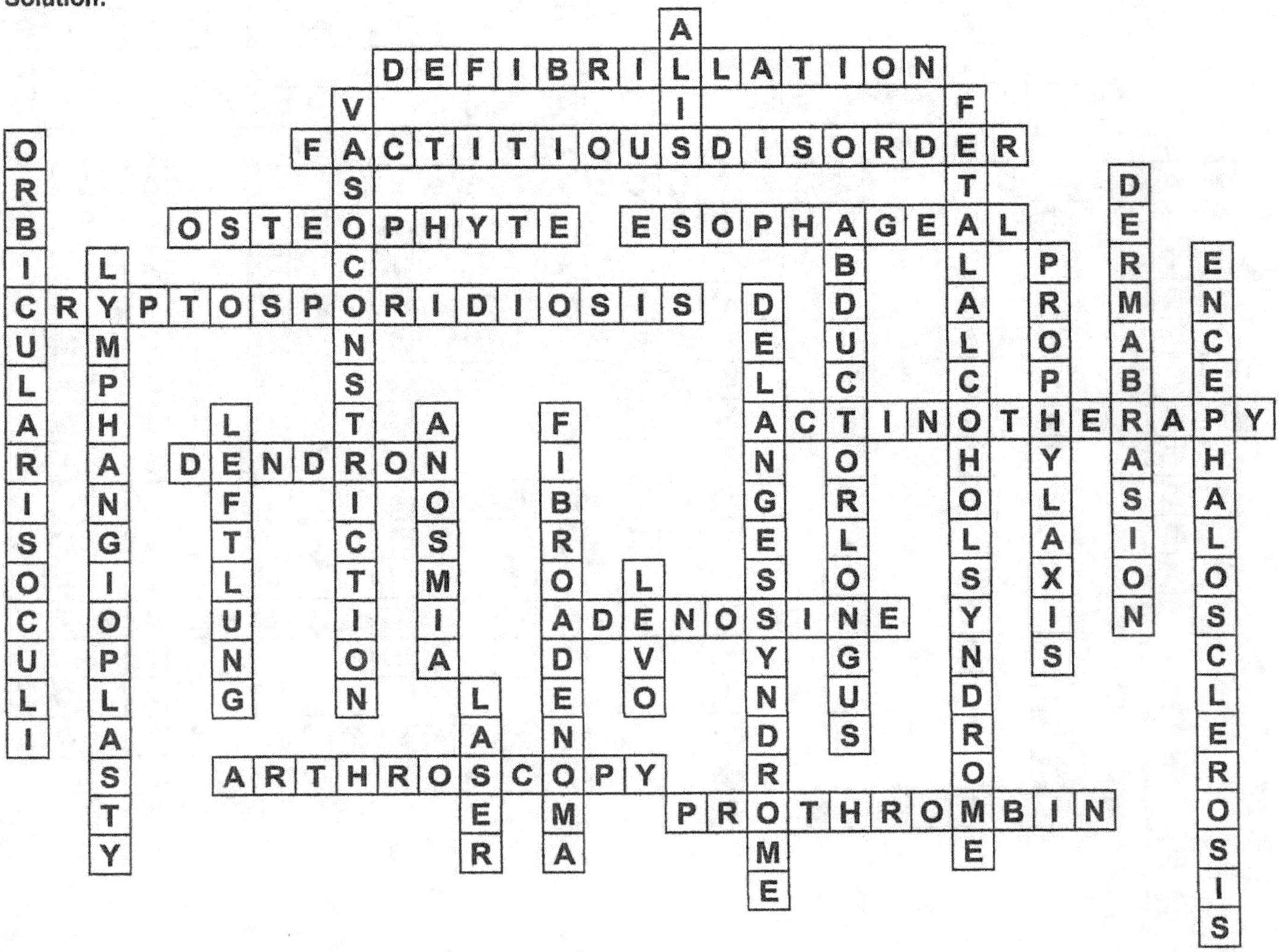

- DEFIBRILLATION
- FACTITIOUS DISORDER
- OSTEOPHYTE
- ESOPHAGEAL
- CRYPTOSPORIDIOSIS
- DENDRON
- ARTHROSCOPY
- PROTHROMBIN
- ADENOSINE
- ACTINOTHERAPY
- ORBICULARIS OCULI
- VASCONSTRICTION
- LYMPHANGIOPLASTY
- FETAL
- DERMABRASION
- ENCEPHALOSCLEROSIS
- LEFT LUNG
- ANOSMIA
- FIBROADENOMA
- LASER
- LEVO
- PROPHYLAXIS
- DELANGE SYNDROME
- ABDUCTOR LONGUS
- TALC
- ALCOHOL SYNDROME

Solution:

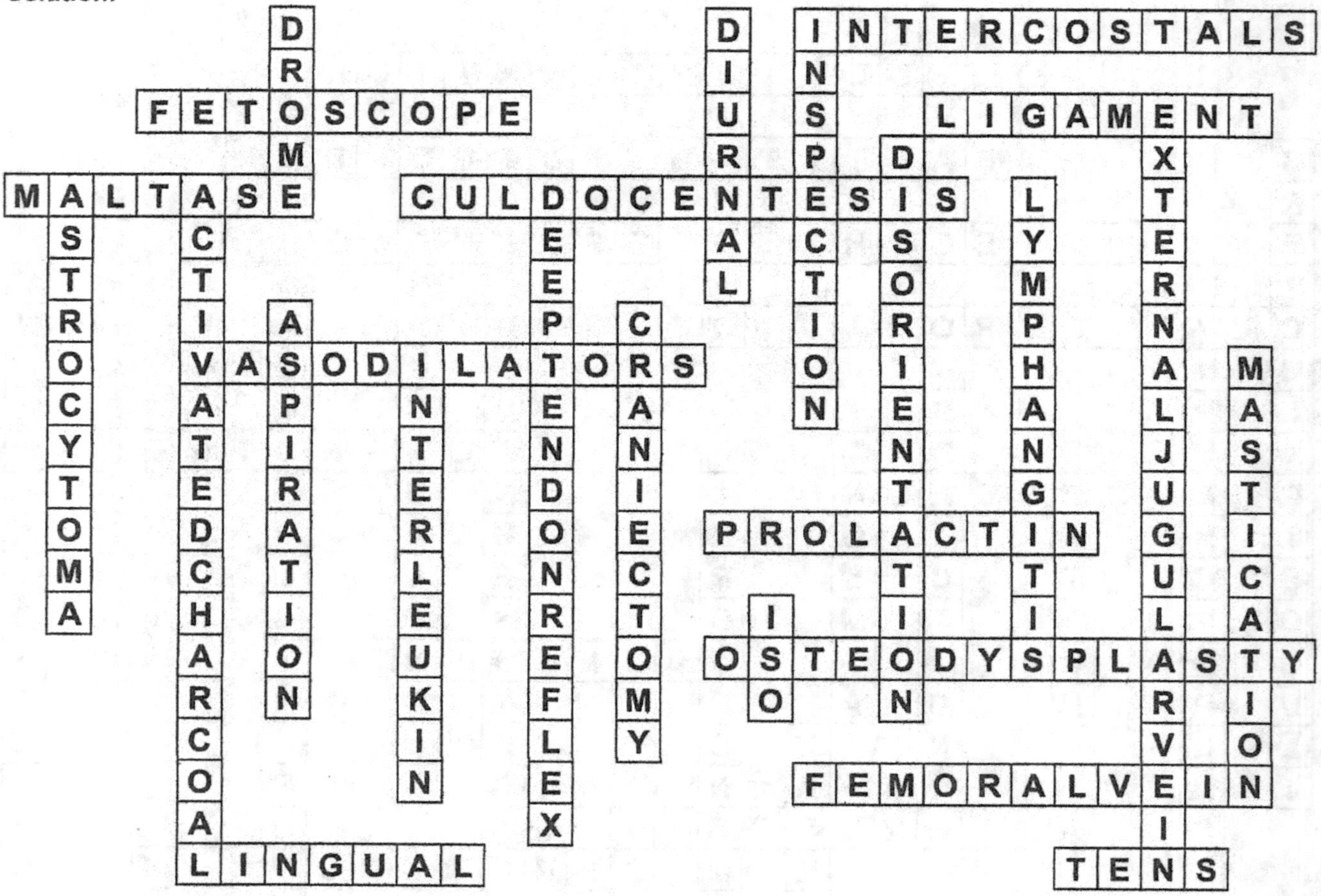
DROME
DIURNAL
INTERCOSTALS
INSPECTION
FETOSCOPE
LIGAMENT
MALTASE
CULDOCENTESIS
DISORIENTATION
LYMPHANGITIS
EXTERNALJUGULARVEIN
ASTROCYTOMA
ACTIVATEDCHARCOAL
ASPIRATION
DEEPTENDONREFLEX
CRANIECTOMY
VASODILATORS
INTERLEUKIN
MASTICATION
PROLACTIN
ISO
OSTEODYSPLASTY
FEMORALVEIN
LINGUAL
TENS

Solution:

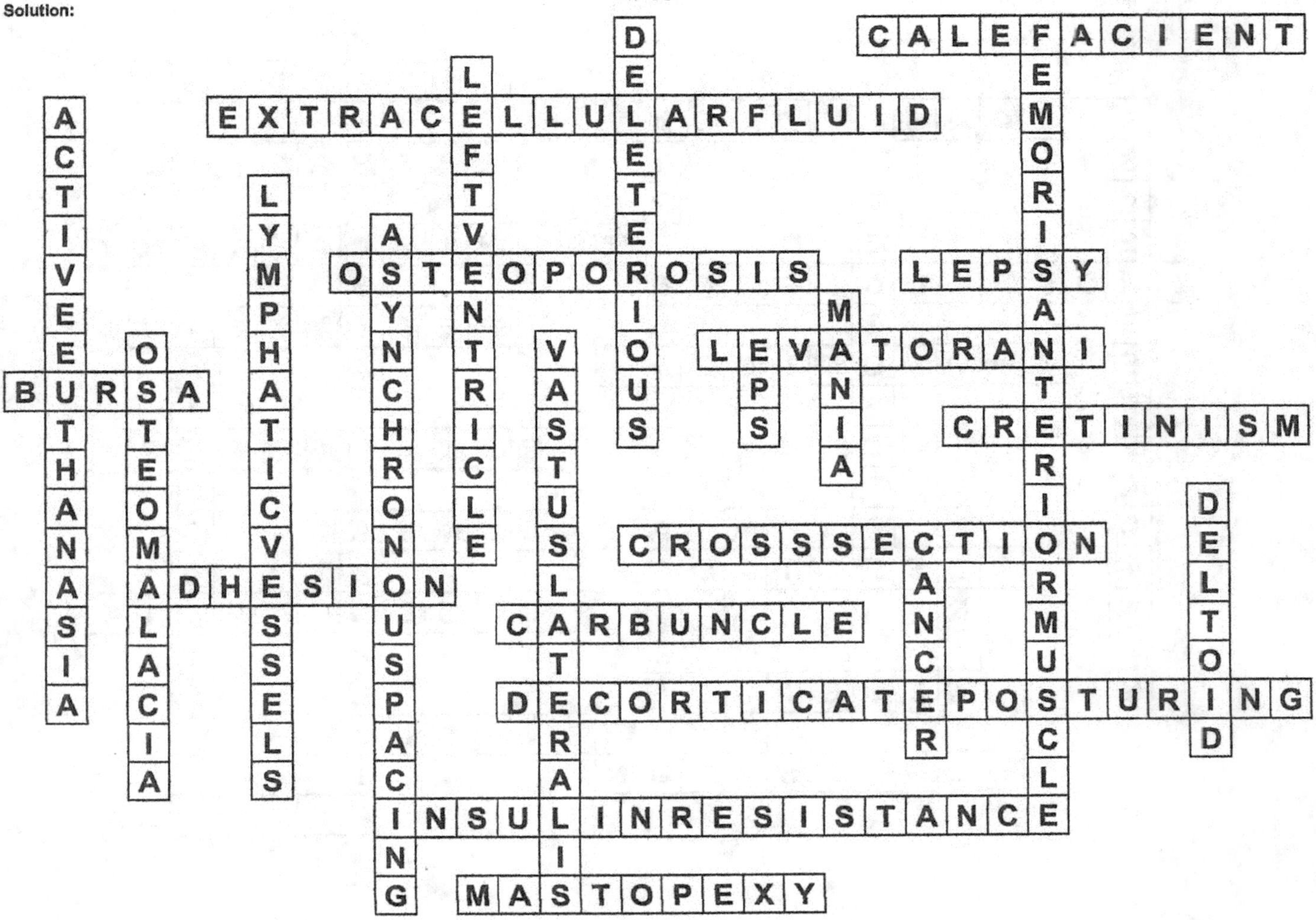

CALEFACIENT

EXTRACELLULARFLUID

ACTIVEEUTHANASIA

OSTEOPOROSIS

LEPSY

FEMORIS

OSTEOMALACIA

BURSA

LYMPHATICVESSELS

LEFTVENTRICLE

ASYNCHRONOUSPACING

DELETERIOUS

LEVATORANI

MANIA

LPS

CRETINISM

ANTERIORMUSCLE

CROSSSECTION

DELTOID

VASTUSLATERALIS

ADHESION

CARBUNCLE

CANCER

DECORTICATEPOSTURING

INSULINRESISTANCE

MASTOPEXY

Solution:

66

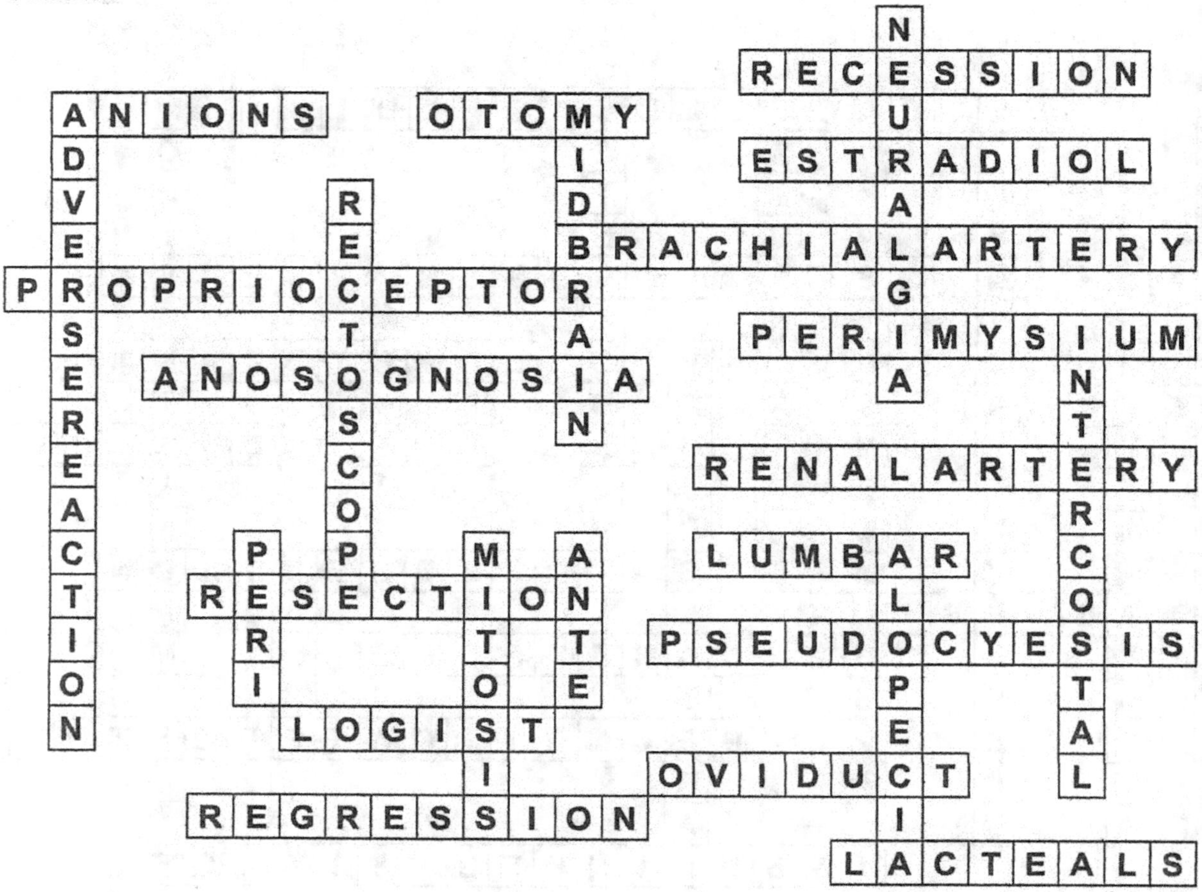
NEURALGIA
RECESSION
ANIONS
OTOMY
ESTRADIOL
BRACHIALARTERY
PROPRIOCEPTOR
PERIMYSIUM
ANOSOGNOSIA
RENALARTERY
LUMBAR
RESECTION
PSEUDOCYESIS
LOGIST
OVIDUCT
REGRESSION
LACTEALS
ADVERSEREACTION
RECTOSCOPE
MIDBRAIN
INTERCOSTAL
PERI
MITOSIS
ANTE
ALOPECIA

Solution:

67

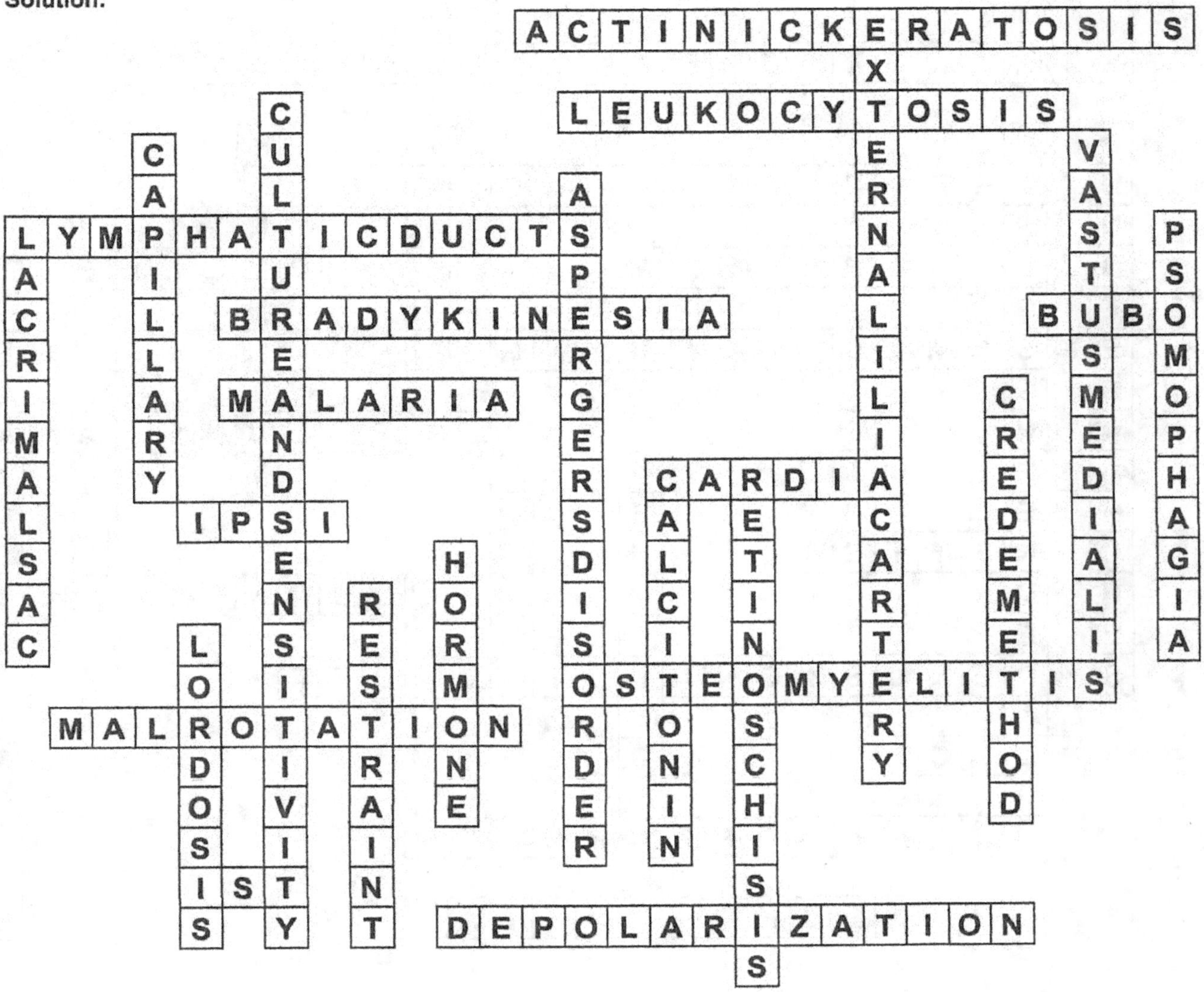
ACTINICKERATOSIS
LEUKOCYTOSIS
LYMPHATICDUCTS
BRADYKINESIA
MALARIA
BUBO
CARDIA
IPSI
OSTEOMYELITIS
MALROTATION
IST
DEPOLARIZATION
EXTERNALILIACARTERY
CULTUREANDSENSITIVITY
CAPILLARY
LACRIMALSAC
ASPERGERSDISORDER
VASTUSMEDIALIS
PSOMOPHAGIA
CREDEMETHOD
CALCITONIN
RETINOSCHISIS
HORMONE
RESTRAINT
LORDOSIS

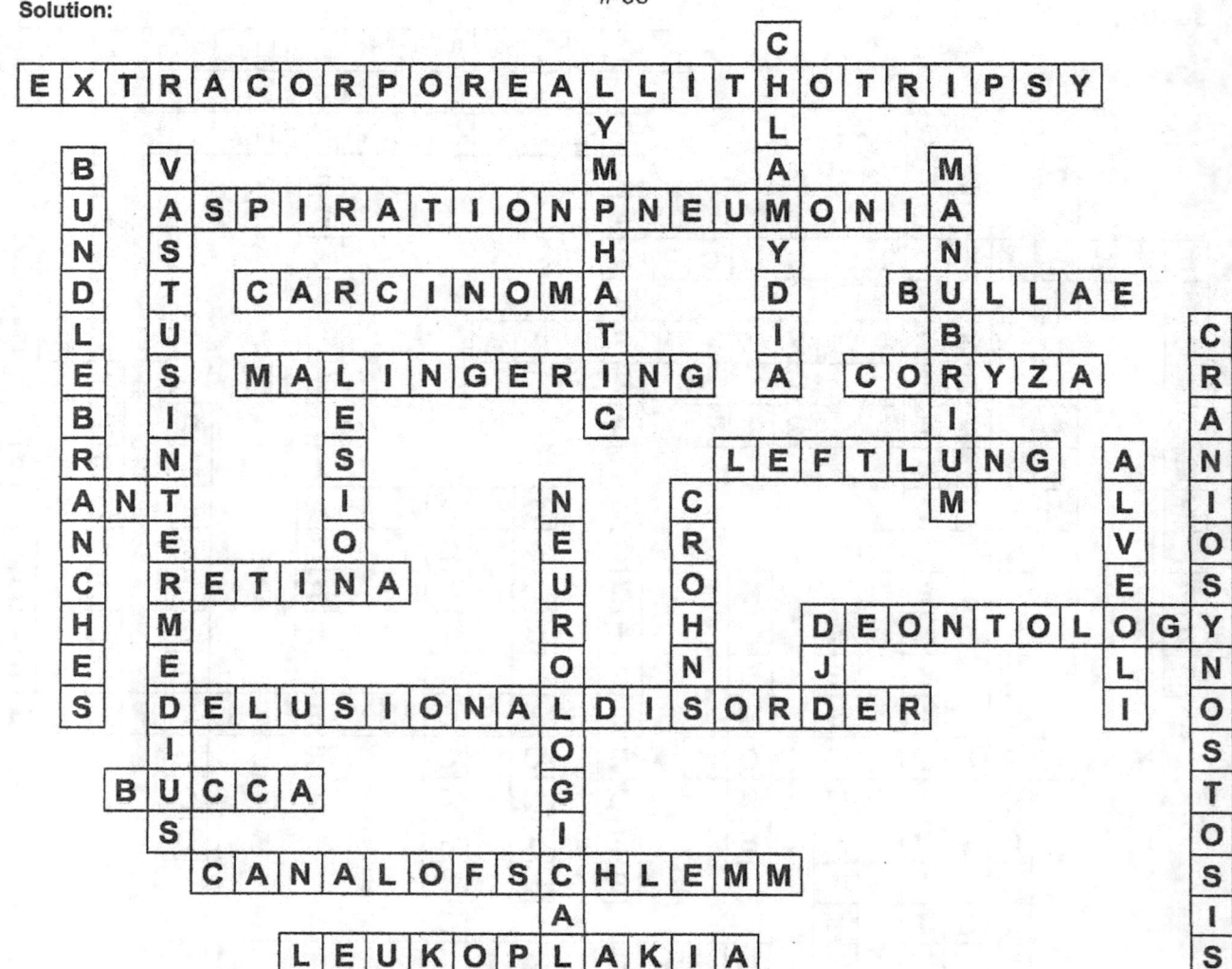

Solution:

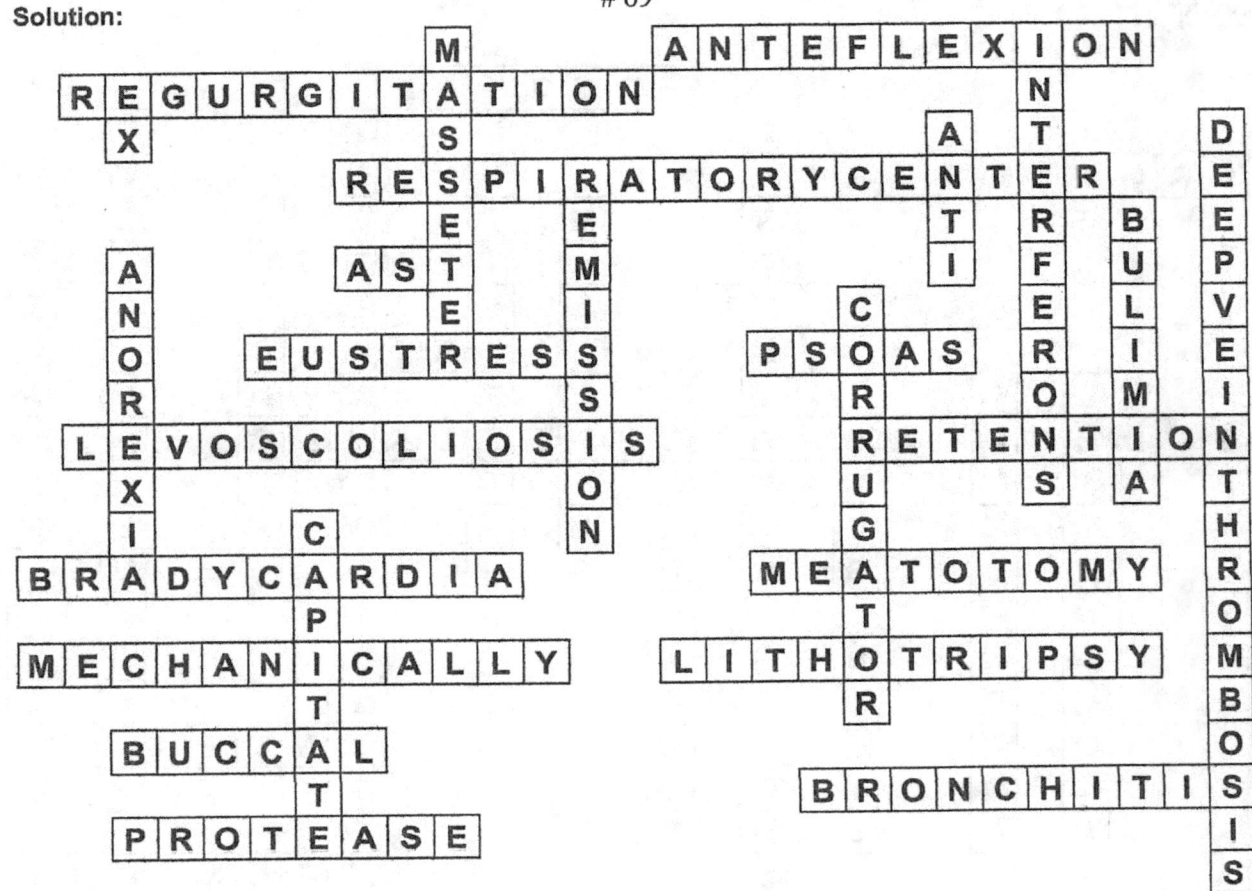

Solution:

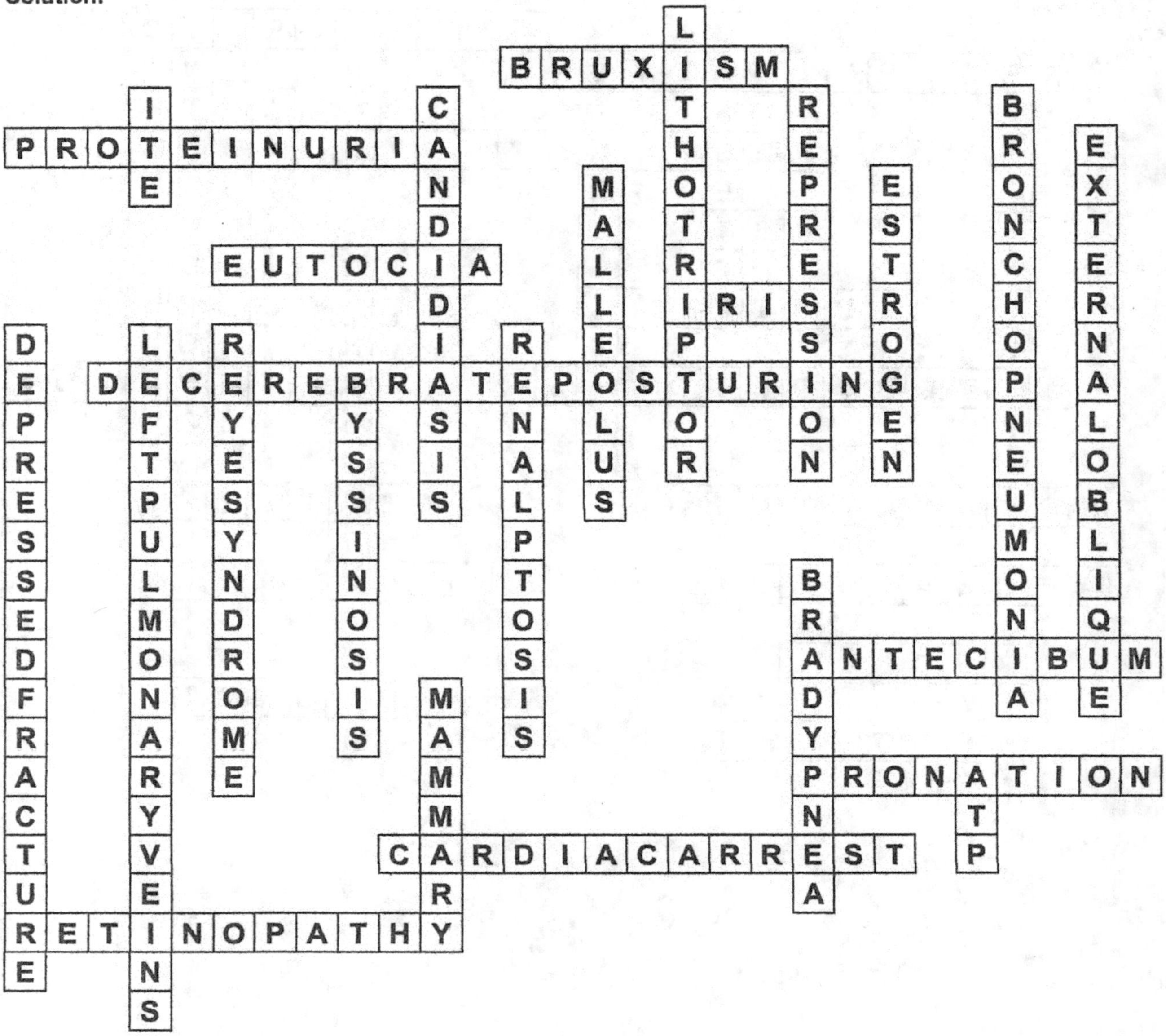

70

BRUXISM

PROTEINURIA

EUTOCIA

DECEREBRATEPOSTURING

ANTECIBUM

PRONATION

CARDIACARREST

RETINOPATHY

Down words (as letters in grid):
- LITHOTRIPTOR
- CANDIDIASIS
- REPRESSION
- ESTROGEN
- BRONCHOPNEUMONIA
- EXTERNALOBLIQUE
- ITE
- MALLEOLUS
- IRIS
- DEPRESSEDFRACTURE
- LEFTPULMONARYVEINS
- REYESYNDROME
- DYSSINOSIS
- RENALPTOSIS
- MAMMARY
- BRADYPNEA

71

Solution:

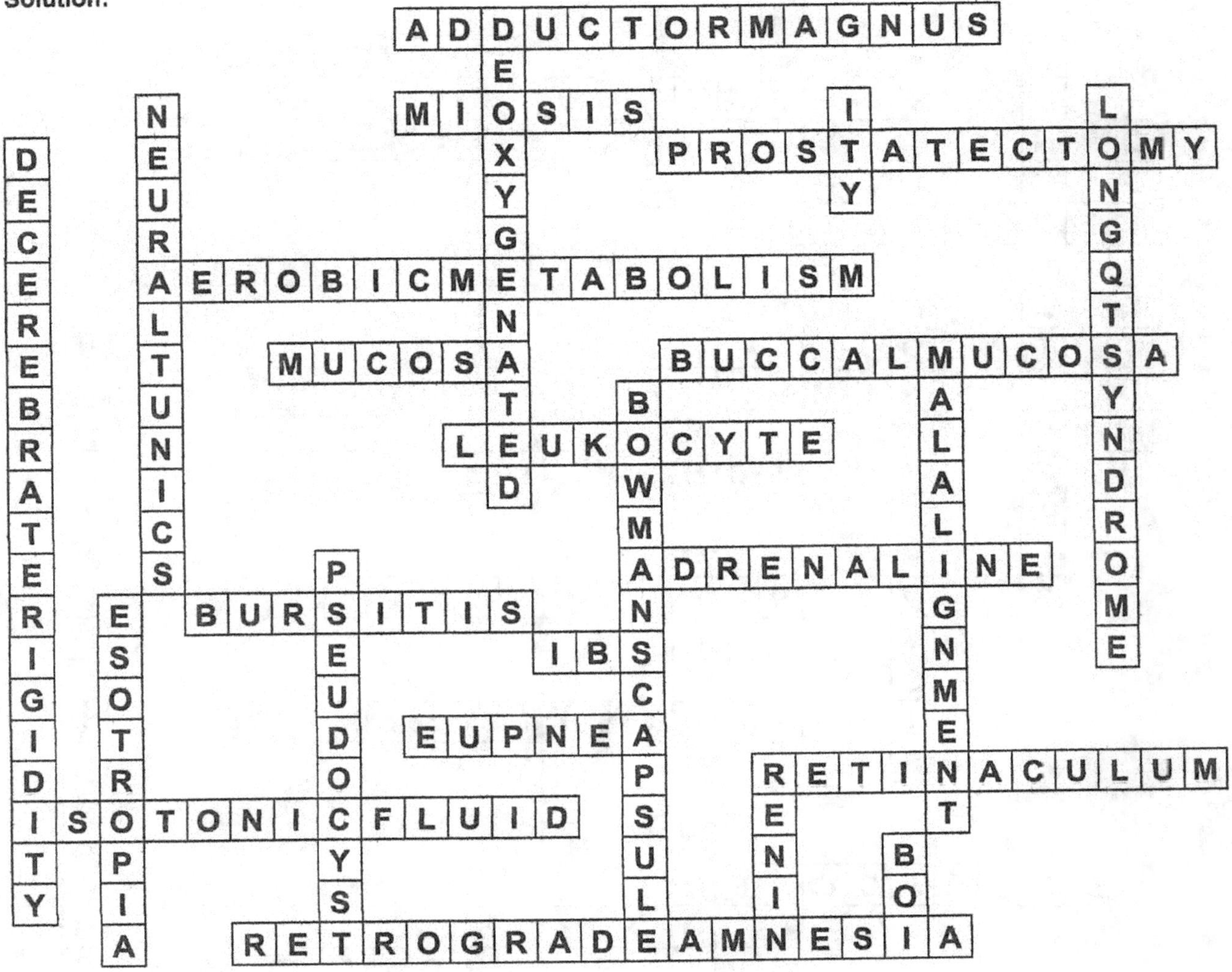
ADDUCTORMAGNUS
MIOSIS
PROSTATECTOMY
AEROBICMETABOLISM
MUCOSA
BUCCALMUCOSA
LEUKOCYTE
ADRENALINE
BURSITIS
IBS
EUPNEA
RETINACULUM
ISOTONICFLUID
RETROGRADEAMNESIA
DEOXYGENATED
NEURALTUNICS
DECEREBRATERIGIDITY
ITY
LONGQTSYNDROME
BOWMANSCAPSULE
MALALIGNMENT
PSEUDOCYSTS
ESOTROPIA
RENIN
BOA

Solution:

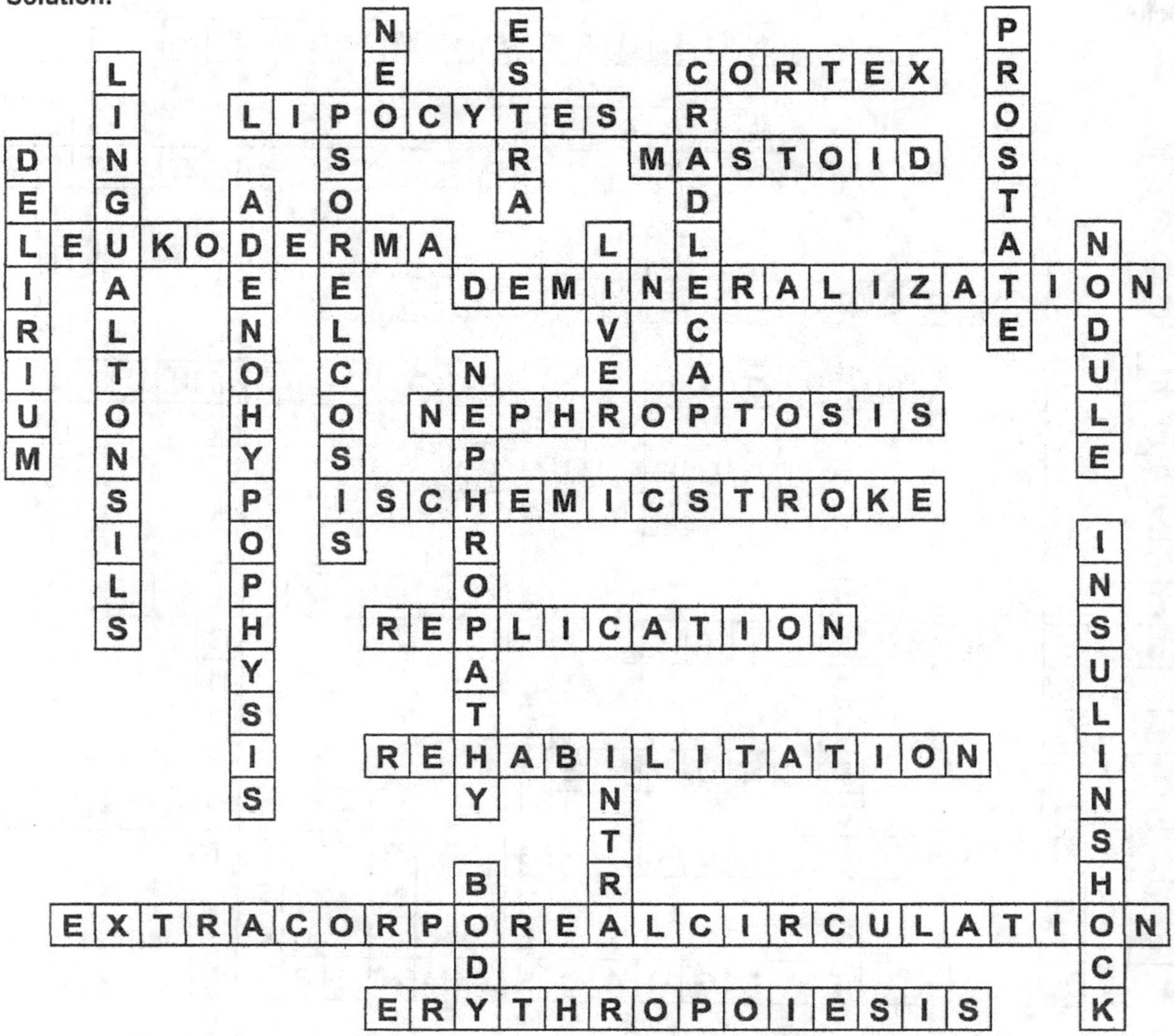

72

A completed crossword puzzle grid containing the following words:

- LINGUAL
- LIPOCYTES
- DELIRIUM
- LEUKODERMA
- CORTEX
- MASTOID
- PROSTATE
- NODULE
- DEMINERALIZATION
- NEPHROPTOSIS
- ISCHEMICSTROKE
- REPLICATION
- REHABILITATION
- INSULINSHOCK
- EXTRACORPOREALCIRCULATION
- ERYTHROPOIESIS
- NEPHROPATHY
- LIVECALCA
- ESTRARA
- CRADLL
- ADENOHYPOPHYSIS
- ISOSOMELCOSIS
- TONSILS
- BODY
- CENTR

Solution:

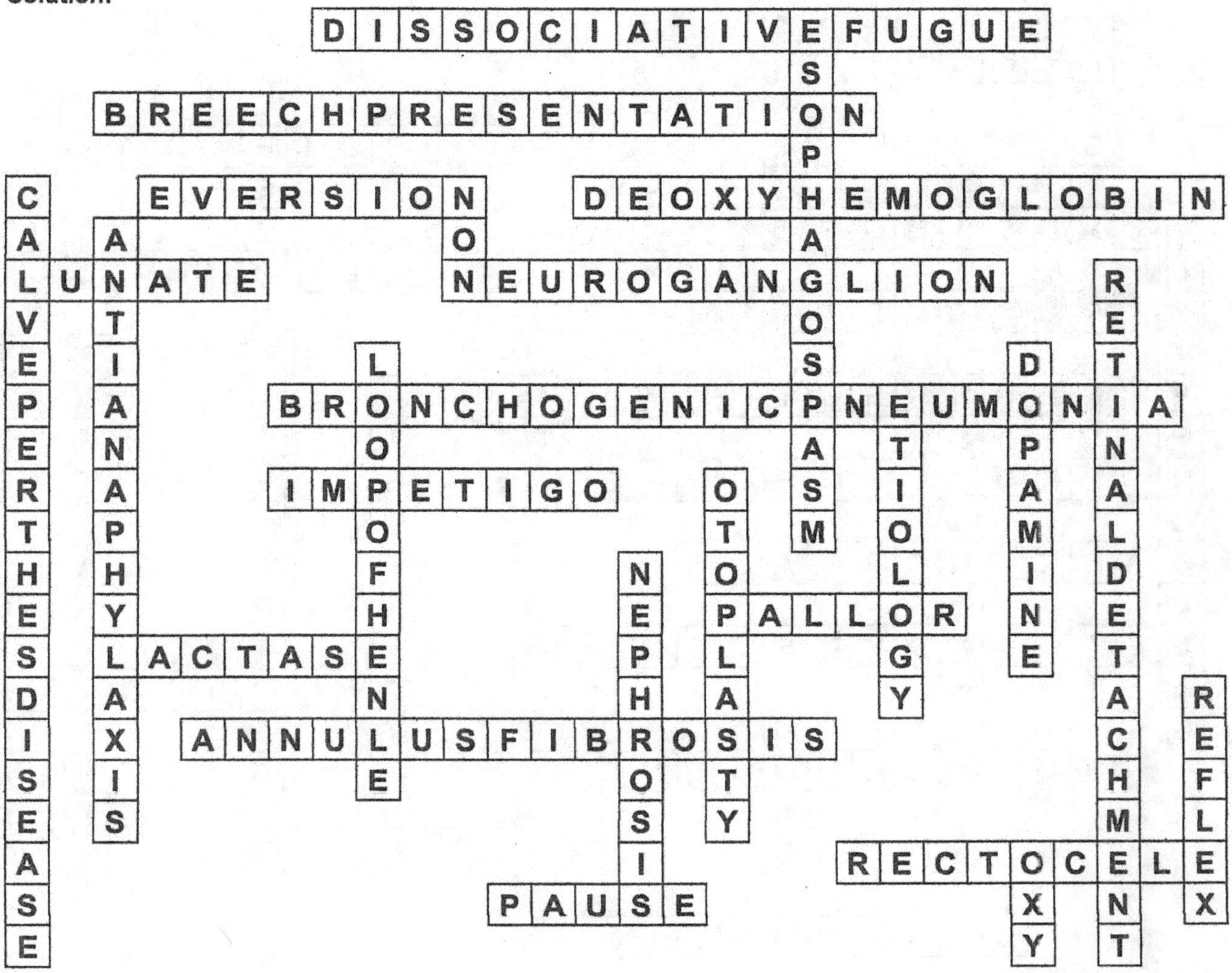
DISSOCIATIVEFUGUE
ESOPHAGOSPASM
BREECHPRESENTATION
EVERSION
NON
DEOXYHEMOGLOBIN
CALVEPERTHESDISEASE
ANTIANAPHYLAXIS
LUNATE
NEUROGANGLION
RETINALDETACHMENT
LOOPOFHENLE
DOPAMINE
BRONCHOGENICPNEUMONIA
ETIOLOGY
IMPETIGO
OTOPLASTY
NEPHROSIS
PALLOR
LACTASE
ANNULUSFIBROSIS
REFLEX
RECTOCELE
OXY
PAUSE

Solution:

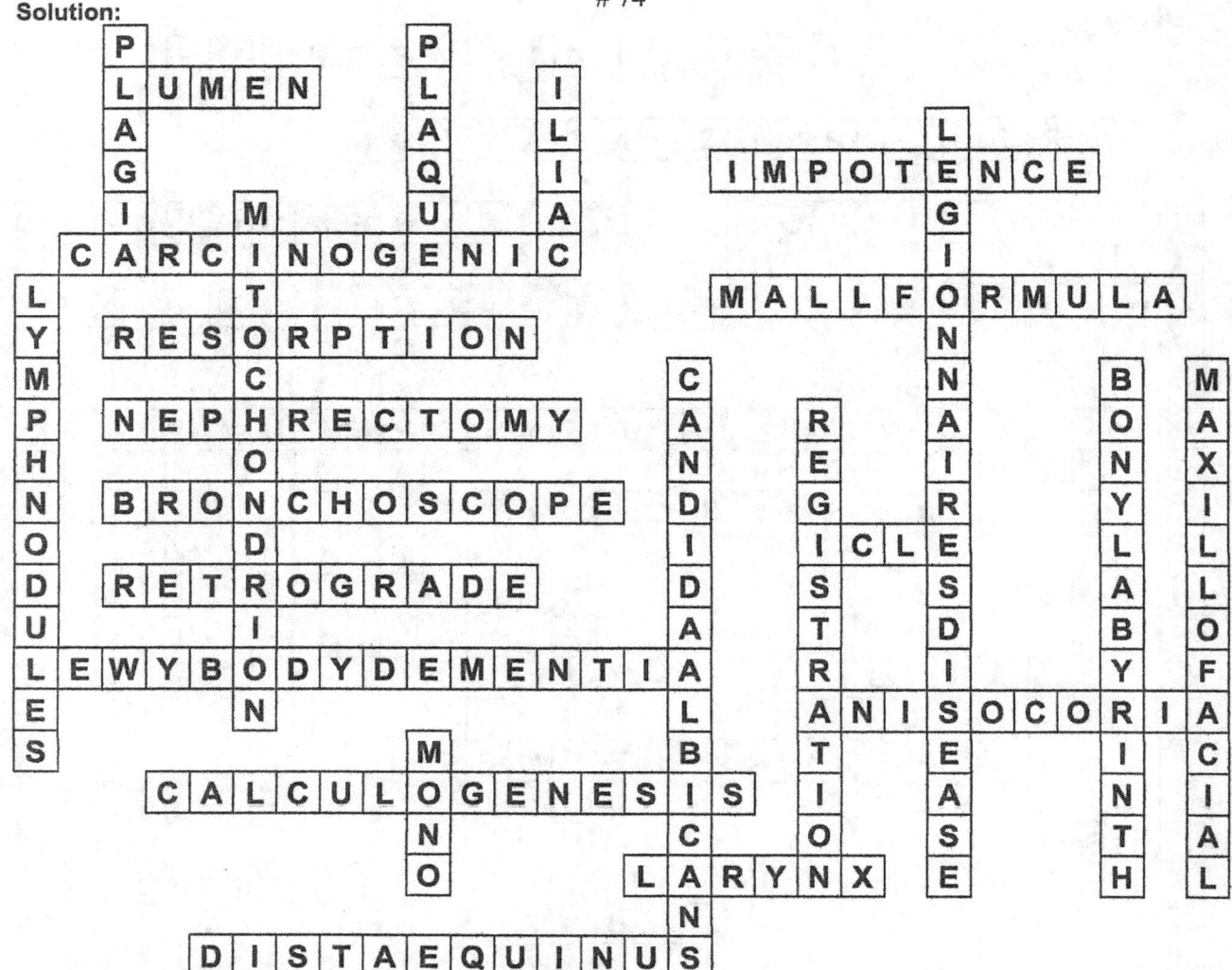

Solution:

75

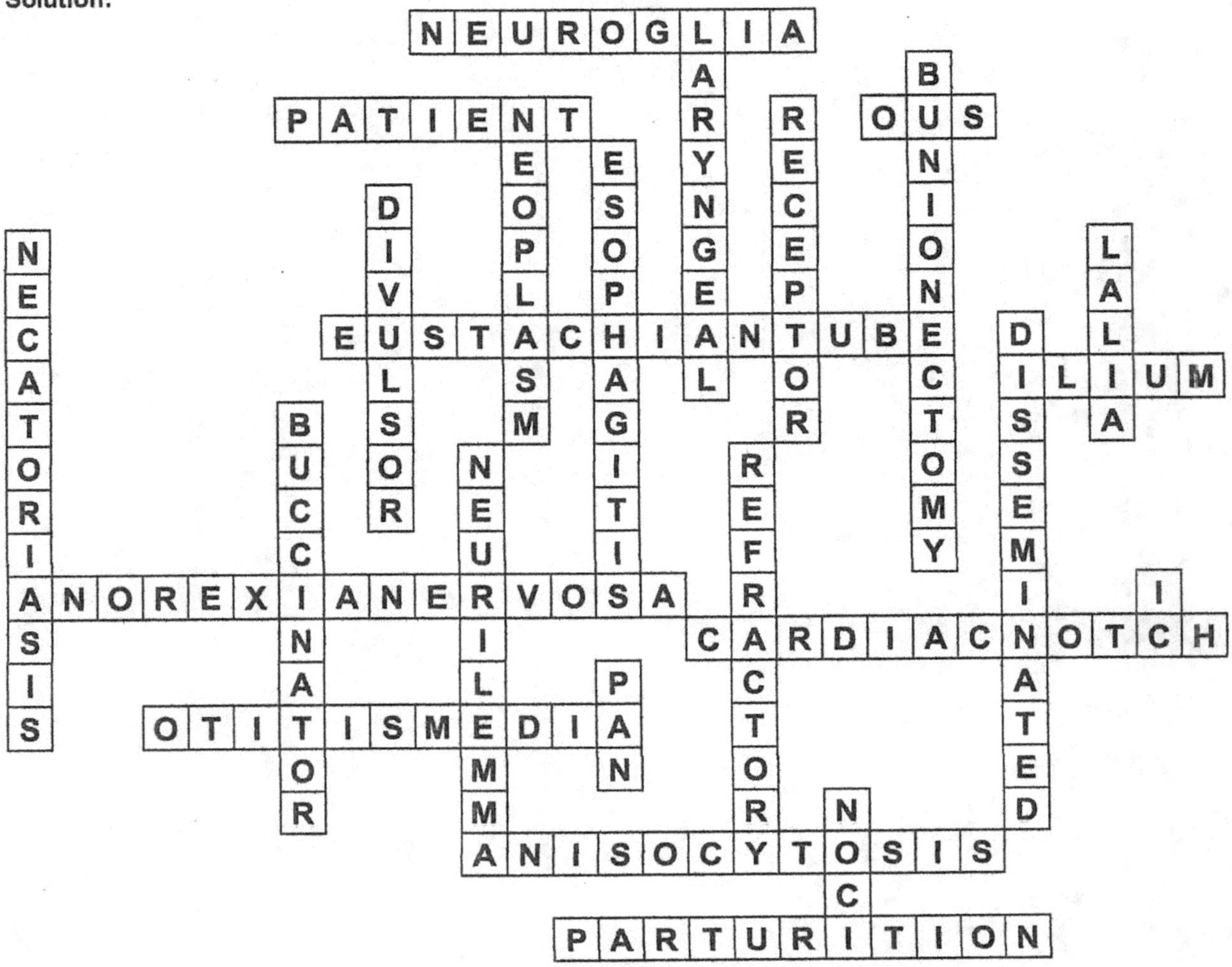
NEUROGLIA
PATIENT
OUS
EUSTACHIANTUBE
ILIUM
ANOREXIANERVOSA
CARDIACNOTCH
OTITISMEDIA
ANISOCYTOSIS
PARTURITION
LARYNGEAL
BUNIONECTOMY
RECEPTOR
NEOPLASM
ESOPHAGITIS
DIVULSOR
LALIA
DISSEMINATED
NECATORIASIS
BUCCINATOR
NEURILEMMA
REFRACTOR
PAN
IT
NOC

NOTES

NOTES

NOTES

NOTES

NOTES